T0331952

DEVELOPMENTAL NEUROPSYCHIATRY

DEVELOPMENTAL NEUROPSYCHIATRY

PROFESSOR ERIC TAYLOR

Emeritus Professor of Child and Adolescent Psychiatry,
Institute of Psychiatry, Psychology and Neuroscience (IoPPN),
King's College London, UK;
Honorary Consultant, South London and Maudsley NHS Trust, UK

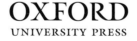

Great Clarendon Street, Oxford, OX2 6DP,
United Kingdom

Oxford University Press is a department of the University of Oxford.
It furthers the University's objective of excellence in research, scholarship,
and education by publishing worldwide. Oxford is a registered trade mark of
Oxford University Press in the UK and in certain other countries

© Oxford University Press 2021

The moral rights of the author have been asserted

First Edition published in 2021

Impression: 1

All rights reserved. No part of this publication may be reproduced, stored in
a retrieval system, or transmitted, in any form or by any means, without the
prior permission in writing of Oxford University Press, or as expressly permitted
by law, by licence or under terms agreed with the appropriate reprographics
rights organization. Enquiries concerning reproduction outside the scope of the
above should be sent to the Rights Department, Oxford University Press, at the
address above

You must not circulate this work in any other form
and you must impose this same condition on any acquirer

Published in the United States of America by Oxford University Press
198 Madison Avenue, New York, NY 10016, United States of America

British Library Cataloguing in Publication Data
Data available

Library of Congress Control Number: 2020949250

ISBN 978–0–19–882780–1

DOI: 10.1093/med/9780198827801.001.0001

Printed in Great Britain by
Bell & Bain Ltd., Glasgow

Oxford University Press makes no representation, express or implied, that the
drug dosages in this book are correct. Readers must therefore always check
the product information and clinical procedures with the most up-to-date
published product information and data sheets provided by the manufacturers
and the most recent codes of conduct and safety regulations. The authors and
the publishers do not accept responsibility or legal liability for any errors in the
text or for the misuse or misapplication of material in this work. Except where
otherwise stated, drug dosages and recommendations are for the non-pregnant
adult who is not breast-feeding

Links to third party websites are provided by Oxford in good faith and
for information only. Oxford disclaims any responsibility for the materials
contained in any third party website referenced in this work.

To the reader

Multi pertransibunt et augebitur scientia

(Many will journey through, and knowledge will be increased)

Daniel xii 4; Francis Bacon, *Novum Organum*

PREFACE

·······································

THE world of the mental health disciplines has come through some remarkable changes. My first experiences, in the early 1960s, were in an era of institutional treatment and care in the UK. Sometimes, this was horribly cruel; occasionally, kind and visionary. Its replacement, by 'normalizing' community programmes, was very necessary and welcome—but is not yet complete. Recent years have seen starvation of services in the UK for child mental health, specialist education, social care, and community resources such as day centres.

Nevertheless, there is much to admire. Most of those with intellectual disability, epilepsy, or autism have lives that are much less constrained by isolation and segregation than they used to be. Many of those with attention deficit hyperactivity disorder (ADHD) are treated with compassion rather than coercion. Guideline developments have encouraged the use of interventions with evidence for value. The lessons of multiple morbidity are familiar to many, especially those working in the fields of intellectual disability.

At several points in my professional life, I have wished for a book such as this. When moving into a new sphere of clinical work, I have looked for unified accounts of the psychiatric, psychological, neurological, medical, social, and educational issues guiding clinical understanding. When starting on a new line of research enquiry, I have sought accounts that would give an appreciation of reliable knowledge together with acknowledgement of what is not yet securely known. I have therefore tried to provide introductory information about the neuropsychiatric conditions themselves, the neurological and genetic influences that can impact psychiatric presentations, and the social and personal contexts in which they unfold.

It is not, however, the book I would have written back then. Modern understanding recognizes that these 'neurodevelopmental disorders' are complex, variable, dimensional, overlapping, and frequently coexistent. I have tried to do justice to this. The book includes short accounts of the typical development and pathology of some key functions whose alterations can underlie some forms of psychopathology. These altered functions, however, do not crystallize into currently demarcated diagnostic entities, but can be influenced by a variety of brain changes and can characterize several types of behavioural and emotional upset.

For the spectra of ADHD, autism, tic disorders, learning disability, and the psychotic disorders of young people, there are descriptions of their coexistence with other conditions as well as the differences from them. The effects of brain disorders on mental life are similarly considered and the consequences for development into adult life drawn out. Influences from genetic and environmental differences between people are described, separately and together, for the light they shed on how psychiatric conditions can arise and how they develop over time. Considerations of pathogenesis and intervention often have to be correspondingly transdiagnostic, focusing on needs rather than indications by diagnoses.

Scientific knowledge is holding out promises of transforming the field. In time, a level of knowledge will develop that should allow it to be organized by mechanisms of dysfunction rather than traditional diagnosis. We can already glimpse significant portions of the causal pathways that link environmental risks (such as the quality of the prenatal environment and subsequent parental care) to their impact on neural function and gene expression.

Service developments are already profiting from the research lessons of high prevalence, dimensional distribution, and frequent overlap of developmental conditions. There is an emphasis on the promotion of resilience and on identifying pathways towards well-being. Clinical diagnosis continues and is valuable, but its goal now is not the perfection of diagnosis for its own sake but to allow treatment to be personalized. Diagnostic schemes retain a humbler—but useful and traditional—purpose of standardizing practice and allowing communication. Biomarkers are extending in numbers, but their roles are often in predicting a variety of outcomes, not only in making existing diagnoses more convenient and objective.

Clinical and behavioural accounts might well come to be supplemented with coherent stories about how changes at one level of discourse (be it molecular, neuroanatomical, neurophysiological function, or psychological process) would translate into progressively higher levels.

In the event, however, a thoroughly reductionist account does not, at present, seem either likely or desirable. Developmental neuroscience has certainly advanced greatly, but so far the main impact on practice has been intangible: a sense of comprehensibility and optimism. A complex, dynamic story is unfolding. We recognize that interactions between common genetic influences and the physical and psychosocial environment guide human brain development in crucial early stages. We know that the results are still seen in later mental life and influence the development of child, adolescent, and adult psychopathology. There is, nevertheless, much that remains in dispute about the exact causal pathways involved and, correspondingly, about good quality in assessment and intervention for individuals. Where there is scientific consensus, I have tried to give an account of it, citing meta-analyses (when possible) rather than details of the primary research findings. Readers seeking up-to-date accounts of the rapid research advances should follow the science through reviews such as the 'Annual Reviews' in the *Journal of Child and Adolescent Psychiatry and Psychology*.

ACKNOWLEDGEMENTS AND THANKS

I have had the privilege of seeing the remarkable advances in the world of mental health by working in most of the fields covered by the following chapters and with most of the disorders and interventions. The people with whom I have worked, and the families and schools involved, have taught me much of what is here. I should emphasize especially:

The massive contribution of Sir Michael Rutter, FRS for his vision of a comprehensive research agenda—spanning neurobiological, cognitive, and social factors—as well as his personal support and kindness.

The supportive environment of the Institute of Psychiatry and the Maudsley Hospital made it possible to combine clinical and research work even when the topics were out of fashion. I do not think it would have been possible elsewhere in the country at that time. Work at St Piers College with Professor Besag greatly advanced my understanding of epilepsy.

I owe a great debt to my academic and clinical supervisors, trainees, and colleagues over the years. Many of them have come to be in more than one of these categories. I hope they will understand if I do not try to list all their names.

The research programmes on which I engaged have been supported, in recent years, by funding from the Medical Research Council, the Wellcome Trust, South London & Maudsley NHS Trust, the National Institutes of Mental Health (USA and UK), the NHS Research & Development Executive, the Mother and Child Foundation, European Union Framework 7, the Croucher Foundation, the MacArthur Foundation, and the Mental Health Foundation. These associations have also led to some collaborations with distinguished researchers that have advanced my understanding.

I should emphasize the aids to my understanding from working with advocacy groups including Andrea Bilbow and her colleagues at ADDISS, James Cusack and his colleagues at Autistica, and Benny Refson and her colleagues at Place2Be. People with neurodevelopmental issues, and their caregivers and supporters, have influenced me to write this book.

The editorial assistance given by Lauren Tiley and her colleagues at the Oxford University Press has improved the book a good deal, and I am grateful.

Contents

ABBREVIATIONS

3di	Developmental, Dimensional, and Diagnostic Interview
AAS	anabolic androgenous steroid
ABA	applied behaviour analysis
ABAS	Adaptive Behaviour Assessment System
ABC	Autism Behaviour Checklist
ACT	acceptance and commitment therapy
ACTH	adrenocorticotrophic hormone
ADHD	attention deficit hyperactivity disorder
ADI	Autism Diagnostic Interview
ADOS	Autism Diagnostic Observational Schedule
AED	antiepileptic drug
AIDS	acquired immune deficiency syndrome
ALD	adrenoleukodystrophy
ANMDA	anti-N-methyl-D-aspartate
ANS	autonomic nervous system
AQ	autism spectrum quotient
ART	antiretroviral therapy
ASCOT	a severity characterization of treatment (scale)
ASD	autism spectrum disorder
ASDI	Asperger Syndrome Diagnostic Interview
ASQ	Autism Screening Questionnaire
ASRS	Adult ADHD Self-Report Scale
BCI	brief cognitive impairment
BD	bipolar disorder
BECTS	benign childhood epilepsy with centrotemporal spikes
BMD	body dysmorphic disorder
BMI	body mass index
BPRS	Brief Psychiatric Rating Scale

CA1	a region of the hippocampus ('cornu ammonis' was an earlier term)
CAPA	Child and Adolescent Psychiatric Assessment
CBCL	Child Behaviour Checklist
CBIT	comprehensive behavioural intervention for tics
CBRS	Comprehensive Behaviour Rating Scale
CBT	cognitive behavioural therapy
CD	conduct disorder
CELF	clinical evaluation of language fundamentals
CGAS	Children's Global Assessment Scale
CHB	challenging behaviour
CHP	Challenging Horizons Programme
CLAS	child life and attention skill
CMV	cytomegalovirus
COS	childhood-onset schizophrenia
CP	cerebral palsy
CPT	continuous performance test
CSF	cerebrospinal fluid
CSWS	continuous spike-waves in slow-wave sleep
CT	computerized tomography
CY-BOCS	Children's Yale–Brown Obsessive-Compulsive Scale
D2	dopamine type 2 receptor
DAMP	disorder of attention, motor control, and perception
DAT	dopamine transporter
DAWBA	Development and Well-Being Assessment
DCD	developmental coordination disorder
DHA	docosahexaenoic acid
DICA	Diagnostic Interview for Children and Adolescents
DISC	Diagnostic Interview Schedule for Children
DISCO	Diagnostic Interview for Social and Communication Disorders
DLD	developmental language disorder/delay
DMDD	disruptive mood dysregulation disorder
DMN	default mode network
DRD4	dopamine-4 receptor
DSM	Diagnostic and Statistical Manual (of the American Psychiatric Association)

DUSP6	dual-specificity phosphatase 6
EBAD	emotional, behavioural, and autonomic dysregulation
ECG	electrocardiogram
ECT	electroconvulsive therapy
EEG	electroencephalogram
EF	executive function
EOCOE	early-onset childhood occipital epilepsy
EOS	early-onset schizophrenia
EPA	Environmental Protection Agency
EPA	eicosapentaenoic acid
EPS	extrapyramidal symptoms
ERP	exposure with response prevention
ESSENCE	early symptomatic syndromes eliciting neurodevelopmental clinical examinations
FAS	fetal alcohol syndrome
FGA	first-generation antipsychotic (drug)
FISH	fluorescent in situ hybridization
fraX	fragile-X
FT4	free thyroxine
GABA	gamma-aminobutyric acid
GARD	Genetics and Rare Diseases Information Center
GHB	gamma hydroxy butyrate
GLD	generalized learning disability/difficulty
GPRD	General Practice Research Database
GTR	Genetic Testing Registry
G-WAS	genome-wide association studies
HA	hyperactivity
HA-IMP	hyperactivity-impulsiveness
HIV	human immunodeficiency virus
HKD	hyperkinetic disorder
HLA	human leukocyte antigen
HOPS	homework, organization, and planning skills
HPA	hypothalamic–pituitary–adrenal
IA	inattentiveness/inattention
ICD	International Classification of Disease (of the World Health Organization)

ICECY	International Classification of Function, Disability, and Health for Children and Young People
ID	intellectual disability
IDD	intellectual developmental disorder
IIH	idiopathic infantile hypercalcaemia
IQ	intelligence quotient
KABC	Kaufman Assessment Battery for Children
KBIT	Kaufman Brief Intelligence Test
K-SADS	Kiddie Schedule for Affective Disorders and Schizophrenia
LDX	lisdexamfetamine
LKS	Landau–Kleffner syndrome
LSD	lipid storage disease
MBD	minimal brain damage
M-CHAT	Modified Checklist for Autism in Toddlers
MLD	metachromatic leukodystrophy
MMR	mumps, measles, rubella
MPH	methylphenidate
MRI	magnetic resonance imaging
MTA	multimodal treatment study of children with ADHD
MVA	motor vehicle accident
NA	noradrenaline
NC	narcolepsy
NCBI	National Center for Biotechnology Information
NICE	National Institute for Health and Care Excellence
NIMH	National Institute of Mental Health
NMDAR	N-methyl-D-aspartate receptor
NMS	neuroleptic malignant syndrome
NNH	numbers needed to harm
NNT	numbers needed to treat
NOS	not otherwise specified
NPV	negative predictive value
NVLD	non-verbal learning disability
OCD	obsessive-compulsive disorder
O/CP	oppositional/conduct problems

ODD	oppositional-defiant disorder
PAM	positive allosteric modulator
PANDAS	paediatric autoimmune neuropsychiatric disorders associated with streptococcal infections
PANNS	Positive and Negative Symptom Scales
PANS	paediatric acute-onset neuropsychiatric syndrome
PBS	positive behaviour support
PCC	posterior cingular cortex
PDA	pathological demand avoidance
PECS	Picture Exchange Communication System
PKU	phenylketonuria
PLD	pragmatic language disorder
PPV	positive predictive value
PRT	pivotal response treatment
PTSD	post-traumatic stress disorder
PUTS	Premonitory Urge for Tics Scale
PWS	Prader–Willi syndrome
QTc	corrected Q-T interval
RDoC	research domain criteria
REM	rapid eye movement
SCD	social communication disorder
SCD	sickle cell disease
SD	standard deviation
SDQ	Strengths and Difficulties Questionnaire
SED	severe emotional dysregulation
SEL	social and emotional learning
SGA	second-generation antipsychotic (drug)
SLD	specific learning difficulty/disorder
SLE	systemic lupus
SLI	specific language impairment
SMD	stereotypic movement disorder
SMD	standard mean deviation
SNAP	Swanson, Nolan, and Pelham (Questionnaire)
SORCS3	sortilin-related VPS10 domain containing receptor 3

SPI-CY	Schizophrenia Proneness Instrument: Child and Youth Version
SRI	specific reading impairment
SSPE	subacute sclerosing panencephalitis
SSRI	selective serotonin reuptake inhibitor
SUD	sudden unexplained death
SWAN	Strengths and Weaknesses of ADHD Symptoms and Normal Behaviour Rating Scale
T3 and T4	tri-iodothyronine and thyroxine
TAU	treatment as usual
TLE	temporal lobe epilepsy
TS	Tourette syndrome
TS	tuberous sclerosis
TSH	thyroid-stimulating hormone
VCFS	velocardiofacial syndrome
VMAT	vesicular monoamine transporter
WAIS	Wechsler Adult Intelligence Scale
WBS	Williams–Beuren syndrome
WHO	World Health Organization
WISC	Wechsler Intelligence Scale for Children
WPPSI	Wechsler Preschool and Primary Scale of Intelligence
YGTSS	Yale Global Tic Severity Scale

(Acronyms to identify genes (such as *IKBKAP*, a gene on chromosome 9) are not treated as abbreviations for the purpose of this list.)

CHAPTER 1

....

SCOPE AND PRINCIPLES OF NEUROPSYCHIATRY IN THE YOUNG

....

1.1 FREQUENCY AND IMPACT OF NEURODEVELOPMENTAL PROBLEMS

....

MANY of the psychological problems in young people originate in altered brain function. Autism spectrum disorder (ASD), attention deficit hyperactivity disorder (ADHD), movement disorders, language problems, and learning disabilities show changes in neurological and cognitive processes. They are usually classified and described as separate neuropsychiatric disorders.

Developing research and clinical experience, however, have made it clear that the conventional classifications do not tell the whole story. The 'separate disorders' in fact very often occur together in the same person. The potential causes (genetic and environmental risks) often coexist too. Further, the 'separate disorders' often exist as dimensions of dysfunction, continuous with the ordinary range of variation in the typically developing population. Further still, they present challenges that alter with development and interact with the physical and social environment.

This book acknowledges the complexity of the modern understanding and the issues it raises for clinical and educational practice. It addresses questions of how to recognize, understand, and help the multiple difficulties confronting affected children and adolescents in their journey into adult life.

The various disorders share, in differing combinations, some alterations of neurocognitive function that can have adverse effects on development. This sharing accounts for some of the high rates of coexistence between disorders. Accordingly, Chapter 2 will identify and describe the development of some of the key neurocognitive functions, and the ways in which they can be perturbed.

This is not to say that individual disorders such as ADHD, ASD, learning difficulties, and chronic tics are pointless exercises in medicalization. On the contrary, they remain very useful tools for thought and communication. They are widely acceptable, including to families and children, and allow direct links between research and clinic. They entail major impact through childhood and adolescence into adult life. The individual diagnoses are very common and increasing in prevalence. ADHD and ASD take pride of place for the speed of such increase.

1.1.1 Attention deficit hyperactivity disorder (ADHD): prevalence and increase

ADHD is a common and controversial diagnosis. It is being diagnosed with increasing frequency. In the USA, the National Health Interview Survey reports frequently on parent accounts of how many children are being diagnosed and treated. ADHD, as diagnosed by a physician or other healthcare professional in the USA, has become increasingly common over the last 20 years. The rate in 3- to 17-year-olds rose there from the already high value of 6.1% in 1997–1998 to 10.2% in 2015–2016 (Xu et al., 2018).

Many observers have queried whether these very high and accelerating rates represent local administrative concerns or an increase in the true prevalence of problems. Meta-analyses of studies reporting the rates of ADHD when standardized diagnostic procedures are followed offer no evidence to suggest a recent increase in the number of children in the population who meet the criteria (Polanczyk et al., 2014). Variations seem to reflect methodological details, especially whether or not the impact on social function is taken as a diagnostic criterion.

Western European countries have also seen high rates for ADHD, which may reflect recent increases in community concern and professional recognition. An epidemiological survey in Germany found the prevalence of ADHD at ages 7–17 to be 5% for symptom presence, 2.2% for full diagnosis, and 1% for hyperkinetic disorder (Döpfner et al., 2008). Administrative prevalence (the rate at which the diagnosis is given in practice) was 4.8% at ages 3–17 (Huss et al., 2008), 5% at ages 7–12, and 1.3% at ages 13–19 (Schlander et al., 2007). In France, a representative population survey found that 3.5% of children had been treated for inattention and/or hyperactivity (Lecendreux et al., 2011). The research prevalence there was also 3.5%, though the two groups were not identical.

In the UK, there was a modest increase in recognized ADHD during the 2000s. Analysis of a primary care database indicated that administrative prevalence in children aged 6 to 17 had risen from a very low rate of 0.19% in 1998 to 0.51% in 2009 (Holden et al., 2013). The rise could well have reflected the impacts of NICE (National Institute for Health and Care Excellence) guidance, public awareness, and continuing professional education. Since 2007, however, prevalence and incidence appear not to have increased and may even have fallen a little. A slight recent fall probably reflected the way in which austerity had diminished resources (see also Chapter 3, Section 3.6).

In 2008/2009, the Millennium Cohort Study in the UK enquired as to whether a doctor or healthcare professional had ever told parents that their child had ASD and/ or ADHD. Out of 14,043 children, 1.4% reportedly had ADHD (Russell et al., 2014).

This was still lower than the research estimate of prevalence in children aged 8 to 12, ascertained from a representative population survey in 1999, of about 2.5% (Ford et al., 2003). The conservative implication is that more than half of the affected children at any one time had *never* been identified as such—or at least that, if they were, the information did not reach the family.

1.1.2 Autism spectrum disorder (ASD): prevalence and increase

In the case of autism, there has also been a massive expansion of the number of cases diagnosed. In the USA, the National Health Interview Survey has found that the percentage of children aged 5 to 17 years reported to have ever been diagnosed with autism rose from 0.1% in 1997 to 1.2% in 2013. Between 2014 and 2017, the rates of reported autism ranged from 2.3% to 2.8%. Specific learning disabilities remained fairly steady over that period, at about 8.2%. In all, some 15% of America's children are currently being diagnosed with a neurodevelopmental disorder (EPA, 2019).

In educational contexts, too, autism has been on the increase. Cohort curves from schools' administrative returns suggest dramatic increases in autism diagnoses in the USA. The rates rose from 3 per 100,000 in 1982 to 18 per 100,000 in 1990 (Newschaffer et al., 2005). Current estimates are of at least 120 per 100,000 (see Chapter 1, Section 1.2.4).

Outside the USA, there is a comparable impression of rapid increase in the number of diagnosed cases. In the UK, the perception that autism spectrum conditions were much more common than previously recognized was tested in an epidemiological survey (Baird et al., 2006). It had indeed become a frequent condition, affecting some 1.2% of children. The increase had happened at the same time as a broadening of the concept and the diagnostic criteria (as described in Chapter 4, Section 4.1.1). This can explain some of the increase, but it is controversial whether it explains all of it (King & Bearman, 2009). The true rates may be even higher. Many countries, including the UK, underdiagnose the problems.

In addition to ADHD and ASD, there is a known high incidence of chronic tics, Tourette disorder, and learning deficits (Chapter 5). Neurodevelopmental disorders play a role in the genesis of adult-onset psychiatric conditions such as schizophrenia (Chapter 4, Section 4.2.5). Early brain disorders include epilepsy, cerebral palsy, and the outcomes of head injury and encephalopathies (Chapter 6). They share the qualities of early onset and continuing, fluctuating psychological challenges.

Most of these conditions can reduce the quality of life. They entail risks for academic underachievement, poor peer and family relationships, physical health problems including early death, mental illness, and underemployment. These adverse outcomes and the influences on them are considered in Chapter 10. The origins of these conditions are often in genetic and environmental influences (Chapter 7). There are many kinds of psychological and pharmacological help available (Chapters 8 and 9). In spite of this, however, a good deal of disability is still encountered, and some of it is avoidable (Chapter 10).

The increasing recognition of the importance of brain-based mental health conditions calls for a well-trained workforce in psychiatric, paediatric, and educational services targeting the problems of children and young people.

The relationships between neurological and psychiatric change are complex. The field has changed from a set of rare disorders to a group of common conditions that frequently coexist, merge gradually with extremes of typical development, and share some principles.

1.2 PRINCIPLES OF NEURODEVELOPMENTAL PSYCHIATRY

1.2.1 Neurodevelopmental disorders are defined clinically, not pathologically

Psychiatry has advanced, in part, using medical metaphors. Categories, syndromes, and diseases have all proved to be useful concepts. In physical medicine, the endless variety of ways in which the body can go wrong have been simplified into categorical units of classification.

Syndromes and diagnoses are key forms of medical categories. They combine many individual problems in various ways. A 'syndrome' is a shorthand description of a symptom profile. If it is tied to a known cause it is called a 'disease'. Medical syndromes have developed historically from several sources. Sometimes, careful clinical observers have recognized distinct profiles of problems and their names have persisted in eponymous syndromes. Sometimes, statistical enquiry has demonstrated clusters of problems such as those of anxiety and depression. Sometimes, advances in measurement have revealed that apparently disparate clinical problems are unified by a common physiological change. For instance, headache, shortness of breath, and palpitation could all be recognized as results of raised blood pressure, once the technique of measurement had been introduced. Enquiry could then describe the range of problems that shared this physiological change, and the syndrome of hypertension was born. This was not yet a 'disease'; that would imply a common set of causes, and in fact there are many causes, ranging from kidney disease to polygenic inheritance and diet.

Psychiatry did not until recently have a biological measure as the equivalent of the blood pressure recording device. Physiological and anatomical measurements of the brain did not advance to the point of being useful descriptions of individuals. Psychometric testing yielded associations between some of the symptom patterns and test results, but none were close enough to generate a different typology in the way that

Table 1.1 Common neurodevelopmental disorders and how they came to be recognized

Disorder	Influences on recognition
ADHD	Response to stimulants; statistical clustering
Autism	Classic description (Kanner); cognitive change; association with epilepsy
Tourette	Classic description (Gilles de la Tourette)
Intellectual disability/learning disorders	Psychometric testing
Schizophrenia/bipolar disorder	Classic descriptions (Kraepelin, Bleuler); courses over time

blood pressure measurement did. There was nevertheless a hope that the careful description of symptoms, course over time, familial patterns, and response to treatment would yield groups with a syndrome-like ability to predict physiology, causes, and treatment response. Sometimes this has worked—up to a point. Table 1.1 indicates the commonest currently recognized neurodevelopmental disorders and the historical reasons for the use of the diagnostic concepts.

Clinical concepts of psychiatric disorders have arisen in various ways. Sometimes, treatment responses have been able to unify clinical characteristics (as with medication for ADHD). Sometimes, striking clinical descriptions have proved to be robust and to predict psychological test results (as in autism). Sometimes, the course over time has defined different groupings of problems (e.g. schizophrenia and bipolar).

Historically, the idea of minimal brain damage (MBD) (later, dysfunction) included many of the disorders in childhood. MBD was intended to describe several common patterns of behaviour that were thought to imply an underlying neurological disease. The idea, however, collapsed when research focused on people with neurological disease or damage, and showed the great variety of mental manifestations and the extent of overlap with non-neurological mental disorders (Rutter et al., 1970).

1.2.2 Neurodevelopmental disorders tend to coexist

It is still useful to recognize differences between disorders, not least in conveying understanding and planning treatment. Nevertheless, the disorders as currently recognized have a good deal in common, as set out in Box 1.1.

Some conditions (e.g. bipolar disorders and schizophrenias) share many of the features listed in Box 1.1, but not all of them. Some others can now be defined neurologically rather than by psychological presentation (e.g. Rett syndrome, fragile-X, fetal alcohol syndrome) (and are described in Chapters 6 and 7). Accordingly, it is perhaps not surprising that the presence of one condition is often accompanied by another. For

---

Box 1.1 Characteristics of neurodevelopmental disorders*

- Neurocognitive alterations
- Male predominance
- Frequent coexistence
- Strong genetic influences
- Associations with epilepsy and brain disease
- Early onset
- Continuity over time, often with fluctuation

* The frequent characteristics that are commonly (but not universally) associated with neurodevelopmental problems, rather than other changes of mental health.

---

instance, many of those with ASD meet diagnostic criteria for ADHD as well; and vice versa. Anxiety states are very common in ASD. Most people with ADHD have additional diagnoses. Tics, obsessions, and ADHD are often found together. Hallucinations and delusions are common in many problems of mental health as well as the various types of psychosis. Detailed accounts will be found in later chapters. In particular, each section describing a syndrome will include consideration of its recognition and presentation in the presence of others.

1.2.2.1 *Reasons for coexistence of disorders*

The simultaneous presence of several diagnoses ('multiple morbidity') can come about in several ways. Some are artefactual: the coexistence is to be found in clinics but not in the general population, and therefore is unlikely to have a biological basis. Referral and selection bias are often responsible.

Referral bias would come about if, for instance, a clinic is known to have a special interest (say, in treating people with both chronic tics and ADHD). Professionals from a wide area would therefore be more likely to refer patients to it if they show both conditions. The clinic will therefore have a higher association between the conditions than would be seen in the population. Similarly, patients with severe and multiple problems might be seen in primary care as in great need of specialist service. Referral to a neuropsychiatry clinic might follow, and lead to an over-representation of patients with multiple problems.

Within a clinic, *selection bias* can also lead to an apparent association that does not apply to the conditions in the population. This is not dependent upon health beliefs by professionals. Berkson (1946) showed that the ratio of multiple diagnoses to single diagnoses in a clinic will always be greater than in the general population. This is a matter of conditional probability and selection only. Two independent disorders become conditionally dependent given that at least one of them occurs. The conditional probability of a disorder occurring, given that it or the other disorder occurs, is inflated.

It is higher than the unconditional probability, because selection has excluded cases where neither occurs.

Berksonian considerations can also lead to misleading conclusions about negative associations within a clinic population. Suppose a clinic accepts cases if they show high levels of ADHD or Tourette features or both. Among the cases accepted by the clinic, a clinical professional might well observe that the ones with more ADHD symptoms would on average have fewer tics (and vice versa), even if these traits were uncorrelated in the general population. The average ADHD case at the clinic would actually be more prone to tics than the average person in the population. However, the clinic's selection policy means that it has stringently high demands. The apparently negative correlation is an effect that arises *within* the clinic: the non-ADHD people who the clinic accepts will have had even more tics to pass the selection hurdle.

1.2.2.1.1 *Difficulties in diagnostic definitions*
Sometimes an apparent tendency for diagnoses to coexist comes about because the wording of the diagnoses is imprecise. 'Impulsiveness', for instance, is part of the definition of severe emotional dysregulation, bipolar disorder, and some personality disorders, as well as ADHD.

Diagnostic definitions may struggle to represent a multidimensional reality in categorical terms. Many people with a single diagnosis of ASD may also have a subdiagnostic but significant level of ADHD features. The coexistence of disorders may then not be fully reflected in the coexistence of diagnoses.

1.2.2.1.2 *Substantive reasons for coexistence*
The coexistence of neurodevelopmental disorders with each other and with other mental afflictions can also result from their history and biology in the general population.

One problem may be the result of another, often indirectly, as when conduct and oppositional disorders appear in the course of ADHD, or the disadvantages of ASD lead to high levels of anxiety. One disorder may masquerade as another, for instance if the social withdrawal of shy children with language disorder is mistaken for ASD. Different disorders may have risk factors in common, as when a head injury causes both ADHD and a motor syndrome. A distinct third condition may give rise to features of both. Intellectual deficit includes many of the features of all the specific learning disabilities.

1.2.3   Brain changes versus supposed causes

The forms of neurodevelopmental disorders reflect the various brain dysfunctions and personal reactions to them rather than the initiating causes. The psychological effects of brain damage and disease are very variable. Alterations of function are influenced by the neural circuits involved rather than the cause of damage to them. Brain changes associated with various dysfunctions are considered in Chapter 2. Few specific brain changes are known to be associated with specific psychiatric syndromes, but have often been sought. Resulting knowledge is considered in the sections on 'risks' in the chapters on individual psychiatric syndromes (Chapters 3, 4, and 5). Looking at the issue in a different way, the effects of specific types of brain damage on mental function are considered in Chapters 6 and 7.

Genetic influences are important and have helped to define the idea of neurodevelopmental disorders. Nevertheless, according to present knowledge, psychiatric presentation and precise genetic cause are not closely linked. The genetic influences are strong, but have proved to be very numerous, very overlapping between psychiatric syndromes, and very diverse (see Chapter 7, Section 7.5). Admittedly, there are several exceptions in which a defined genetic change or environmental exposure produces a characteristic syndrome. Such conditions, exemplified for instance by Prader–Willi and Lesch–Nyhan syndromes, will be considered in Chapter 7, Sections 7.3 and 7.4.7. Individually, they are rare; collectively, they account for a significant minority of cases. In general, however, most known genetic changes with major effects (e.g. 22q11 deletion) produce a wide range of problems. Bodily changes are often specific, mental changes not. Tuberous sclerosis, for instance, can be diagnosed from characteristic physical changes, but not from the psychological changes. The mental manifestations are protean and overlap with those resulting from other brain conditions.

Most of the known environmental causes also have widespread and varied effects. Injury to the developing brain is certainly capable of causing a wide range of mental presentations; but according to current knowledge, the range is so wide and so nonspecific that presentations with brain damage cannot be clearly separated from those without. As an example, fetal alcohol exposure can produce so characteristic a pattern of physical changes that the cause can be inferred from the appearance of the face and other features. Even here, however, the psychological effects are not by themselves specific enough to make the diagnosis.

It may of course be that the apparent non-specificity of mental sequelae is the consequence of inadequate precision in measuring them. Recently, the advent of effective neuroimaging has offered the opportunity to analyse clinical problems at the level of brain anatomy and physiology. So far, this has been for group findings only. However, the possibility of applying the same concepts to individuals will give a different set of answers and questions. It should be possible to measure, rather than infer, that an individual has a particular combination of fronto-striatal dysfunctions in the control of behaviour, emotions, and cognition. Perhaps they would still be described as 'ADHD', and that concept might still guide the simpler levels of practice, but specialists would fractionate the individual components into a new typology. Spectacular advances in genetics offer a linked possibility of identifying fundamental causes. A long-term research programme at the National Institute of Mental Health (NIMH) in the USA is already seeking the knowledge to replace clinical diagnoses with 'research domain criteria (RDoC)' based on biomarkers (Insel, 2014). The search is likely to illuminate our understanding of the pathogenesis of disorders.

An immediate practical implication is that it is seldom possible to divine the precise cause from mental features alone. Nevertheless, it is often possible to be clear that the causes include brain dysfunction, even if the exact dysfunction is not yet known.

1.2.4 Mental features of developmental disorders show continuous levels of severity

The disorders described in the international and American classifications have in the past been considered as distinct categories with clear differentiation from normality. The features which define them, however, have proved to occur in a continuum. There are progressively fewer cases at greater levels of severity.

Table 1.2 indicates the approximate prevalence of the validated diagnoses and their broader spectra from population surveys in developed countries. Beyond the recognized conditions, however, there are related subclinical conditions that merge with the ordinary variability of people. Tics, for example, are very common as transient features of typically developing children. Tourette disorder is uncommon but defined by the severity and frequency of the tics. In a similar way, the category of 'hyperkinetic disorder' has been defined by greater pervasiveness of the same features of impulsiveness and inattention that are diagnostic of broadly defined ADHD. There is no sign of any major qualitative change. The social communication problems and rigidity of people in the spectrum of autism are probably similar in kind to those in people without a diagnosis who are identified as 'geeks' or 'nerds' in common conversation.

Table 1.2 Narrow and broad definitions and their approximate prevalence

Disorder	Prevalence	Core features
Hyperkinetic disorder? ADHD	1% 5%	Varying degrees of inattention, restlessness, and impulsiveness
Autism Autism spectrum disorders	0.3% 1.2%	Varying degrees of social communication problems and insistence on sameness
Tourette Chronic motor tics	0.1%–1%? 3%?	Sudden, unwanted, repetitive movements
Reading problems Specific reading impairment	16% 4%	Reading worse than in most children Reading worse than predicted by other cognitive abilities
'Dyslexia'?	4%?	Reading impaired by neurological or phonological problems?

Rates are taken from expert reviews and meta-analyses described in other chapters, and are not definitive.

? indicates marked scientific disagreements about the definition or its frequency.

In the case of later-arising disorders such as schizophrenia and bipolar disorder, the distinction from typical development is somewhat more secure; but even in these examples the boundaries of disorder are hard to draw. 'Psychotic' features such as hallucinations and delusions are increasingly recognized in people who do not have diagnosable illness.

Both conceptual and practical difficulties consequently arise in making the categorical diagnoses based on symptoms alone. The demarcation from typical development is uncertain and often controversial. There are no biological markers to draw on. No points of rarity at increasing levels of severity can usually be discerned. As a result, diagnostic schemes such as DSM-5 set a boundary at the point where there is 'impairment' resulting from the symptoms (American Psychiatric Association, 2013). In practice, this is often a critical point for decisions about how widely the diagnosis is to be applied. 'Impairment' is often a feature of the environment as much as of the person (see this chapter, Section 1.2.8).

1.2.5 Many changes in early brain development have multiple effects on mental function

In early development, nerve cell migration and specialization, and synaptic proliferation and culling are prone to perturbation, and the results are likely to be unpredictable.

The progress of myelination through childhood and adolescence allows for more rapid communication between nerve cells and therefore better synchronization. Alterations in this process are likely to have multiple effects. High levels of communication between different parts of the brain are crucial for integrated behaviour. Many of the current findings from neuroimaging psychopathological conditions are related to abnormalities of connection. Fronto-striatal disconnection in ADHD, and local versus generalized processing in autism, are examples of potentially causative changes.

Injury to the developing brain can have results not only on the immediately traumatized area but also on the rest of the brain. Contre-coup and shearing injuries play a part in this; and there is a possibility of hypoxic and other metabolic changes with remote consequences.

There is therefore good reason to expect that people with one kind of neurodevelopmental change will often have others too. Indeed, as considered earlier, this turns out to be the case. These overlaps have often been described as 'comorbidity'. In most branches of medicine, the word has been used to describe the coexistence of two diseases. Unless and until psychiatry has developed to the point where it has *diseases,* the word often implies an understanding that we do not have. At a neurological level, it seems better to recognize that brain changes will often lead to several components of dysfunction. Brain changes will often be multiple; and even single changes will have multiple consequences.

The possibility of distinguishing these components by neurophysiological and neuropsychological methods is likely to become more feasible. Chapter 2 distinguishes several of these components.

1.2.6 Changes with time and social environment

The mental consequences of brain changes can be delayed and change over time, and are mediated, in part, by the social environment. The brain undergoes spectacular changes between birth and adulthood, and continues to change through adult life (Figure 1.1) (Andersen, 2003).

When similar functions are studied both in adulthood and in childhood, the localization of brain activity is often broadly similar, but there can be modifications. Encephalization refers to a progressive trend for frontal structures to be involved in functions previously served by subcortical circuits. Some functions may come to be served by more specific modules as they become more automatic and less effortful than in earlier life. The behavioural and emotional changes that result from altered neurological functions can also change over time, for several reasons. Changes of presentation can be seen most clearly for brain changes with a defined onset, such as birth trauma or postnatal head injury.

Over time there can be recovery of function. There may be compensation as other structures take over the compromised function; or secondary complications if the compensated function involves distortion. There may be new challenges if partial recovery leads to an enhanced level of expectation for social or occupational performance,

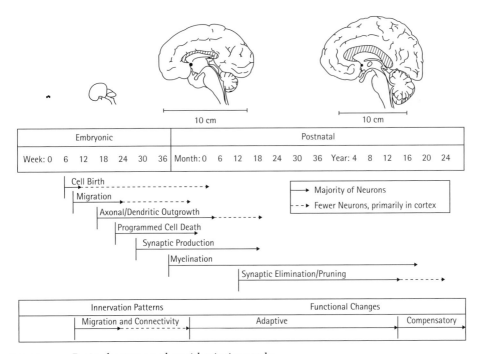

FIGURE 1.1 Brain changes on a logarithmic time scale

Reproduced from *Neurosci Biobehav Rev.*, 27(1–2), Andersen SL, Trajectories of brain development: point of vulnerability or window of opportunity?, pp. 3–18, Copyright (2003), with permission from Elsevier Science Ltd.

and those new challenges may stress different functions. If the environment helps to compensate for impaired functions, there may be less pressure to learn compensatory skills. A specialist school placement for children with autism may reduce anxiety; or an institutionalizing placement may lessen challenges but hold back cognitive development.

Secondary emotional changes may appear as a result of frustrations or threats, and the resulting levels of anger, anxiety, or unhappiness may themselves either worsen or ameliorate the core dysfunctions.

Environmental influences on development can themselves vary with age. The effects of a head injury on cognition are often more general and less specific for children than for adults. Education often provides cognitive stimulation for impaired young people much more systematically than for young adults.

Some of the effects of brain dysfunction can appear only gradually. Schizophrenia can develop after many years of different abnormalities such as language or motor impairments. Temporal lobe epilepsy in childhood and adolescence can lead to hallucinations and delusions in much later life. The mechanisms may well be indirect and complex, but a progression is clear.

In addition to direct age effects on impaired functions, the resulting disabilities can also change over time. People can learn life skills in different ways; they can find niches where their deficits do not matter; they can find helpers. They may also evoke adverse environments. They will certainly encounter a different range of challenges.

1.2.7 Deficit and productive conditions can be distinguished, but can coexist

Neurologists often recognize two broad groupings of conditions resulting from disease and injury. Table 1.3 illustrates the features of each. The distinction is often between cortical lesions with specific cognitive results (such as spatial agnosias) and subcortical conditions with altered behavioural and emotional changes.

Deficits can be found in some early-onset conditions such as cerebral palsy (Chapter 6, Section 6.3). There have been many attempts to reduce neuropsychiatric conditions

Table 1.3 Two types of neuropsychiatric disorder

Systemic ('fundamental')	Modular ('instrumental')
Mood, emotion, motivation	Cognition, language
Productive syndromes	Deficit syndromes
Disconnection rare	Disconnection syndromes
Subcortical	Cortical
Monoamines	GABA, glutamate
Drug effects	Little benefit from drugs

to specific neurocognitive deficits. A set of experimental studies by Beate Hermelin and Neil O'Connor (1970) sought a specific cognitive deficit in autism, and the work was influential in generating distinguished neuropsychological analyses of 'the underlying deficit' in both autism and ADHD. Most would probably now agree that there is no single underlying deficit in either of those conditions.

A hallmark of a dissociated problem would be superior performance under some conditions, for instance the 'autistic advantage' in some cognitive skills. Unusually high performance by autistic people on some psychological tests under certain conditions has long been sought. For instance, some people with autism achieved excellent scores on a visuospatial test of block design requiring matching a very complex pattern to the same pattern, among others, on different sides of a cube (Shah & Frith, 1993). This and similar results are often cited as support of a general theory of weak central coherence in autism (Chapter 4, Section 4.1).

In general, however, unique deficit explanations of neurocognitive problems have so far failed to lead to robust and useful clinical results. Attempts to remediate specific deficits (such as working memory in ADHD; see Chapter 3, Section 3.8) have not yet been successful treatments of the psychiatric condition(s) in which they are found. This may emphasize the heterogeneity of cognitive profiles within a disorder. Chapter 2 describes the development and pathology of some of the key functions, such as attention and communication, that are involved.

1.2.8 Impairment of function does not necessarily imply disability

Terminology about disability has become somewhat confused. Medicine usually distinguishes between impairment and disability.

Impairment refers to the lesion—the loss or abnormality of structure or function. A neurological example would be the loss of brain cells after a stroke. In psychiatry, however, a basic impairment is often hard to define. We will then simply seek to define the functional limitations and await clearer description of underlying anatomical or physiological impairments. Chapter 2 sets out the development of some of the key functions, and the ways in which they can be altered in pathology.

Disability refers to the consequent restriction of life. The word 'disability' has, however, become offensive to many because of its vagueness and the implication that it is a quality of the affected individual solely. In truth, the ability to participate is also a function of society.

The World Health Organization's (WHO's) approach is embodied in the *International classification of functioning, disability and health: children and youth version* (ICF-CY) (WHO, 2007). The wide concept of disability is replaced by three dimensions: impairments of body structures and body functions, of activities, and of participation. *Activity limitations* are the difficulties an individual may have in executing activities—as example, inability to walk. *Participation restrictions* are the restriction of life that

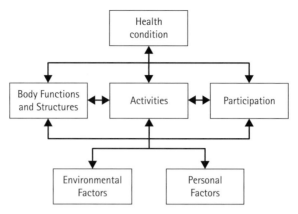

FIGURE 1.2 Conceptual model of International Classification of Functioning, Disability, and Health

Reproduced from World Health Organization, *International Classification of Functioning, Disability and Health*, pp. 18, Copyright (2001), with permission from World Health Organization.

results—in this example, being unable to join in sporting activities and loss of friends (Loe & Feldman, 2007; and see Figure 1.2).

Different countries are implementing the distinctions in different ways. This book will follow the distinction between impairments of functions (as described in Chapter 2) and disability in the sense of participation restrictions. Both need to be recognized in a clinical formulation. Both should come into descriptions of overall severity. A transdiagnostic severity measure suitable for describing children and young people, the Children's Global Assessment Scale (CGAS), was presented by Shaffer et al. (1983). It is widely used for clinical purposes such as helping decisions about the level of support required by an individual.

There can be some tension between models of disorder that include disability as a diagnostic criterion and those that separate diagnosis from a more social model of disability. The American Psychiatric Association's (2007) diagnostic manual (DSM-5), for example, takes a view that is closer to a traditional medical model than to the WHO's more social model outlined earlier. DSM-5 often specifies that there should also be clinically significant 'impairment' in 'social, occupational, or other important areas of current functioning' or 'disability' or 'significant interference'. 'Impairment' in this sense is close to 'participation restrictions' in the international sense. The criteria for making a DSM-5 diagnosis very often require that this 'impairment in social or occupational functioning' is present. (The exception is for Tourette and chronic tics, where the DSM-5 criteria do not require impairment.) If participation difficulties then become a necessary condition for having the disorder, it is hard to discriminate clearly between the clinical features that define (for example) ASD and the problems they impose for everyday life.

In practice, some people have all the symptoms and signs of a syndrome without being limited by them. The spectrum of autism, for instance, will comprise both some individuals with little or no social or occupational disability and high achievement (e.g. in information technology), and other individuals unable to live an unsupported life. Some people with Tourette disorder will be well accepted socially; others are grossly stigmatized. Some people with ADHD symptoms will be well-adjusted and find satisfactory occupational niches (e.g. in sales); others will develop a cycle of failure and antisocial adjustment.

The factors making for good or poor social adjustment will certainly include the severity of functional limitations, such as an inability to concentrate, and the range of other dysfunctions present. There will also be other factors leading to restriction of life. Appropriate education, access to treatment, acceptance by family members, and peer relationships can all contribute to social integration. Improvement of these potential protective factors can improve the quality of life. Public acceptance of people with disability can be greater when there are good role models of high-functioning and productive life. Chapter 10 describes the encounters with the real world that lead to restriction of life, and how they may be modified.

1.2.9 Directing intervention at both altered function and the social consequences

The 'core features' of disorders (i.e. those symptoms central to the concept of the disorder) are often the targets for clinical trials. In the case of drug treatments, regulators often require that the diagnostic criteria for a disorder should be the primary goals of therapy. Sometimes, however, drugs can have marked short-term effects on behaviour changes considered to be central, yet not improve the quality of life overall. Happily, the pharmacological interventions reviewed in Chapter 9 are sometimes helpful in reducing the behaviours and cognitive changes that define ADHD, and the frequency and severity of motor tics in Tourette disorder. They do not always have long-term effects even on symptoms, and this sometimes leads to rejection of their use; but the key consideration in judging them should be their impact on the quality of life.

Similarly, psychological interventions for ADHD are sometimes dispraised because they have little effect on 'core features'. Nevertheless, the same meta-analyses that suggest only small effects of cognitive behavioural therapy (CBT) on impulsiveness have also shown helpful effects in restricting the development of antisocial complications—which are an important part of the complex of problems. Chapter 8 will document the range of methods that should be available.

1.3 CLINICAL IMPLICATIONS

The principles outlined in this chapter will be illustrated by referenced examples in later chapters and will sometimes need to be qualified. There are, however, some general clinical consequences to introduce right away.

Services for each disorder should be able to cope with multidimensional problems. A specialist in one condition should have enough training to be competent over a range of neurodevelopmental conditions and their associated disadvantages (e.g. not solely in autism assessment). In affluent services, a team approach of complementary specialists may be preferred. Even then, there will be issues around communication, meaning that ultra-specialists will need to know enough about the basics of others' practice that they can coordinate effectively.

Diagnoses should not ordinarily be regarded as implying cause. It is therefore better to avoid asking: 'Does he have ADHD or fragile-X?' or 'Does she show autism or early neglect?' Rather, both the clinical presentations and the initiating factors should be recognized.

Severity and probable outcome should usually be defined on the basis of multidimensional psychopathology rather than being confined to the presence of a single diagnosis.

Dimensionality is the rule. The aim of therapy will often be the reduction of symptoms or better coping with them, rather than cure.

Communication between professionals and families should include multidimensional perspectives from the start. Many parents have been confused because the diagnosis appears to change when the profile of disability is fluctuating. Sometimes, multiple diagnoses from different providers have led the family to a lack of confidence in any. When there is confusion between impairment and disability, some educators have come to reject the whole idea of the psychiatric diagnoses as being too 'pathologizing'. Careful person-specific descriptions are often better understood than single diagnoses which encapsulate only a part of the person's problems.

Families and individuals with a disorder should be active participants in drawing up a formulation and a treatment plan.

References

American Psychiatric Association. (2013). *Diagnostic and statistical manual of mental disorders* (DSM-5).

Andersen, S. L. (2003). Trajectories of brain development: point of vulnerability or window of opportunity? *Neuroscience & Biobehavioral Reviews, 27*(1–2), 3–18. https://doi.org/10.1016/S0149-7634(03)00005-8

Baird, G., Simonoff, E., Pickles, A., Chandler, S., Loucas, T., Meldrum, D., & Charman, T. (2006). Prevalence of disorders of the autism spectrum in a population cohort of children in South Thames: the Special Needs and Autism Project (SNAP). *Lancet, 368*(9531), 210–215.

Berkson, J. (1946). Limitations of the application of fourfold table analysis to hospital data. *Biometrics Bulletin, 2*(3), 47–53.

Döpfner, M., Breuer, D., Wille, N., Erhart, M., Ravens–Sieberer, U., & Bella Study Group. (2008). How often do children meet ICD-10/DSM-IV criteria of attention deficit-/hyperactivity disorder and hyperkinetic disorder? Parent-based prevalence rates in a national sample—results of the BELLA study. *European Child & Adolescent Psychiatry, 17*(1), 59–70.

EPA (Environmental Protection Agency). (2019). *Neurodevelopmental disorders*. https://www.epa.gov/americaschildrenenvironment/ace-health-neurodevelopmental-disorders

Ford, T., Goodman, R., & Meltzer, H. (2003). The British child and adolescent mental health survey 1999: the prevalence of DSM-IV disorders. *Journal of the American Academy of Child & Adolescent Psychiatry, 42*(10), 1203–1211.

Hermelin, B., & O'Connor, N. (1970). *Psychological experiments with autistic children*. Pergamon.

Holden, S. E., Jenkins–Jones, S., Poole, C. D., Morgan, C. L., Coghill, D., & Currie, C. J. (2013). The prevalence and incidence, resource use and financial costs of treating people with attention deficit/hyperactivity disorder (ADHD) in the United Kingdom (1998 to 2010). *Child and Adolescent Psychiatry and Mental Health, 7*(1), 34.

Huss, M., Hölling, H., Kurth, B. M., & Schlack, R. (2008). How often are German children and adolescents diagnosed with ADHD? Prevalence based on the judgment of health care professionals: results of the German health and examination survey (KiGGS). *European Child & Adolescent Psychiatry, 17*(1), 52–58.

Insel, T. R. (2014). The NIMH research domain criteria (RDoC) project: precision medicine for psychiatry. *American Journal of Psychiatry, 171*(4), 395–397.

King, M., & Bearman, P. (2009). Diagnostic change and the increased prevalence of autism. *International Journal of Epidemiology, 38*(5), 1224–1234.

Lecendreux, M., Konofal, E., & Faraone, S. V. (2011). Prevalence of attention deficit hyperactivity disorder and associated features among children in France. *Journal of Attention Disorders, 15*(6), 516–524.

Loe, I. M., & Feldman, H. M. (2007). Academic and educational outcomes of children with ADHD. *Journal of Pediatric Psychology, 32*(6), 643–654.

Newschaffer, C. J., Falb, M. D., & Gurney, J. G. (2005). National autism prevalence trends from United States special education data. *Pediatrics, 115*(3), e277–e282.

Polanczyk, G. V., Willcutt, E. G., Salum, G. A., Kieling, C., & Rohde, L. A. (2014). ADHD prevalence estimates across three decades: an updated systematic review and meta-regression analysis. *International Journal of Epidemiology, 43*(2), 434–442.

Russell, G., Rodgers, L. R., Ukoumunne, O. C., & Ford, T. (2014). Prevalence of parent-reported ASD and ADHD in the UK: findings from the Millennium Cohort Study. *Journal of Autism and Developmental Disorders, 44*(1), 31–40.

Rutter, M., Graham P., & Yule W. (1970). *A neuropsychiatric study in childhood*. Heinemann Medical.

Schlander, M., Schwarz, O., Trott, G. E., Viapiano, M., & Bonauer, N. (2007). Who cares for patients with attention-deficit/hyperactivity disorder (ADHD)? *European Child & Adolescent Psychiatry, 16*(7), 430–438.

Shaffer, D., Gould, M. S., Brasic, J., Ambrosini, P., Fisher, P., Bird, H., & Aluwahlia, S. (1983). A children's global assessment scale (CGAS). *Archives of General Psychiatry, 40*(11), 1228–1231.

Shah, A., & Frith, U. (1993). Why do autistic individuals show superior performance on the block design task? *Journal of Child Psychology and Psychiatry, 34*(8), 1351–1364.

World Health Organization. (2007). *International classification of functioning, disability and health: children & youth version* (ICF-CY).

Xu, G., Strathearn, L., Liu, B., Yang, B., & Bao, W. (2018). Twenty-year trends in diagnosed attention-deficit/hyperactivity disorder among US children and adolescents, 1997–2016. *Journal of the American Medical Association Network Open, 1*(4), e181471.

CHAPTER 2

....

DEVELOPMENT AND PATHOLOGY OF KEY FUNCTIONS

....

2.1 BRAIN ORGANIZATION

THE brain is an exceptionally complicated system of connections. During pregnancy, a fetus develops about a quarter of a million nerve cells, on average, every minute. At birth, there will be around 100 billion. After birth, there will be some reduction. The connections between them (synapses) will increase and then be reduced and refined as the brain evolves. At maturity, the brain is estimated to have some 100 trillion (or so) synapses. Mathematical analyses indicate the utility of thinking about these patterns of communication in terms of: *modules* serving specialized functions within which there is efficient communication, *hubs* (large-scale modules), and *connectors* allowing for their integration (Bertolero et al., 2018).

Modules can function for psychologically separate functions—such as hearing, vision, motor function, attention, memory, and social understanding. They must communicate well with each other for good adaptive function. For instance, functional interactions between the amygdala and prefrontal cortex mediate both emotional influences on cognitive processes, such as decision making, and cognitive influences on emotion.

Anatomically defined areas of the brain contain nerve cells involved in diverse sets of functions, integrated by communications between networks (Salzman & Fusi, 2010). There is extensive current research on how best to divide separate modules and separate functions. There are many problems, both technical and conceptual, for integrating this research into clinical understanding (see, for instance, Poldrack & Yarkoni, 2016). One of the main conceptual problems is achieving a consensus about how to identify and classify separate functions.

Accordingly, this chapter will describe some key functions that are vulnerable to genetic and environmental changes affecting the brain. Motor function, attention, memory, executive function, communication, social understanding and empathy, reality testing, and emotional regulation will be considered separately. Their development and the consequences in psychopathology will be described as the basis for understanding the complex and overlapping results of brain dysfunctions.

2.2 MOTOR CONTROL

The fetus is very active in the womb. Muscular activity appears as soon as the muscles are innervated. Kicks, movements of trunk and head, arm extensions, movements of thumb to mouth, facial expressions and grimaces are all very common, often in bursts of activity. These spontaneous movements help muscular development. They are not in themselves goal-directed, but generate sensory signals back to the brain, allowing the latter to build a picture of the nature of movement and eventually to develop plans.

After birth and during the first year of life, spontaneous movements continue at a very high rate and become more coordinated. The stages in this process are often described. At 6 weeks of postnatal life, the baby will start to lift their head from a prone position; at 20 weeks, to roll over; at 6 months, to sit without support; at 12 months, to take first steps; and so on. Many charts are available to describe the 'motor milestones' in detail, and many clinicians are taught to elicit and observe them. They have been a source of reassurance and delight to many parents. They can also be misleading.

The 'stage charts' can seem to illustrate an invariant progression in all 'normal' children, while in fact there is a considerable range. They can seem to support a universal system, though in fact they are usually based on a narrow range of cultural backgrounds, and an examiner would be well advised to use local norms. Their 'staging' can underestimate the variability within children—the first time a child sits is often followed by days and weeks in which they can no longer do so. The stage charts can seem to promote a mechanistic idea of specific muscular sequences being programmed in the brain. In fact, the muscular activity required to raise the leg of a 12-month-old is different in kind from that called for by the lesser weight and length of the neonate's limbs. The process is one of adaptation and flexibility. It represents the evolution of plans and monitoring for movement. Completely different plans may be employed for a single purpose: as when children will bottom-shuffle for a while rather than crawl or walk.

The spontaneous movements are soon used for intentional activity. Arm flapping when a toy is presented turns into reaching movements and eventually contacting it. Object-related play, like other kinds of play, is not at first directed to the achievement of a goal but still serves as a system in which intentional and goal-directed activity can arise. For instance, at 3 to 5 months, children make finger–thumb movements that are very similar to the pincer grip used later in development to pick up small objects.

In later development, motor acts become more coordinated and efficient. Unnecessary movements are reduced. For instance, 'mirror movements', in which the unoccupied hand reflects those of the active hand in young children, decrease with maturity. Planned movements are correspondingly more effective. Reaching for a toy, for example, is transformed over the second and third years of life from a jerky process of movement and correction into a smooth action, coordinating elbow, wrist, and fingers into a rapid movement that slows down as it approaches the toy. The full development of grip and manipulation of objects will not be complete until adolescence, and will depend on learned strategies, voluntarily applied plans, and opportunities to practise. Motor skills will be subject to local and cultural influences.

Through motor control, the child develops independence and the ability to explore the world. It allows richer cognitive development, clearer speech and communication, facial expression of emotion, and is important for social interaction.

2.2.1 Alterations in motor function

There is marked variation between individuals in the level of motor control attained at any specific age. Clumsiness can occur for several reasons, the commonest being the immaturity described as 'developmental coordination disorder (DCD)'. DCD is considered further in Chapter 5, Section 5.2.1. Other specific causes are listed in Box 2.1. Detection requires the clinician to be alert to the possibilities and to refer for neurological or other medical investigation. Indications such as progressive worsening or asymmetrical involvement of the body should be signals for further investigation.

2.2.2 Qualitative differences in motor development

Some altered patterns of movement are not simply immaturities and are not typical of any age. Paralyses, weaknesses, and abnormal postures are considered under cerebral palsy (Chapter 6, Section 6.3).

Unwanted movements are also quite common and contribute to functional impairment.

2.2.3 Repetitive movements

Repetitive movements are of several types. Stereotypies (with or without self-injury), rituals, compulsions, and tics should be distinguished, though they can shade into one another.

2.2.3.1 *Stereotypies*

Stereotypies are defined (e.g. in DSM-5) as 'repetitive, seemingly driven, and apparently purposeless motor behaviour' (American Psychiatric Association, 2013). Some of this definition needs qualifying. 'Seemingly driven' should not be taken to allow speculation from the examiner about the internal state to become a diagnostic criterion. 'Apparently purposeless' should not discourage one from seeking its functional importance. It may be modifying arousal level, or reducing anxiety, or creating predictability, or forming a

Box 2.1 Disorders involving clumsiness

Associated with localized neurological disorder

Upper motor neurone lesions
- Cerebral palsy, tumours, traumatic damage, hydrocephalus

Ataxias
- Cerebellar disorders, posterior fossa tumours, vestibular disorders

Peripheral nerves/muscles
- Hereditary sensorimotor neuropathy
- Muscular dystrophies, mitochondrial myopathies

Associated with intellectual disability

Coordination immature, but in line with developmental age

Genetic syndromes
- Many, including Rett, Angelman, and Wilson diseases

Associated with systemic disorders

Skeletal/ multisystem
- Friedreich ataxia

Connective tissue abnormality
- Ehlers–Danlos syndrome, hypermobility

Sensory problems
- Visual and hearing impairments

distraction from unpleasant sensations, or serving an intent to self-injure. Quite often children, and adults too, enjoy performing them. Indeed, DSM-5 modified the wording from the previous '*non-functional*', presumably with this in mind.

Stereotypies have in common that the activity is highly predictable in pattern, intensity, and location. Examples include body rocking, head banging, hand/arm flapping, lip smacking, rubbing surfaces, and head nodding. They are not preceded by the urge to act that is often a part of a tic; and they are more consistent over time than are tics. Motor stereotypies start early—before age three in one series—in contrast to tics, which usually have a later onset (Mahone et al., 2004). They are frequent in ordinary development, being shown by at least 7% of children.

A clinical diagnosis such as *stereotypic movement disorder* (SMD) is only applied if the movements cause distress, injury, or interference with other activities (Barry et al., 2011). Very often they do not. Most children learn to treat them as private quirks and confine them to situations where they are alone or in the presence of people who they can trust not to mock them. (When this is the case, they are often regarded simply as 'mannerisms'). As with other neurodevelopmental continua, the behaviours themselves do not have a clear defining line to indicate abnormality. Accordingly, the need for a medical approach may appear only for the social reason of unpleasant reactions by other people. That situation may change if sound biological markers appear, to predict the expected later course.

The presence of stereotypic movements, short of an SMD diagnosis, may still need to be recognized explicitly for other reasons. They may be the presentation of other problems that need to be diagnosed, or they may be obscuring the presence of other problems. They may be falsely suggesting the presence of autism, or they may need to be differentiated from compulsions, tics, postictal automatisms, or paroxysmal dyskinesias. They are typical of Rett syndrome (especially, midline hand-wringing) and fronto-temporal degeneration. They are also often found in other conditions associated with intellectual disability. Descriptions of anti-N-methyl-D-aspartate receptor encephalitis stress stereotypies as one of the features.

Stereotypic movements are very common in young people with sensory disabilities. For instance, most blind children show them to some extent. Such movements are also more common in restrictive environments with little stimulation. This has invited speculation that they serve to provide a higher level of sensory stimulation. This cannot be the whole story, for they typically appear when children are excited, as well as at times of boredom. Perhaps they can be seen, sometimes, as modulators of arousal. The commonest methods of managing SMD are through the modification of environmental stimulation, for example by the provision of pleasurable and stimulating activities.

No single explanation will suffice. There is often a story of family members being affected in similar ways, though molecular genetic studies and neuroimaging have not yet given a clear account. Persistence or otherwise can be influenced by learning, especially by contingent reward. Reduction of high levels of SMD can be achieved by the withdrawal of other people's attention—both positive and negative—with the aim of extinguishing the learned component (Chapter 8, Section 8.4).

Severe levels of SMD can disrupt development. Learning and social life can be markedly disadvantaged. The advent of self-injury is particularly serious and may require similar approaches to those used for the problems of harmful repetitive behaviour in autism spectrum disorders.

2.2.3.2 *Rituals*

Some repetitive behaviours are complex, involving many motor actions.

Young children very often follow set patterns of activity in repetitive ways. Some are clearly comforting: thumb sucking and head banging tend to be more marked when children are tired or stressed, and interrupting them is distressing.

Complex rituals tend to arise about the age of 2 years, increase for a short while, and then decline after the age of 4 years. At ages 2 to 4 years, they are very common. Parent reports suggest about 62% of children show them (Evans et al., 1997). Most carry little or no pathological significance—like walking only on the pavement cracks. They may well have a function of creating predictability in the experienced world, or increasing time spent with parents. After that age range, it is harder to see entrenched ritual behaviours as normative, and they start to be associated with anxiety and shy temperaments. They can represent attempts to cope with high anxiety, a direct expression of anxiety, or a cause of anxiety if other people disapprove.

2.2.3.3 *Compulsions*

Some intrusive ritual movements are accompanied by a sense that they are irrational and unwelcome. These are compulsions. They can occur either with or without obsessions (intrusive thoughts). They have mostly been studied as a part of obsessive-compulsive disorders (OCD), of which they are often the first sign to be noticed.

Compulsions are not rare. Estimates of population prevalence are influenced by age and level of definition taken. The 1999 British Child Mental Health Survey suggested a rate of 0.25% at ages 5 to 15 years (Heyman et al., 2001). The rate increased after puberty, towards adult levels.

They typically come to light during the early years of schooling. The first such movements to appear often involve excessive and stereotyped cleaning, such as lengthy handwashing. Sometimes there is a trigger, such as a respiratory infection that starts a cough which becomes chronic and compulsive. Counting, checking, and touching rituals and preservations of symmetry are also frequent forms. They are often being used to ward off fears of terrible events or harm to others, and some sufferers come to take these fears as veridical. Most, however, understand the fears very well as irrational, and keep them secret, often with great difficulty and effort.

Developmentally, compulsions tend to persist, and single compulsions tend to be joined by others. Early onset, coexistent tics, and emotional problems all predict a more persistent course.

In individual children, they can occur together with non-obsessive rituals or in succession. One boy, for instance, had, at the age of three, a fixed interest in the edges of the pages in books. By the age of six, this had become a repetitive, slow thumbing through the pages and, later, counting the pages in a fixed way. Later still, by the age of eight, when he was assessed professionally, the counting ritual was maintained by a dread that, if not done with complete accuracy, other people reading the book would be poisoned. Such a progression raises unsolved questions about whether the anxieties accompanying ritual behaviours are a reaction to their presence, a cause of them, or both. The association between tics and compulsions raises similar queries and is discussed further in Chapter 5 (Section 5.1.5).

2.2.3.4 *Tics*

Tics are sudden, rapid, recurrent, non-rhythmic motor movements or vocalizations. They are usually short fragments of ordinary movements. Eye blinking, throat clearing, head jerks, and shoulder shrugs are among the early ones, but any part of the body can come to be affected and the course is not constant. Complex tics tend to emerge later and can appear more purposive, such as hand gestures or hopping. Some tics involve the muscles of vocalization and produce sounds such as squeaks, shouts, and grunts. The presentation can be altered by voluntary efforts to turn the tic into a comprehensible action.

Tics are very often accompanied by a sensory premonition, commonly experienced as an urge to carry out the act. This urge can have an obsessional quality, with a compulsion to carry out the tic repeatedly in order to get it 'just right'. The urge, and the ability to suppress a tic by an act of will, are often seen as being on the borderline between the voluntary and the involuntary. Nevertheless, the urges are not themselves voluntary, and suppressing them is effortful and temporary.

It can be difficult to distinguish tics from other kinds of stereotyped movement. It can be very difficult in autism spectrum disorders. Problems in communication may remove the usual clues of sensory urges. The distinction may have to be made based on the forms of movement involved. Even this can be difficult in the case of complex tics involving many parts of the body and appearing purposive. A filmed record may make the diagnosis easier.

Tics fluctuate greatly according to every timescale measured, from the course of a day to the long-term changes that occur from week to week and month to month. This phenomenology distinguishes them from the rhythmic, slower movements of stereotypies. The fluctuations in tic frequency and intensity are not predictable. They can be confusing to professionals, in several ways. The diagnosis can be missed if they are not shown at the time of examination. Therapists can mistake spontaneous improvement to be resulting from their efforts. Teachers can be misled into perceiving tics as deliberately disruptive behaviour.

2.2.4 Catatonia

Catatonia describes a distinctive cluster of behaviour changes: echo phenomena, rigidity, speech abnormalities, and withdrawal. These features can better be described as problems of volition rather than motor control. They are described as a psychiatric syndrome in Chapter 4, Section 4.2.10.

2.3 ATTENTION

Attention has been described and studied at least since classical antiquity (Lucretius, 1951). Then, the idea described the steps between sensing and conscious perception. It was not itself a conscious process, but the application of attention enhanced both the intensity of what was perceived and the quality of the response to it. Nowadays, it would better be described as the processes involved in selecting and admitting sensory information to the brain's processing. These are active processes and can be described at levels of behaviour, cognition, and neural activity, which do not all map neatly on to one another.

'Attention' therefore has attracted many definitions and theories. For some, it has been an agent that selects and binds sensory information (Treisman, 1988); for others, one to amplify or reduce sensitivity (Yeshurun & Carrasco, 1999); for yet others, a filter to prevent information overload (Broadbent, 1958). For all, it has been essential to mental activity. The complexity of the world is so great, and our ability to process its information is so limited, that the information must be coded, filtered, and selected if it is to be useful.

2.3.1 Inspection and search

Newborn babies move their sensors to get good quality of information from the outside world. They will turn their heads to the sound of a rattle, thus aligning eyes and ears with the object. Furthermore, they are exploratory and curious in gathering information. A new sound attracts their orientation; as it is repeated the orientation wanes; and if it is changed in quality, they look again. They are active harvesters of information from the start.

Very young children are also systematic in their exploration. They scan a featureless field with wide and jerky eye movements. Then, an edge of high contrast is quickly detected. Coarse eye movements become fine ones, scanning backwards and forwards across the edge.

Search is also captured by novelty—or, to put it another way, infants prefer novelty. When a stimulus is repeated, as in habituation experiments, orientation towards it fades rapidly. As children develop over their first year, they attend preferentially to complex stimuli and irregular patterns. Face-like patterns attract gaze, but shortly afterwards an actual face will be preferred to an abstract design, and then later, the mother's face specifically attracts longer gazes.

There are already considerable individual differences in infancy. These differences are not lasting, yet they predict cognitive function later in childhood. For example, those 6-month-olds with the longest time of gazing at a new object will tend to be those with the lowest IQ in middle childhood. Similarly, infants whose looking time reduces only slowly with repeated presentation (habituation) are also those with a lower IQ between the ages of 2 and 18 years (Kavšek, 2004). This may appear counter-intuitive until one realizes that a short gaze will result from rapid appreciation and memory. Habituation becomes more efficient, and the object will no longer attract orientation.

Inspection time in infancy is therefore partly a measure of the speed of processing information. By the end of the first year, however, a longer inspection time will reflect differences in more complex processes of evaluation.

A general trend after the first year is for inspection times to become shorter. By about 18 months, however, a distorted mask is looked at for longer than a regular one. (Presumably, there is more to investigate about the unexpected stimulus.) Over the next 18 months, systems develop that allow selective engagement with salient, relevant, and novel features of the environment. During the early school years, the capture of attention by what is salient and novel gives way to active and organized plans for searching the visual world.

2.3.2 Covert attention

Some systems of attention do not involve physically moving the sense organs. This 'covert attention' also develops through the first years of life. It is shown, for instance, in laboratory experiments where visual stimuli are presented too briefly for the eyes to move to them. Attention effects can still be seen, for example by modifying the visual presentation to include information about when a target will appear (alerting) and where (orientating). If attention is orientated to one side, information presented on the other side is dealt with more slowly (Posner et al., 2016).

2.3.3 Focused and sustained attention

The intensity of orientating to a stimulus increases with development. Focused attention can be inferred from facial expression, rapid reaction times, slowing of heart rate, and physiological changes of arousal (e.g. EEG, skin conductance).

During the second year of life, focused attention becomes intense but short-lasting. Common observation makes it clear that a toddler's attention is hard to shift from whatever has captured it, but that it is not usually sustained for more than a couple of minutes. By the age of 3 years, it becomes more flexible, and by the age of 4, it is under voluntary control. Children can cope with complex situations, such as the combination of a parent talking and a play activity, by seamless shifts of attention between them.

By the time of entering school, an attention span at one activity of at least 5 minutes can be expected. By the time of secondary school, children will often be expected to maintain sustained attention over periods of half an hour or more. Over these longer periods, focused attention will not be continuously deployed. For one thing, the overt manifestations of attention may not accurately represent covert information processing. A child may be staring intently at the teacher without processing what is being taught. For another, neuroimaging studies have shown that periods of activation of attention-related structures are frequently succeeded by short periods of reduced activation, and activation of other structures—the so-called 'default network'. Mind-wandering is the subjective equivalent.

As schooling proceeds, students are very often expected to maintain focus over periods of many minutes. The apparently simple instruction from a teacher to 'pay attention' usually refers to increasing intensity of focus or maintaining performance over time. These functions can be assessed in various ways. Behaviourally, the facial expression of mental effort and reduction of task-irrelevant activity often influence teachers' judgements. Measures of performance are also used but need to be interpreted in the light of understanding the individual's cognitive ability.

2.3.3.1 *Psychological tests*

Several kinds of psychological test have been developed for measuring focused attention.

'*Readiness to respond*' can be indexed by the extent to which the response to a signal is made faster or more accurate by giving a warning that it is about to appear. If the warning is very close to the signal (less than about a quarter of a second), then there is not enough time for readiness to work, reaction time is slow, and the signal may even be missed entirely. If the warning period is too long (depending on age and gender, but typically more than 7 seconds), then readiness is not maintained and again the reaction to the signal is slow. Readiness over longer periods, sometimes called 'vigilance', is frequently operationalized as a score on a continuous performance test (CPT). This is a repetitive sequence of reaction time signals, typically given over 15 minutes or more, which are unpredictably presented in the course of a larger number of stimuli that do not require a response. This stresses several mental functions. Speed of reaction to the cues, inhibition of responses to non-cues, and sustaining performance over time are all involved. In many versions, memory is also required if, for instance, the signal to respond is the repetition of the preceding stimulus. A rapid decline of performance and speed over time implies more difficulty in sustaining attention.

In general, performance on a CPT increases steadily through the early primary school years. Such tests are readily available commercially, and widely used in clinical practice, often with more clinical reliance placed on them than they can reasonably sustain. Modifications of such tests allow them to be used to assess memory (Section 2.4) and inhibitory function (considered as an aspect of executive functioning in Section 2.5).

In all types of psychological test, focused attention is a function of the demands of the task as well as the individual's capacities. It may seem to fluctuate over the course of development, in several ways:

1) Assigned tasks tend to get harder as children get older, and orientation to them may correspondingly increase to allow more time for processing.
2) Some tasks for older children become more interesting and engaging for the individual, and mental effort becomes rewarding and persistent.
3) Some tasks become too hard or unattractive, and the child switches off and deploys no mental effort.
4) Memory and learning themselves increase, so that tasks become easier and no longer require the same mental effort to achieve them.

2.3.4 Selective attention and distraction

To choose which parts of the outside world to focus on requires that some stimuli are highlighted and others not. Sometimes this can be done by physical properties. A child can respond to an important person's voice, even in the presence of ambient noise, on the basis of its pitch and rhythm. Sometimes, however, selecting stimuli for processing needs a higher level of analysis. Relevance to tasks in hand, and the history of what has proved to be important in the past, come to play a part. When an adult tells a child to 'pay attention' it is not only about intensity, but also a direction towards which aspect of the world is immediately relevant and worthy of selection.

Concentration on one thing in the presence of a mass of unrelated information is a key aspect of attention control. The decision of what is relevant may be imposed from outside (as in traditional classroom learning) or from within (as part of the executive functions of planning and goal setting).

Distractibility is both a behavioural and a cognitive construct. Behaviourally, it is inferred from frequent changes of orientation or from easy interruption of activity by irrelevant external stimuli. Cognitively, it implies a weak ability to ignore irrelevance.

The mere addition of irrelevant stimuli does not consistently worsen performance—it often does so, but for some individuals in some situations, it improves it. When young children are in a quiet room and working on a set task, extraneous noises worsen their performance and they look away from the task more often. Older children (by the end of primary school) are different. Extraneous noise often improves performance on the same kind of test (Higgins & Turnure, 1984).

As children develop, they become increasingly expert at ignoring stimuli that are clearly extraneous to the activity in hand. It is however much harder to ignore stimuli that are embedded in the task in hand. Stroop tests are a case in point. In their original form (from 80 years ago; there are now many), these involve naming the colour of the ink in which words are written, when the word themselves are the names of colours. On this kind of test, performance increases steadily into young adult life. Several processes and brain circuits are involved, not only the ability to focus. The systems involved in resolving conflicts and selecting responses (the anterior cingulate cortex and dorsolateral prefrontal cortex) are also activated.

High-level decision making about what is relevant is required. One way of making the decision is for the individual to be guided by experience. Research in adults has emphasized the extent to which attention is paid selectively to those stimuli that have previously been very predictive. A test of this learning influence is given by, for instance, the Kamin blocking procedure (Kamin, 1969). This involves first a process in which a cue is established as being a good predictor of whether an outcome will follow. Once the individual has learned that it is relevant, a further learning period continues to train them, but now with the addition of a new cue that is also highly predictive of the outcome. Subsequent testing finds that little has been learned about the new cue. It has not been deemed relevant, so does not capture attention when presented alone. The suggestion is that there is an active process of learning what to ignore, and that this is present from the age of about 6 years.

This learning what to ignore will matter when ignoring some aspects helps the learning about others. Children have been tested for their learning on a task—for instance, to remember the positions of cards on which there are animal pictures. On this 'central' task, older children performed better than younger ones. However, if they were subsequently asked about 'incidental' features, such as the colour of the cards on which the different animals had been shown, there was no such improvement with age. Indeed, after the age of about 12 years, performance on the 'incidental' learning gets worse as the children get older (Hagen & Hale, 1973). Selective attention comes at a cost, but the result is greater efficiency. Without it, there is the danger of distorted learning about the world.

The need to deploy attention in order to fulfil a plan, to allocate attention to self-chosen goals, and to monitor one's progress in complex tasks is an achievement of middle childhood and adolescence. It becomes relevant to personality and temperament. Influential research by Rothbart and others (Shiner et al., 2012) has argued that one of the dimensions in behaviour rating scales should be labelled as 'effortful control'. It includes behaviours interpreted as planning, focusing, and sustaining activity over time, evident by toddlerhood and early to middle childhood (Nigg, 2017).

2.3.5   Brain networks for attention and related functions

The brain structures involved in selective attention are both cortical and subcortical. Experiments with mice allow them to be studied by manipulating the activity of different parts of the brain. Harassa and colleagues (Wimmer et al., 2015) found that selection towards stimuli in one sensory mode or another depended on interactions between the prefrontal cortex (determining whether, for instance, visual or auditory signals should be attended to) and the sensory parts of the thalamus that downgrade or upgrade sensitivity to one or the other mode. Human research with functional imaging adds that the amygdala play an important role in attending to emotionally important signals via direct connections with the sensory cortex (Pourtois et al., 2013). It seems that the individual's choices about relevance are matters of motivation and learning—but systems to focus on the relevant and ignore the irrelevant are also key abilities, and require both cortical and subcortical circuits to modulate responsiveness to stimuli.

Knowledge about the brain structures involved in focusing and selecting is increasing. They can better be thought of as distributed networks than closely defined anatomical centres. Several such brain networks involved in the ordinary development of attention and related functions can be distinguished. The systems go beyond the frontal and striatal areas that are usually described. From magnetic resonance imaging, Castellanos and Proal (2012) have described such networks based on connectivity measures in more than a thousand healthy young adults. They distinguished:

- a *frontoparietal network* that guides decision making about where to attend;
- a *ventral attention network* (in areas bounded by the temporoparietal cortex, supramarginal gyrus, frontal operculum, and anterior insula) that monitors for salient stimuli and interrupts activity when appropriate;
- a *dorsal attention network* (including frontal eye fields) underpinning shifts of attention and mediating executive control processes;

- a *visual network* (the occipital and lateral temporal cortex), interacting with the dorsal attention network to suppress attention to irrelevant stimuli and maintain focused attention;
- a *motor network* for activation and timing (involving the motor and sensory cortex, ventral premotor cortex, putamen, thalamus, and cerebellum);
- a *default network*, that is 180 degrees out of phase and negatively correlated with the other networks related to cognitive control.

It is not yet clear exactly how these networks develop or how they relate to cognitive deficits, but the research emphasizes the distributed nature of information processing in the brain. Useful understanding of deviations of attention development will need to take account of a wide range of other abilities.

2.3.6 Alterations of attention in disorders

2.3.6.1 *Alterations in focusing and sustaining attention*

Delays in focusing and sustaining attention are part of general immaturity in brain development. Intellectual disability is associated with a reduced orientating reflex and longer reaction times to simple stimuli. Short attention spans and distractibility are also part of specific learning difficulties, but it is often unclear whether improving attention helps learning. More often, inattentiveness is an understandable reaction to working on tasks that are too difficult for the individual.

Sustaining responsiveness over time can be a problem after damage to the brain, and if attention is blunted (e.g. by sedative drugs). A CPT can be used to detect periodic failures to respond to stimuli. It is helpful in people with epilepsy, to monitor an adverse effect of antiepileptic medication.

Problems in orientation to people are important for social development. Attention is a social behaviour as well as a cognitive function. In the parent–child relationship, looking at each other is rewarding. Children who are slow to develop focused looking will risk being perceived as uninterested by their caregivers and attract less attention from them.

Joint attention ordinarily develops from around 9 to 15 months, and delays are often the first sign of autism spectrum disorder (ASD). Not only do children avoid the other person's gaze or fail to point to something, they do not reference the other or share their interest.

2.3.6.2 *Alterations of selective attention*

Easy susceptibility to distraction is a feature of several kinds of pathology. It may involve a failure of selective attention, but often reflects a voluntary alteration of the direction of attention (see 'Specific learning difficulties', Chapter 5, Section 5.2.3).

2.3.6.3 *Altered breadth of attention*

A very broad strategy of admitting information risks overload. Subjective accounts of some people with schizophrenia emphasize confusion and a sense of being overwhelmed by things that should not matter and should be screened out by the filters of attention. Experimentally, attention to irrelevant cues is enhanced in schizophrenia (Morris et al., 2013). Kamin blocking (see Section 2.3.4) is reduced in schizophrenia, implying that processing resources are diverted to non-relevant information (Jones et al., 1997). Some psychotic symptoms such as auditory hallucinations could be due to alteration of the usual filtering processes by which thoughts are distinguished from real sounds.

Conversely, a very narrow strategy of responding, 'hyperfocus', can be seen in some autistic people, some with attention deficit hyperactivity disorder (ADHD), and some who have suffered frontal damage.

Admission into consciousness of significant material can be impaired in agnosia syndromes where parietal damage leads to a loss of conscious perception even though sensation is intact. This can complicate the motor development of people with cerebral palsy. Dissociative losses of processing sensory information can lead to conditions such as physically unexplained blindness and fugue states (see 'Functional neurological disorders', Chapter 6, Section 6.8).

2.3.6.4 *Alterations of shifting attention*

Moving from one class of stimuli to another can be vulnerable to brain lesions. Disengaging the focus of visual attention from one place, moving it to another, and re-engaging there, can be impaired in parietal lesions and disorders of the midbrain. People with schizophrenia often find it hard to shift attentional set.

2.3.6.5 *Alterations of direction of attention*

Bias of attention towards particular aspects of the world is implicated both as a result and possibly a cause of some types of psychopathology. Possible cues to threatening events, for example, are highlighted in high anxiety and paranoia. People with psychotic features may react excessively to trivial features of the world around them and attach undue salience to them. Preferential attention to potential threats is considered to maintain worry and brooding, and is targeted in some forms of cognitive therapy.

2.3.6.6 *Alterations of mental effort*

Children's ability to deploy attention in order to fulfil a plan, and with effort, is reduced in ADHD. A lack of attention to details, sustaining attention poorly over time, not following through on instructions, avoiding effort, and forgetfulness are all central parts of the condition (see Chapter 3, Section 3.2.3).

Nevertheless, 'attention deficit' is something of a misnomer. At a cognitive level, the condition is not particularly characterized by deficits in focusing, sustaining, or selecting.

Rather, the neurocognitive changes in ADHD are widespread and heterogeneous (see Chapter 3, Section 3.8). Many of the changes (such as delay aversion and default mode activation) reflect differences of style or alterations of motivation rather than 'deficits' in attention development or even executive function.

2.4 MEMORY

Short-term memory retains a large but finite amount of information over periods of a few seconds. It is apparent in a digit span test, in which a list of digits is presented at 1-second intervals and must be repeated by the examinee. By the age of 8 years, most children manage five digits; in adult life, six or seven is usual. This kind of test is often followed by a request for the same digits to be repeated in reverse order. This is harder— usually the span is one less than the straightforward repetition. After about 15 seconds, much less of the information is recalled. It can be extended by rehearsing it, either aloud or covertly, so that it re-enters the system. 'Chunking' also extends the information that is kept (e.g. replacing single digits with meaningful clusters). Working memory is not the same thing; it refers to short-term manipulation of information and is considered under 'executive function'.

Long-term memory retains information that has been selected for the purpose. It can be explicit or implicit. *Explicit* (declarative) memory is that in which facts ('semantic memory'), experiences ('episodic memory'), and concepts are recalled into conscious experience. *Implicit* (procedural) memory is that in which the ability to perform a learned skill is retained without the conscious recall of what was learned.

The transfer of information to an enduring record (engram) takes place over a period of minutes to hours. Protein synthesis is involved and modifies synaptic transmission. The hippocampus and related structures are involved in this consolidation, but the resulting trace, whatever its physical nature, is stored elsewhere in the brain. There is some evidence from adults that procedural memories are stored in basal ganglia, declarative in medial temporal (Squire et al., 2004). Sleep enhances the process. Emotionally positive information is probably more likely than negative to become permanent. The engram is still subject to being degraded by decay and interference from other memories. Intermittent rehearsal (recapitulation) can maintain the trace.

2.4.1 Development of memory

Implicit memory is present from early in development and involves activity in early-developing structures of the brain stem, striatum, and cerebellum. Learning, for instance of language, proceeds with amazing efficiency during the first two years of life, although the context in which it was learned is forgotten. The process responsible is probably the rapid development of myelination, which allows increasingly rapid and therefore more complex communication between nerve cells.

Explicit memory, by contrast, seems to be more dependent on the later maturation of the hippocampus and related structures (Richmond & Nelson, 2007). The system consists of the hippocampal region (CA1 fields, where pyramidal cells are the first region in the circuit and project to the dentate gyrus and subicular complex) and the adjacent perirhinal, entorhinal, and parahippocampal cortices.

Established knowledge, as it increases and becomes increasingly well organized, allows more efficient coding of new memories. By the age of 2 years, episodic memory allows conscious recall of experiences. Memories from this age can be confused with false images and memories. They are susceptible to suggestion, making them less trustworthy. During the early school years, autobiographical memories become more coherent, probably because they can now be recapitulated and therefore strengthened. They can also be modified. After the age of about 7 years, children learn how to memorize. They use strategies such as conscious rehearsal and conceptual organization of what they should learn. Events from after the age of 10 years are relatively easy to remember correctly. During adolescence, there is continuing development of conscious knowledge about memory and deliberate use of strategies.

2.4.2 Alterations of memory

Amnesia can follow from localized damage to the hippocampus. Young people affected in this way have major problems in storing and recalling memories of past events. They can still learn new skills and show otherwise intact cognition.

In otherwise high-functioning people with ASD, there is often diminished memory for social or emotional events. Other, non-personal memories are mostly intact and appropriate to IQ. Experimental studies of memory in autism tend to present a picture of problems with material requiring complex information processing, but intact or superior ability to recall simpler material such as lists of random words or recall of locations where objects have been presented (Boucher et al., 2012; Williams et al., 2006). Free recall of meaningful stimuli can be poor, especially in young people with ASD who also show intellectual disability.

Memory problems can exist on their own or in combination with other developmental difficulties. On their own, they can be associated with problems in the classroom and learning difficulties (Alloway et al., 2009). They overlap with the inattentive dimension of ADHD (Holmes et al., 2014). Both include:

- weaknesses in working memory
- poor academic progress in reading and mathematics
- difficulties in following instructions
- problems with learning activities that require both storage and processing
- behaviours suggesting a short attention span and distractibility.

2.5 EXECUTIVE FUNCTION

Executive function (EF) is closely related to attention. It comprises a set of ways in which one's responsiveness, memory, thoughts, and actions are controlled to achieve goals and solve problems. It is not a unitary process, but a complex of abilities in which working memory, inhibitory control, and cognitive flexibility figure prominently. Different authorities take the term EF to mean different sets of abilities and sometimes include nearly all the supposed functions of the frontal lobes including planning and self-monitoring. Most would concentrate specially on working memory, inhibition, and cognitive flexibility. Their underpinning by distributed brain networks has been emphasized in Section 2.3.

Developmental research suggests that EFs emerge early in development, usually being established in simple form by about 4 years, and that they continue to develop into adolescence, with adult-level performance on many standard tests of EF being reached at about 12 years of age, and performance on some measures continuing to change into early adulthood. This developmental course runs parallel to the slow growth of the pre-frontal cortex. Visu–Petra et al. (2014) suggest a developmental process in which EFs depend on the speed of processing information (measured for instance by reaction time). The idea is that speed increases through development and allows larger numbers of neural networks to be coordinated.

2.5.1 Working memory

Problem solving often requires a system in which a limited amount of information can be registered for a short period and transformed into something available for cognitive processing. For example, children may need to keep a string of numbers in mind while they are deciding which is largest. Baddeley and Hitch (1974) described separate systems in short-term memory: a *phonological loop* and a *visuospatial scratchpad* feed into an *executive system* that supervises and controls the contents and is involved especially in their manipulation. An *episodic buffer* works across sensory modalities to provide a temporary store of limited capacity in which information can be coded into chunks, facilitating entry into long-term memory.

The amount of information that can be manipulated and reasoned about increases steadily from preschool to adolescence. Complex memory tasks involving some manipulation of what has been remembered start to be achievable from the age of about 4 years. Difficulties often show up in academic settings.

Working memory is problematic in ADHD, ASD, and learning impairments. It has attracted remedial attention. A controlled trial of educational remediation of working memory, in children selected for poor working memory specifically, was effective in the sense that working memory scores were improved (Dunning et al., 2013). Indeed, the improvement could still be detected a year later. It did not, however, improve performance in other types of cognitive test, and it did not help academic progress or ADHD.

2.5.2 Inhibition

There are many kinds of inhibition in mental life, from the suppression of socially inappropriate acts to the reduction of emotional expression (Nigg, 2000). Indeed, inhibition of alternative responses is probably necessary in every skilled act and every successful choice. It is so broad and general a requirement, and achieved in so many ways, that to regard it as a single function would be misleading. Rather, neuropsychiatry uses a variety of concepts of 'inhibition' for different purposes, from understanding overflow movements in coordination disorders to attempting to explain uncontrolled aspects of cognition, response selection, obedience to social rules, overemotional states, and impulsiveness.

Cognitive inhibition is the exclusion of some information from processing—as when irrelevant features of the environment are ignored (see 'Selective attention and distraction', Section 2.3.4). It is necessary, for instance in the 'false belief' tests considered under theory of mind, where the memory of a scene must be suppressed in the interest of understanding how the same scene has looked to somebody else. This ability is present from about the age of 4 years and increases steadily until adult life.

Response inhibition is the suppression of a prepotent response so that a more considered one can be made, or that conflicts between responses can be resolved. It is often assessed by modified CPTs (described earlier as measures of sustaining attention). They are repetitive and speeded tests of stimuli requiring responses. The modification to test inhibition comprises an instruction not to respond to some of the stimuli. In 'go, no go' tests, most of the stimuli presented do require a response, but infrequent signals scattered among them signify that the response must be withheld. In 'stop' tests, the instruction not to respond comes after the signal, and provides an even stronger test of the ability to inhibit responding.

Inhibitory function can be judged as the individual's capacity and willingness to delay a response—and thereby to allow more time for reflection and correct selection of a response. This capacity to reflect is indexed by, for instance, the matching familiar figures test (Kagan et al., 1964). In this difficult task, a target picture is presented, and the person being tested must choose which one out of a set of subtly varying pictures is identical to the target. The target needs to be compared with the reference set on several dimensions of colour, shape, and positioning of components. As a result, most children need to give themselves plenty of time to solve it (depending on the exact form, more than 10 seconds). If they give themselves too little time, they are likely to make mistakes and are then classified as 'impulsive'. From the age of 7–8 years upwards, children become slower and more accurate in their performance on this sort of test. There are quite stable individual differences, and the least impulsive children also tend to be those who use the most efficient and systematic search strategies and are the best performers on continuous performance tests.

Emotional inhibition is a key aspect of emotional regulation. Problems in inhibition include both excessive and defective control. Children with high levels of inhibition are often anxious and vulnerable to developing emotional problems. By contrast, those whose style is most impulsive may have problems in conforming to social rules and expectations.

2.5.3 Cognitive flexibility

Flexibility is especially useful when the rules of how to cope with a situation change. It is often studied experimentally through the ability to shift focus. For instance, an experimenter might present a set of objects to be sorted that could be arranged either by colour or by shape, and children's performance is then classified by their tendency to perseverate, after a change of rule, on the first rule given. Most children are poor at shifting until they are aged about 4 years. Thereafter, performance depends on the complexity of the task and on individuals, between whom there is considerable variation.

Difficulties of cognitive flexibility can be reflected in coping poorly with transitions and changes, sticking to routines, having fixed special interests, and interacting unhappily with unpredictable situations such as play with peers (Strang et al., 2017). The resulting rigidity is a key component of, but not restricted to, individuals falling within the autism spectrum.

2.5.4 'Hot' and 'cold' executive functions

Many experts distinguish between 'hot' and 'cold' types of EF. Most laboratory tests mentioned, such as rapid responses to screen signals, are rather abstract, or 'cold'. They are served by the dorsolateral prefrontal cortex, connecting with circuits involving the thalamus, dorsal caudate nucleus, hippocampus, and posterior temporal cortex. 'Hot' functions, by contrast, come into play when there are strong incentives, as is often the case in motivated and social behaviour. They tend to be more involved with orbitofrontal parts of the prefrontal cortex, connecting with the limbic system and amygdala.

2.6 SOCIAL INTERACTION AND UNDERSTANDING

Social understanding is acquired in the course of interactions with other people. We make relationships with others right from the start of life. The developmental strand of understanding them involves learning, emotional life, and experiences of relating to others (Carpendale & Lewis, 2004).

2.6.1 Social relationships

Parent–child relationships work in both directions from early life. Infants cry; parents respond both to the situation and the urgency of its expression in ways coloured by their own mental state; infants respond to parental distress. By the third month of life, the infant is sharing in positive relationships. Infants smile, parents respond, and that response is gratifying to the child. The child initiates sequences of activity, and often mirrors the parent's actions and responses.

Social interaction is rewarding. Infants look at faces, or pictures of faces, more than they do to similar pictures shown upside-down or distorted. Direct gaze from another person elicits more gaze from the infant. If mothers 'freeze' and keep an expressionless face, infants will get angry or distressed. Social interactions become even more reciprocal with age. Mirroring actions are followed by gestural and vocal conversations. After about the fourth month, vocal responses and interactive games come to the fore. The child is often the initiator and indicates that they want games to continue. The process of socialization is different in different cultures, as caregivers respond selectively—some favouring vocal interaction over play with toys, some expecting obedience rather than initiative. Turn-taking, in one form or another, becomes a great source of fun.

With developing ability to move around, the child is capable of more independence. The parent is the force for security in the child's exploration of the world. Secure attachment allows greater degrees of exploration away from the secure base provided by the primary caregiver. Rules appear.

In social referencing, a child in an uncertain or confusing situation will look at the caregiver for clues on what is going on and how they should react. The emotional tone of the mother's response will be reflected in the child's. By about 18 months, the acquisition of names for objects will be assisted by the child working out what the parent is looking at when they name something. By about 24 months, they will share recollections of events and narratives about them. This will also inform the child's understanding about social rules in general. Social interactions become generalized to a wider range of people.

Relationships with siblings cast other children in the family in the role of playmates, rivals, and teachers. After about 3 years, conversations with siblings (if any) become more frequent, at the expense of conversations with parents. Some forms of talk are much common between siblings than between children and adults—for instance, fantasy and jokes. The more equal nature of most sibling relationships creates both more conflict and more understanding of siblings' beliefs and attitudes and how they shape behaviour.

Peer relationships involving children outside the immediate family also create the opportunity and the need for more complex understanding, including that of group norms and rules. Infants from about 3 months reciprocate eye gaze with others of the same age.

Toddlers initiate and respond to social overtures from one another and develop turn-taking rules. In the third year of life, the social milieu of peers extends considerably. How one joins a group, and how one learns the rules of games, both lead to acceptance or otherwise by the group. It usually works best for children to observe group play before joining and to take their cue about the rules of the game from others.

Social connectedness is intrinsically rewarding. By the age of 3 years, toddlers prefer to get a reward when it is given by humans rather than mechanically. If the choice is to get a food reward by either working collaboratively with another child or by working independently, they strongly prefer collaboration (Rekers et al., 2011). (Incidentally, human children are more social than chimpanzees of comparable maturity in this kind of set-up.) Toddlers behave less helpfully to others if the rewards for cooperating are material gain rather than social praise (Warneken & Tomasello, 2008). Interaction with other people is, for typically developing children, its own reward.

2.6.2 Social understanding

Social understanding helps children to adjust their behaviour to the social context, and to share imaginative play with others. Consistent styles of interaction such as shyness and assertiveness emerge. Abilities for communication (Section 2.8) further influence the acquisition of friends, the resolution of conflicts, and resistance to bullying.

Individual differences emerge in the understanding of other people. Young people's cognitive abilities mature to a level where they can, for instance, work out strategies for dealing with interpersonal conflict (see Section 2.9). They come to differentiate between their self and others, and to recognize others' states of mind. They develop strategies for influencing other people, based on both experience and ideas about others' reactions to them.

2.6.2.1 *Theory of mind*

'Theory of mind' refers to the ability to explain, predict, and interpret behaviour by attributing mental states—such as desires, beliefs, intentions, and emotions—to oneself and to other people. Developmental research has used ingenious behavioural testing measures to track the ability of children and young people to pass false-belief tasks, false-appearance tasks, and deception.

A typical false-belief test presents a child with a scene of two people in a room. The first person hides an object and then leaves the room. The other person moves the object to a different place. When the first person comes back to the room, the child who has watched the whole scene is asked where the first person will look for the object. Correct answers need the child to have understood what is in the first person's memory—that they will not know about the change of location and so will look where they hid it. By late preschool, most will have reached this understanding. Before then, they will say that the first person will look to the place to which the object has been moved and actually is. By the age of 4 years, there are consistent findings on neural activity during this sort of false-belief test. Sabbagh et al. (2009), for example, found localized EEG activity in the dorsal medial prefrontal cortex and right temporal–parietal juncture. The alpha activity varied between individual children and was positively associated with their performance.

Even before that age, infants can have a rudimentary appreciation when tested more subtly with length of eye gaze. Delays in the ability can reflect either problems of congenitally deaf children in understanding the language or, in autism, a more fundamental difficulty in understanding other people's thoughts and beliefs (Tager-Flusberg & Joseph, 2005).

Deciding who to trust is another kind of situation where children can be shown, experimentally, to understand what is in other people's minds. By the time they enter school, children are more likely to believe a person who has previously given them correct information than someone who has provided false information.

2.6.2.2 *Empathy*

Empathy is another function relying on and contributing to social understanding. It entails both the ability to understand other people's subjective experiences and the concern with and for other people that will lead to prosocial behaviour and a sharing of their emotions. In the second and third years of life, nearly all toddlers react to others' distress with some helping behaviour such as a hug or a sad expression (Zahn–Waxler et al., 1992). As children get older, this develops into verbal expressions of sympathy ('sorry') and enquiry about the reason ('what's wrong?') This may well be taking the form of the comforting acts and words they have experienced themselves.

Prosocial behaviours such as these proceed in parallel with emotional sharing through the school years. Comparisons of monozygotic and dizygotic twins indicate some heritability, and there is some stability of individual differences through childhood—but it is not yet clear how far these amount to consistent personality traits. There is also some evidence that greater synchrony, more attachment security, and greater warmth between mother and child in early childhood are associated with greater affective empathy in the child later. High levels of cognitive and affective empathy contribute to social competence and to internalizing rules of conduct.

There is some evidence for a neural basis of empathy (Fan et al., 2013). Amygdala responsiveness to images of other people's distress seems to correlate with children's behavioural responsiveness.

2.6.3 Alterations of social interaction and understanding

Children vary in the extent to which social connectedness is intrinsically rewarding, and therefore in the knowledge about other people that they acquire. Those who are more interested in making friends are likely to have more opportunities to develop their understanding of them and, in turn, to relate more fully. The more that children are restricted in opportunities to interact and relate—whether because of external constraints or self-imposed isolation—the less chance they have to talk about mental states and the experiences of other people.

Poor scores in theory of mind tests often go together with changes in tests of face processing, motor imitation, working memory, phonological processing, and other tests of executive function (Kaiser et al., 2010). Recognition of faces is an early-arising ability, and difficulties here could have developmental consequences for the other aspects of delayed social understanding. In ASD, impairments of social understanding start early, with reduced imitation of adult facial gestures and scant signs of response to another person's distress or fear (Sigman et al., 1992). They are not typical of people with intellectual disability (ID) or ADHD alone.

The cognitive and affective aspects of empathy do not always vary together. Extreme difficulties in understanding other people's thoughts characterize many autistic people, who can still be very caring to others in distress. High levels of the unemotional adjustment seen in psychopathy or 'conduct disorder with limited prosocial emotions' in DSM-5 are accompanied by an unusual lack of emotional sharing. Such individuals can nevertheless be very good indeed at predicting and manipulating other people.

Several brain areas have shown signs of atypical development in people with impaired social understanding. As an example, Pelphrey and Carter (2008) described differences from typical development in the orbitofrontal and medial frontal cortex, amygdala, and inferior frontal gyrus.

2.7 REALITY TESTING, IMAGINATION, AND PRETENCE

Pretend play emerges early, typically around 18 months (Piaget, 1962). By the age of 28 months, children understand when adults are pretending. They do not expect that an imaginary tea party will actually wet them if the pretend tea is spilled. They do nevertheless competently play along and generate the consequences that would follow in the real world. They can create a mental representation of a pretend episode and use that representation to guide their own pretend actions and language (Harris et al., 1993).

Three- to five-year-old children understand that make-believe situations do not exist in the real world and do not behave as if they do (Harris et al., 1991). This ability to understand make-believe has much in common with the ability to understand other people's mental states. It allows the development of spontaneously generated pretend play, for instance in the creation of imaginary friends or animated toys. Imagination is of great importance in the mental life of children.

This raises questions about the nature of beliefs that do not correspond with reality. What accounts for their development? How do non-veridical sensory experiences come to be recognized as such, rather than as true accounts about the real world? How do hallucinations and delusions come about? Is an imaginary friend an hallucination or a pretend game, and how and when does it change from one to the other? The answers are not known. It may be that the sense of agency is critical, and perhaps can be lost in pathology. It may be that a make-believe set of mental states is separately tagged as such unless the mechanism is deficient in some way. It may be that volition is the key to distinguishing which actions are one's own rather than the result of inserted thoughts. Lewis and Boucher (1988) found that children with ASD can indeed pretend *if* they are prompted. Any deficit is in the spontaneous production of pretend play.

2.7.1 Alterations of reality testing

Distortions of reality testing can appear in several psychiatric conditions and are often called 'psychotic'.

- *Hallucinations* are sensory perceptions in the absence of external stimuli. Auditory and visual modalities are the commonest, but smell, taste, and bodily sensation are also frequently involved.
- *Delusions* are false beliefs, held irrationally and not in keeping with the rest of the culture. They include beliefs that one is being followed or persecuted or has a special importance in the world.
- *Perceptions of self* can be distorted into a nihilistic or grandiose self-image. In depersonalization, there is a sense of being altered or unreal, or not being the volitional agent of one's actions.
- *Passivity phenomena* are altered experiences of one's thoughts and volitions, inserted into one's mind or extracted from it by external agencies, or available for other people to experience directly.
- *Derealization* is an altered experience of the external world (e.g. that it is unreal or menacing).

Altered experiences such as these are common in children. In one study, using 8,000 children's replies to direct questioning, two-thirds of 9- to 11-year-olds in London described at least one (Laurens et al., 2012). The vast majority of such experiences are transient and resolve spontaneously within a few weeks or months. They typically come at times of anxiety and/or stressful events. In children before the age of 7 years, thoughts can often be described as 'voices' and dreams as 'visions'. Some vivid hallucinations—for instance, the presence of imaginary friends—are associated with desirable traits such a strong imagination or superior performance in tests of theory of mind.

The qualities of any hallucinations, and especially their impact on the young person's life, will often help in deciding whether they need to be investigated. Their frequency, duration, intensity, and controllability (e.g. by distraction) are usually good guides. The level of insight into their unreality, and any distress in reaction to them, will help to guide how seriously other people should take them. Their meaning in relation to socio-cultural factors needs to feature in a judgement about their possible significance. Ethnic differences are well-known in adults (Earl et al., 2015), and similar differences are seen in children.

The clinical significance of delusions can be judged also from their form. It is not so much the lack of correspondence with reality that makes them pathological as the irrationality with which they are held. Relatives' explanations may show that unusual beliefs are in fact shared. When there is religious or magical content, then a community leader can be a good guide as to whether the beliefs are out of keeping with those of the community. Special care will be needed when the clinician is culturally distant from the patient. It is not usually enough for her/him to rely on theoretical knowledge of the patient's presumed culture: many subcultures and variants exist. Rather, s/he should ask for explanations of the shared belief systems.

Even though altered reality experiences are common in children, they are not necessarily trivial. Drugs such as cannabis (Chapter 7, Section 7.9.11) should always be suspected when psychotic-like features need investigation. Sometimes, the features are part of an emotional or behavioural disorder, including depersonalization disorder, or part of the consequences of abusive experiences in childhood, including posttraumatic stress disorder. Sometimes, autistic people report experiences that never actually happened.

Epilepsy can include unusual experiences, especially when the temporal lobes, limbic system, and sensory cortex are involved. Narcolepsy, too, can produce hallucinations on falling into sleep or awaking from it.

A main concern often expressed by the young people and their caregivers is that they are going mad or, more specifically, that the abnormal experiences are the beginning of schizophrenia. Diagnosis and the need for intervention are considered in 'Premorbid conditions and prodromes' in Chapter 4, Section 4.2.5.

2.8 DEVELOPMENT AND PATHOLOGY OF COMMUNICATION

2.8.1 Language and speech

Newborn babies already have considerable competencies that will later be used for speech. The cochlea, auditory nerve, and cochlear nucleus are well adapted to analyse the sounds of consonants. Babies can recognize patterns of sound well before they recognize meaning. Auditory development allows some basic abilities fundamental to communication: for instance, in preferring to orientate to speech rather than mere noise, to their mother's speaking voice rather than that of strangers, and to speech in their mother language rather than a foreign one.

By about 3 months, infants are cooing, and by about 6 months, they are babbling. This stage comes even in those who are deaf, and probably represents learning how to use the lips, tongue, larynx, and lungs. Refinement into word-like sounds comes later, often at about 12 months in those with ordinary hearing.

First words are often simplified versions, sometimes to the point where only parents can understand them. They are attached to meanings through social referencing. The caregiver uses joint attention and shared eye gaze to show, for instance, the animal referred to as 'dog'. As the number of words increases, it can be challenging to keep them separate. Often a word will be used in an overgeneralized way (e.g. 'dog' being used for any animal); sometimes, undergeneralized (e.g. 'dog' only for one specific animal). Furthermore, word patterns start to be recognized (e.g. 'my dog', not 'dog my'), often after a period of experimentation. Acquiring the knowledge of putting words together is guided by experience and is a beginning of grammar.

Intonation and pauses also come to be used in regular ways, and to convey meaning (e.g. a rising intonation to convey that a question is being asked). The first words are typically labels for familiar things and people, social words ('bye-bye'), and words indicating states ('here', 'now'). In the second year of life, children are learning what words are for (especially, to communicate).

There follows a remarkable explosion in the number of words with consistent meanings. Furthermore, after (about) the third birthday, the meanings of words are classified and generalized. Words higher in the hierarchy of meaning (e.g. 'animal' over 'dog') are used flexibly and increasingly correctly. Verbs follow different rules from nouns. Young children can generate plurals (e.g. 'wugs') even for a nonsense word ('wug') they have never heard before. They recognize the classes of words that behave differently semantically (e.g. 'more food' rather than 'foods'; but 'dogs' rather than 'more dog').

Rules about word order very soon come to be used correctly in the convention of the local language (e.g. 'dog eat' not 'eat dog'). Successful use of grammar can involve complex judgements and memory. Inflections of verbs, for instance, require not only the knowledge of a rule (for instance, in the English language, the addition of 'ed' at the end of a verb to signal the past tense—e.g. 'walked') but also awareness of when to use it (not, for instance, when an auxiliary verb has done the same job, as in 'did walk'). More complex grammatical constructions (such as negatives, prepositions, auxiliary verbs, passive constructions, joined sentences, relative clauses) follow steadily, with the simplest constructions first. Individual differences in the consistency and accuracy of using grammatical rules appear. Cultural and subcultural variations need to be understood and distinguished from abnormality.

For many languages, charts are available showing the typical ages at which features of language appear. They can be used to assess immaturity. Standardized tests of language are available in some countries and should be given priority in recognizing the presence of delays.

In early development, parents' knowledge of the child may yield very valuable information about key stages for language. The MacArthur Communicative Development Inventory is a well-standardized checklist based on the observations and recollections of parents (Fenson et al., 1993, 1994).

2.8.2 Function of language

There are many functions of language, often expressed in rather different styles. Needs, for instance, can be put in different ways: 'Please can I have some cherries', 'It would be nice to have some cherries', 'Those cherries look very nice'. More subtle and indirect expressions can be misunderstood if taken literally by a listener who does not understand. Communication can be adapted to the listener: 5-year-olds will use simpler language in talking to a 2-year-old than to a contemporary. Taking turns in conversation can express reciprocality with the other person. Formal and 'correct' language is sometimes expected in the classroom but would be unsettling in the playground. Peacemaking in conflicts and deception call for different verbal styles. People who are more advanced in communication than others use language more flexibly in the service of different functions. This is called the pragmatic use of language,

Even so brief a sketch emphasizes that language acquisition involves many other lines of development—sensory integrity, motor control, attention, social understanding, and learning all contribute. All of them need to be considered in a full evaluation of children with substantial difficulties in communication.

2.8.3 Sign language

Gesture and intonation accompanying speech are used from the start of language acquisition to intensify utterances or add significance—for instance, to show what is intended as a joke.

Language develops in very similar ways in children who do not hear or speak—if they are living with people who use a sign language. The milestones of single-sign and two-sign expressions appear at similar ages to those indicated earlier for typical development. Grammar often uses hands, arms, and face to indicate relationships (such as who did what to whom), through positions in physical space rather than word sequences. Signed languages are naturally all different, and can convey rich propositions and poetic beauty. Families using a sign language see themselves as a minority rather than a disabled group.

2.8.4 Alterations of language development

Problems in communication arise in various ways (Box 2.2). Many children show difficulties in using language effectively. Some find it hard to communicate because their speech is slurred or indistinct. They try to communicate, and they understand what other children are saying, but are frustrated by their inability to make themselves understood.

Box 2.2 Primary communication problems

Language

Production
- Vocabulary
- Grammar
- Discourse (conversation, narrative, exposition; formal v. vernacular)

Comprehension

Language-related academic problems: reading, writing, spelling

Non-verbal: gesture, facial expression, signing

Social

Autism spectrum disorders

Pragmatic language/social communication disorder

Selective mutism

Speech

Speech sound
- Articulation: dysarthria, phoneme substitution, intelligibility
- Voice: shouting, whispering
- Perception of speech

Fluency
- Stammering
- Cluttering
- Verbal dyspraxia
- Tics

Other children may have no difficulty in articulating clear speech but what they produce is immature. They use fewer words and simpler grammar than others of their own age, so they seem younger than they really are. Some can express themselves fluently but struggle to understand what is said to them. It makes them appear to be inattentive, and they often fall behind other children socially and academically. Yet others can use language well when dealing with events and their personal interests, but struggle to understand what other children are trying to tell them and lose interest in communicating with them. Even with adults, they may find it hard to make themselves understood because they do not comprehend what the others need to know.

Some children have difficulties in all the aforementioned areas of speaking clearly, using vocabulary and grammar well, comprehending others, and making social use of language. Difficulties often coexist with each other and with other problems of development. Clinicians should consider whether communication problems are primary or secondary to other impairments (e.g. deafness). Box 2.2 lists the range of primary problems.

The recognition of significant problems is usually based on standardized tests of competence in communication and detecting that an individual child is not advancing to the expected stages. Failing that, clinicians' and educators' observations of conversation, narrative and exposition, and repeating speech can yield a similar, if less precise, result.

The terminology is rather variable. A distinction is often made between 'delay' and 'disorder'. The idea of 'disorder' has historically often been operationalized as a discrepancy between language ability and non-verbal IQ. Scientifically, there is little to support the practice. Children with verbal–non-verbal discrepancy have similar linguistic profiles to those whose non-verbal IQ is similar to their language test scores. Such children have, if anything, a better outcome in later life; they do not respond differently to remedial teaching (Bishop, 2003).

Practically, therefore, the effect in clinics and schools of restricting special provision to those with a good non-verbal IQ is discriminatory. It risks withholding provision from those who need it most and could use it best. The effect, however, of eliminating the distinction could be an unfulfilled increase in demand. It remains a potent source of misunderstanding between clinical and educational professionals. The DSM-5 definition of 'developmental language disorder' has abandoned the practice of referencing against non-verbal IQ. It includes only a requirement that it 'cannot be attributed to intellectual disability or global developmental delay' (American Psychiatric Association, 2013).

Spoken (or signed) language is the foundation for the written word. Children with delays in producing language are at risk for problems with reading. New skills are also needed. The visual image of a letter has to be linked to the sound, so good registration and clear analysis of the sounds ('phonemic awareness') help in recognizing print. At a further stage, the decoding of print into sound ('phonics') needs to become rapid and automatic for reading to become fluent. Rhyming games rely on understanding the sounds and their relationship to the way they are written. Accurate spelling is easier in languages with regular relationships between how words are written and how they are pronounced (the English language being notorious for its inconsistency).

Decoding, however, is not the only kind of cognitive skill that is needed: some children can read aloud rapidly and accurately but fail to understand what they have read. Reading comprehension is a major aspect of literacy and is aided by good spoken or signed language—including high-level linguistic skills such as figurative language, fantasy, and making inferences about what happens in a story. Executive function skills such as working memory are also involved.

Learning to read is a key attainment for progress in education. Different educational and linguistic traditions take a variety of approaches to understanding how difficulties arise in learning to read. However, they have in common that they recognize that general intelligence and adequate instruction are not sufficient to guarantee adequate literacy. This is the heart of the concept of 'dyslexia', described in Chapter 5, Section 5.2.3.

2.9 EMOTIONAL REGULATION

Emotion (mood, affect) is a key part of mental development, both typical and in those with impaired cognitive functions. The negative emotions (anger, depression, anxiety) make difficulties for the impaired if they are displayed to excess. Excessive anger (irritability) is unpleasant for young people and unwelcome to caregivers.

Emotional regulation refers to an individual's ability to modify an emotional state so as to promote adaptive, goal-orientated behaviours. Reappraisal of stimuli and contexts is an important part, as is the inhibition of overt expression. *Emotional dysregulation* refers to immaturity or deviation of regulation and to control being overwhelmed by intense experiences. It is described in more detail in Section 2.9.2.

Figure 2.1 follows Wessa and Linke (2009) to give an account of the stages of emotional response to a stimulus. In the case of anger, the stimulus will usually be an indication of an impending threat or frustrating non-reward. The amygdala signal this even before attention is engaged. The brain's full response will follow, with allocation of attention and admission to detailed processing. Processing progresses to the appraisal of the signal's significance, recall of its reinforcement history, and awareness (Rolls, 2005). At this point (see the right-hand edge of Figure 2.1), there is the opportunity to control the behavioural response. This is largely achieved through circuits (involving the orbitofrontal cortex) that integrate the response with the current contingencies, determining what behavioural reactions are practical and favoured.

2.9.1 Control of anger

The control of anger in typical development is a story of increasing voluntary regulation (see Box 2.3). It is partly a function of the integrity of control circuits to inhibit activity in structures initiating emotional arousal (the amygdala and hypothalamus). It also requires input from reward history, cognitive appraisal of context, and social relationships.

2.9.1.1 *Infancy*

Soothing by caregivers is in reaction to infants' expressions of needs and distress. It is initially achieved by physical comfort, feeding, stroking and rocking, and distraction. Modelling is also used when a parent displays a moderate level of comparable distress and then reduces it. At a later stage, verbal intervention can both be soothing and convey a labelling of the mood state: 'I know, you're all cross, never mind'.

Infants also find ways to comfort themselves, for instance with thumb sucking. Repetitive activities such as head banging can start as self-comforting but later become excessive and problematic. After the first months, direction of attention becomes a

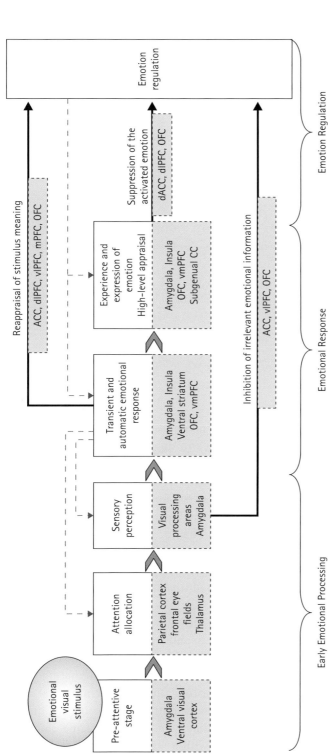

FIGURE 2.1 Successive and recurrent mechanisms in emotional processing. Broken arrows indicate different emotion regulation strategies at different time points during emotional processing.

OFC, orbitofrontal cortex; mPFC, medial prefrontal cortex; vmPFC, ventromedial prefrontal cortex; vlPFC, ventrolateral prefrontal cortex; dlPFC, dorsolateral prefrontal cortex; dACC, dorsal anterior cingulate cortex; CC, cingulate cortex.

Reproduced from *Int Rev Psychiatry*, 21(4), Wesse and Linke, Emotional processing in bipolar disorder: Behavioural and neuroimaging findings, pp. 357–67, Copyright (2009), with permission from Taylor & Francis.

Box 2.3 Early stages of anger regulation

Infancy

Soothing by caregivers

Repetitive self-stimulation

Attention directed away from provoking stimulus

Preschool

Effortful self-control

Tantrum consequences

Development of covert hostility

School age

Masking anger

Rule learning, culture

Problem solving

Gender differentiation

---

means of emotional regulation. Children can now be seen to look away from moderately frustrating situations. By contrast, situations arousing fear typically cause attention to be strongly focused on the scary object.

These active responses by young children are both emotional reactions and methods of coping. They are followed by less overt distress (Buss & Goldsmith, 1998). Children at 6 months who make less use of such tactics as looking away are also the ones whose anger can most readily be aroused (Calkins & Fox, 2002).

Great emphasis has sometimes been placed on the availability of comforting in the first years as a determinant of later emotional resilience (e.g. Gottman et al., 1996). Empirical observation in Western cultures has suggested a rather complex pattern of relationships between parental reactions to distress and later emotional competence by the child. A longitudinal study found little or no relationship between the ways in which mothers reacted to children's emotions after disappointment, at 18 months, and the children's emotional resilience at 5 years (Spinrad et al., 2004). There was also little evidence for parental reactions predicting the child's use of self-regulation. There was a contrasting finding for children at a slightly later stage. At 30 months, their parents' response strategies—soothing, distracting, explaining, questioning—did indeed predict how much the same children, at 5 years, reacted to frustrating non-reward with a strategy such as self-distraction. The children had learned something about emotional competence. If, however, parents had previously responded by making up for the disappointment—'OK, you can have the toy after all!'—then, at 5 years, the children were more likely to respond to disappointment with overt anger.

2.9.1.2 *Preschool*

The classic expression of negative emotion at this age is the tantrum (Box 2.4). This is composed of both anger and distress—usually anger first, and crying and comfort seeking later. It is both an individual passion and a social event. Parental reactions range from early recognition, comfort, and removal of provocation, to some level of punishment, intended to reduce tantrums in the future.

Toddlers are often oblivious of consequences once a tantrum is established and forget it afterwards. This has clinical consequences: first, a rage can be misinterpreted as a seizure; second, it is pointless to reason during a tantrum; third, delay can help. A tantrum is often followed later by a period of remorse during which a child can appreciate explanations and suggestions for the future.

After about 15 months, children are typically developing more ways of controlling their emotions as they acquire a wider range of cognition, language, and motor skills. Parental regulation is still important, and children still soothe themselves, but effortful inhibitory self-control comes to the fore. By 18 months, there is less thumb sucking and much more self-distraction and complex social referencing. Children recruit their caregivers as a source of assistance and mutual regulation of emotion (Diener & Mangersdorf, 1999). Inhibitory control is also developing at this age, and the child's ability to hold back immediate overt responses starts to play a part.

Children are starting to be able to describe their states verbally ('Ellie cross') and to link their feelings to their external causes. They understand the consequences better and acquire the ability to use the behaviours of anger not only to express irritation,

---

Box 2.4 Influences on tantrums

The persistence and frequency of tantrums in early childhood are influenced by:
- the extent to which they succeed in achieving their goal,
- the form of parental discipline,
- the emotional availability of parent(s),
- the extent to which discipline is perceived by the child as unfair,
- the models of anger that the children see in their milieu,
- the level of encouragement of anger (e.g. by parents in conflict with each other or siblings stirring),
- the levels of frustration to which the children are exposed,
- the extent to which they have been shown how to recognize their anger and in what ways to express it.

but to control other people. They learn to talk with their caregivers about what makes them cross and how that affects other people. Constructive coping with anger-provoking situations becomes increasingly possible: they develop, for example, skills in compromising with other children when their interests conflict. The greater the use of attentional control and constructive coping, and the less the emotional intensity of anger, the less likely the children are to use abusive language or to run away from the situation (Fabes & Eisenberg, 1992).

The continuum between ordinary and excessive irritability means that assessing anger-based behaviour is necessary in many of the presentations of neurodevelopmental disorders. Box 2.5 indicates considerations of when tempers should be considered as excessive. Assessment should include whether the level of irritability is beyond the usual range. Can it be attributed, entirely or in part, to the same influences operating on typically developing children? Does neurological dysfunction play a part in generating it?

Covert and prolonged anger, even in the absence of overt tantrums, is also a feature at this stage of development. It is linked to children's perception and appraisal of how they are treated. Strong feelings of resentment are typically linked to feeling unfairly dealt with, or coerced, or humiliated. A sense of helplessness can contribute to sullen and inarticulate anger, as can the imposition of conflicting rules that make it impossible to be correct. Misconceptions can arise—for example, the perception of unavoidable misfortune as being maliciously intended, or of a parent as being hostile or neglectful when, in fact, this represents misrepresentation by another parent (parental alienation).

2.9.1.3 *School age and adolescence*

After the transition into school, or from around the age of five, young people are increasingly capable of hiding their anger. They can appraise situations potentially arousing anger, recognize the early signs in themselves, and make decisions about how to respond. They learn what the expression of anger can achieve and what the costs are—for

---

Box 2.5 When are tempers excessive?

In an observational study of preschool children, involving 50 minutes of play and different tasks, Wakshlag and colleagues (2012) found that the more disruptive children's tempers were more likely to be:

- *Intense*: loud, active, strong, and forceful movements
- *Easily elicited*: could occur after only slight provocation
- *Progressive*: rapidly escalating to a crescendo
- *Pervasive*: observed during several different tasks
- *Persistent*: slow to recover and needing adult attention to resolve

instance, in the ways that other children react. Children also come to understand the social rules and context—for example, that what is acceptable to a boy may be different from that for a girl.

2.9.1.4 *Mood swings in adolescence*

Adolescence is famously a time of unstable mood, at least for some young people. Depression, anxiety, and anger are all likely to be subject to intense and rapid shifts in reaction to events—even more so than in younger children or adults. Casey et al. (2010) linked this to neural events. Frontal cortical regions are developing and exerting increasing control. Subcortical structures, however, are mature at an earlier age. Therefore, some adolescents have a preponderance of subcortical limbic (amygdala) activity over the controlling influences of prefrontal cortical regions. This is a potential mechanism for heightened emotionality during adolescence.

Empirical findings have not been wholly consistent, but some research supports the idea of the cortex and limbic system maturing at different rates. For instance, 50 subjects aged 10 to 24 received functional magnetic resonance imaging (MRI) while they viewed and rated emotionally neutral, negative, and positive pictures (Vink et al., 2014). Activity in the subcortical structures of the amygdala and hippocampus decreased with age. The opposite was found in the ventrolateral prefrontal cortex. Frontal activity when viewing emotionally salient stimuli increased with age and became more coupled to subcortical structures.

2.9.2 Alterations of emotional regulation

Simple immaturity in the progress of self-control can have consequences in psychiatric problems. Rapidly fluctuating emotions challenge self-control. Children and young people are then often referred to as showing 'instability' or 'lability'. Individual differences are also marked and the concept of 'emotional dysregulation' is applied.

Emotional dysregulation is a dimensional trait encompassing:

- emotional expressions and experiences that are excessive in relation to social norms and developmental level;
- rapid, poorly controlled shifts in emotion;
- anomalous allocation of attention to emotional stimuli;
- irritability (inappropriate levels of reactivity), unpredictable mood changes, hot temper, temper tantrums, tearfulness, low frustration tolerance.

Irritability has special importance for people with neurodevelopmental syndromes. It can be a dominant factor in disrupting home and social relationships. Box 2.6 indicates the wide range of recognized psychiatric conditions in which irritability plays a major part.

Box 2.6 Excessive anger in psychiatric disorders

Accompanied by other negative mood changes (misery, anxiety)

Depression

Post-traumatic stress disorder (PTSD)

Disruptive mood dysregulation disorder (DMDD)

Borderline personality ('emotionally unstable personality disorder')

Accompanied by positive mood changes (euphoria)

Bipolar I (episodes lasting 7 days or more)

Bipolar II (episodes lasting 4–7 days)

Bipolar NOS (short episodes; if < 2 days can be synonymous with disruptive mood
dysregulation disorder)

Accompanied by other mental health problems

ADHD

Substance misuse

Autism spectrum

Oppositional–defiant disorder

Accompanied by neurological problems

Traumatic brain injury

Organic brain disease

Pseudobulbar palsy

Epilepsy

Sleep-related abnormalities (including gene syndrome)

Dementias

Occurring in isolation

Secondary to drug use, diet, maltreatment

Intermittent explosive disorder

The multiple influences on development give rise to a continuum of severity, and the point at which it becomes impairing for the individual, or intolerable to others, will depend very much upon the context in which it occurs. Some aspects of treatment (see Chapter 8, Section 8.7) depend upon encouraging the positive influences promoting regulation.

2.10 Autonomic nervous system (ANS)

The sympathetic and parasympathetic nervous systems are often overlooked by those giving advice on the neurodevelopmental disorders. They are often seen as peripheral and concerned with 'lower' functions such as the control of breathing, sweating, heart, and respiration. There is also, however, a central autonomic system involving brain areas from the medial frontal and insula to the amygdala, hypothalamus, and midbrain (Axelrod et al., 2006). It is involved in the expression of emotional responses. Children with impaired ANS function may, for instance, cry emotionally but without tears and, therefore, puzzle their caregivers.

Autonomic changes are part of the response to stress and infections that can influence emotional development, as described in Chapter 7, Section 7.6. They are often described in ASD and especially in Rett syndrome. They can be part of some epileptic seizures. Familial dysautonomia (Riley–Day syndrome) is a recessively inherited syndrome resulting from mutations in the IKBKAP gene on chromosome 9. It is more or less confined to Ashkenazi Jews, and conveys serious risks to life. Insensitivity to pain is a frequent finding.

References

Alloway, T. P., Gathercole, S. E., Kirkwood, H., & Elliott, J. (2009). The cognitive and behavioral characteristics of children with low working memory. *Child Development*, 80(2), 606–621.

American Psychiatric Association. (2013). *Diagnostic and statistical manual of mental disorders* (DSM-5).

Axelrod, F. B., Chelimsky, G. G., & Weese-Mayer, D. E. (2006). Pediatric autonomic disorders. *Pediatrics*, 118(1), 309–321.

Baddeley, A. D., & Hitch, G. J. (1974). Working memory. In G. H. Bower (Ed.), *The psychology of learning and motivation* (pp. 47–89). Academic Press.

Barry, S., Baird, G., Lascelles, K., Bunton, P., & Hedderly, T. (2011). Neurodevelopmental movement disorders–an update on childhood motor stereotypies. *Developmental Medicine & Child Neurology*, 53(11), 979–985.

Bertolero, M. A., Yeo, B. T., Bassett, D. S., & D'Esposito, M. (2018). A mechanistic model of connector hubs, modularity and cognition. *Nature Human Behaviour*, 2(10), 765.

Bishop, D. V. (2003). Specific language impairment: diagnostic dilemmas. In L. Verhoeven & H. v. Balkom (Eds.), *Classification of developmental language disorders: theoretical issues and clinical implications* (pp. 309–326). Lawrence Erlbaum.

Boucher, J., Mayes, A., & Bigham, S. (2012). Memory in autistic spectrum disorder. *Psychological Bulletin*, 138(3), 458

Broadbent, D. E. (1958). *Perception and communication*. Pergamon.

Buss, K. A., & Goldsmith, H. H. (1998). Fear and anger regulation in infancy: effects on the temporal dynamics of affective expression. *Child Development*, 69(2), 359–374.

Calkins, S. D., & Fox, N. A. (2002). Self-regulatory processes in early personality development: a multilevel approach to the study of childhood social withdrawal and aggression. *Development and Psychopathology*, 14(3), 477–498.

Carpendale, J. I., & Lewis, C. (2004). Constructing an understanding of mind: the develop-ment of children's social understanding within social interaction. *Behavioral and Brain Sciences*, 27(1), 79–96.

Casey, B. J., Jones, R. M., Levita, L., Libby, V., Pattwell, S. S., Ruberry, E. J., Solima, F., & Somerville, L. H. (2010). The storm and stress of adolescence: insights from human imaging and mouse genetics. *Developmental Psychobiology*, 52(3), 225–235.

Castellanos, F. X., & Proal, E. (2012). Large-scale brain systems in ADHD: beyond the prefrontal–striatal model. *Trends in Cognitive Sciences*, 16(1), 17–26.

Diener, M. L., & Mangelsdorf, S. (1999). Behavioral strategies for emotion regulation in toddlers: associations with maternal involvement and emotional expressions. *Infant Behavior and Development*, 22, 569–583.

Dunning, D. L., Holmes, J., & Gathercole, S. E. (2013). Does working memory training lead to generalized improvements in children with low working memory? A randomized controlled trial. *Developmental Science*, 16(6), 915–925.

Earl, T. R., Fortuna, L. R., Gao, S., Williams, D. R., Neighbors, H., Takeuchi, D., & Alegría, M. (2015). An exploration of how psychotic-like symptoms are experienced, endorsed, and understood from the National Latino and Asian American Study and National Survey of American Life. *Ethnicity & Health*, 20(3), 273–292.

Evans, D. W., Leckman, J. F., Carter, A., Reznick, J. S., Henshaw, D., King, R. A., & Pauls, D. (1997). Ritual, habit, and perfectionism: the prevalence and development of compulsive-like behavior in normal young children. *Child Development*, 68(1), 58–68.

Fabes, R. A., & Eisenberg, N. (1992). Young children's coping with interpersonal anger. *Child Development*, 63(1), 116–128.

Fenson, L., Dale, P. S., Reznick, J. S., Bates, E., Thal, D., & Pethick, S. (1994). Variability in early communicative development. *Monographs of the Society for Research in Child Development*, 59, 1–173.

Fenson, L., Dale, P. S., Reznick, J. S., Thal, D., Bates, E., Hartung, J. P., Pethick, S., & Reilly, J. S. (1993). *MacArthur Communicative Development Inventory: users guide and technical manual*. Singular Publishing Company.

Gottman, J. M., Katz, L. F., & Hooven, C. (1996). *Meta-emotion: how families communicate emotionally*. Erlbaum.

Hagen, J. W., & Hale, G. A. (1973). The development of attention in children 1. *ETS Research Bulletin Series*, 1973(1), 1–37.

Harris, P. L., Brown, E., Marriott, C., Whittall, S., & Harmer, S. (1991). Monsters, ghosts and witches: testing the limits of the fantasy—reality distinction in young children. *British Journal of Developmental Psychology*, 9(1), 105–123.

Harris, P. L., Kavanaugh, R. D., Wellman, H. M., & Hickling, A. K. (1993). Young children's under-standing of pretense. *Monographs of the Society for Research in Child Development*, i–107.

Heyman, I., Fombonne, E., Simmons, H., Ford, T., Meltzer, H., & Goodman, R. (2001). Prevalence of obsessive–compulsive disorder in the British nationwide survey of child mental health. *British Journal of Psychiatry*, 179(4), 324–329.

Higgins, A. T., & Turnure, J. E. (1984). Distractibility and concentration of attention in children's development. *Child Development*, 55, 1799–1810.

Holmes, J., Hilton, K. A., Place, M., Alloway, T. P., Elliott, J. G., & Gathercole, S. E. (2014). Children with low working memory and children with ADHD: same or different? *Frontiers in Human Neuroscience*, 8, 976.

Jones, S. H., Hemsley, D., Ball, S., & Serra, A. (1997). Disruption of the Kamin blocking effect in schizophrenia and in normal subjects following amphetamine. *Behavioural Brain Research*, 88(1), 103–114.

Kagan, J., Rosman, B. L., Day, D., Albert, J., & Phillips, W. (1964). Information processing in the child: significance of analytic and reflective attitudes. *Psychological Monographs: General and Applied*, 78(1), 1–37.

Kamin, L. J. (1969). Predictability, surprise, attention and conditioning. In B. A. Campbell & R. M. Church (Eds.), *Punishment and aversive behaviour* (pp. 279–296). Appleton–Century–Crofts.

Kaiser, M. D., Hudac, C. M., Shultz, S., Lee, S. M., Cheung, C., Berken, A. M., Deen, B., Pitskel, N. B., Sugrue, D. R., Voos, A. C., Saulnier, C. A., Ventola, P., Wolf, J. M., Klin, A., Vander Wyk, B. C., & Pelphrey, K. A. (2010). Neural signatures of autism. *Proceedings of the National Academy of Sciences of the United States of America*, 107(49), 21223–21228.

Kavšek, M. (2004). Predicting later IQ from infant visual habituation and dishabituation: a meta-analysis. *Journal of Applied Developmental Psychology*, 25(3), 369–393.

Laurens, K. R., Hobbs, M. J., Sunderland, M., Green, M. J., & Mould, G. L. (2012). Psychotic-like experiences in a community sample of 8000 children aged 9 to 11 years: an item response theory analysis. *Psychological Medicine*, 42(7), 1495–1506.

Lewis, V., & Boucher, J. (1988). Spontaneous, instructed and elicited play in relatively able autistic children. *British Journal of Developmental Psychology*, 6(4), 325–339.

Lucretius. (1951). *On the nature of the universe*. (R. Latham, Trans.). Penguin Books

Mahone, E. M., Bridges, D., Prahme, C., & Singer, H. S. (2004). Repetitive arm and hand movements (complex motor stereotypies) in children. *Journal of Pediatrics*, 145(3), 391–395.

Morris R., Griffiths. O., Le Pelley, M. E., Thomas W., & Weickert, T. W. (2013). Attention to irrelevant cues is related to positive symptoms in schizophrenia. *Schizophrenia Bulletin*, 39(3), 575–582.

Nigg, J. T. (2000). On inhibition/disinhibition in developmental psychopathology: views from cognitive and personality psychology and a working inhibition taxonomy. *Psychological Bulletin*, 126, 220–246. https://doi.org/10.1037/0033-2909.126.2.220

Nigg, J. T. (2000). On inhibition/disinhibition in developmental psychopathology: views from cognitive and personality psychology and a working inhibition taxonomy. *Psychological Bulletin*, 126, 220–246. https://doi.org/10.1037/0033-2909.126.2.220

Nigg, J. T. (2017). Annual research review: on the relations among self-regulation, self-control, executive functioning, effortful control, cognitive control, impulsivity, risk-taking, and inhibition for developmental psychopathology. *Journal of Child Psychology and Psychiatry*, 58(4), 361–383.

Pelphrey, K. A., & Carter, E. J. (2008). Charting the typical and atypical development of the social brain. *Development and Psychopathology*, 20(4), 1081–1102.

Piaget, J. (1962). *Play, dreams and imitation in childhood*. Routledge.

Poldrack, R. A., & Yarkoni, T. (2016). *Annual Review of Psychology*, 67, 587–612.

Posner, M. I., Rothbart, M. K., & Voelker, P. (2016). Developing brain networks of attention. *Current Opinion in Pediatrics*, 28(6), 720–724.

Pourtois, G., Schettino, A., & Vuilleumier, P. (2013). Brain mechanisms for emotional influences on perception and attention: what is magic and what is not. *Biological Psychology*, 92(3), 492–512.

Rekers, Y., Haun, D. B., & Tomasello, M. (2011). Children, but not chimpanzees, prefer to collaborate. *Current Biology*, 21(20), 1756–1758.

Richmond, J., & Nelson, C. A. (2007). Accounting for change in declarative memory: a cognitive neuroscience perspective. *Developmental Review*, 27(3), 349–373

Rolls, E. T. (2005). *Emotion explained*. Oxford University Press.

Sabbagh, M. A., Bowman, L. C., Evraire, L. E., & Ito, J. M. (2009). Neurodevelopmental correlates of theory of mind in preschool children. *Child Development*, 80(4), 1147–1162.

Salzman, C. D., & Fusi, S. (2010). Emotion, cognition, and mental state representation in amygdala and prefrontal cortex. *Annual Review of Neuroscience, 33*, 173–202.

Shiner, R. L., Buss, K. A., McClowry, S. G., Putnam, S. P., Saudino, K. J., & Zentner, M. (2012). What is temperament now? Assessing progress in temperament research on the twenty-fifth anniversary of Goldsmith et al. *Child Development Perspectives, 6*(4), 436–444.

Sigman, M. D., Kasari, C., Kwon, J. H., & Yirmiya, N. (1992). Responses to the negative emotions of others by autistic, mentally retarded, and normal children. *Child Development, 63*(4), 796–807.

Spinrad, T. L., Stifter, C. A., Donelan–McCall, N., & Turner, L. (2004). Mothers' regulation strategies in response to toddlers' affect: links to later emotion self-regulation. *Social Development, 13*(1), 40–55.

Squire, L. R., Stark, C. E., & Clark, R. E. (2004). The medial temporal lobe. *Annual Review of Neuroscience, 27*, 279–306.

Strang, J. F., Anthony, L. G., Yerys, B. E., Hardy, K. K., Wallace, G. L., Armour, A. C., Dudley, K., & Kenworthy, L. (2017). The Flexibility Scale: development and preliminary validation of a cognitive flexibility measure in children with autism spectrum disorders. *Journal of Autism and Developmental Disorders, 47*(8), 2502–2518.

Tager-Flusberg, H., & Joseph R. M. (2005). How language facilitates the acquisition of false belief understanding in children with autism. In J. W. Astington & J. A. Baird (Eds.), *Why language matters for theory of mind* (pp. 298–318). Oxford University Press: New York.

Treisman, A. (1988). Features and objects: the fourteenth Bartlett memorial lecture. *Quarterly Journal of Experimental Psychology, 40*(2), 201–237.

Vink, M., Derks, J. M., Hoogendam, J. M., Hillegers, M., & Kahn, R. S. (2014). Functional differences in emotion processing during adolescence and early adulthood. *Neuroimage, 91*, 70–76.

Visu–Petra, L., Stanciu, O., Benga, O., Miclea, M., & Cheie, L. (2014). Longitudinal and concurrent links between memory span, anxiety symptoms, and subsequent executive functioning in young children. *Frontiers in Psychology, 5*, 443.

Wakschlag, L. S., Choi, S. W., Carter, A. S., Hullsiek, H., Burns, J., McCarthy, K., … & Briggs-Gowan, M. J. (2012). Defining the developmental parameters of temper loss in early childhood: implications for developmental psychopathology. *Journal of Child Psychology and Psychiatry, 53*(11), 1099–1108.

Warneken, F., & Tomasello, M. (2008). Extrinsic rewards undermine altruistic tendencies in 20-month-olds. *Developmental Psychology, 44*(6), 1785.

Wessa, M., & Linke, J. (2009). Emotional processing in bipolar disorder: behavioural and neuroimaging findings. *International Review of Psychiatry, 21*(4), 357–367.

Williams, D. L., Goldstein, G., & Minshew, N. J. (2006). The profile of memory function in children with autism. *Neuropsychology, 20*(1), 21.

Wimmer, R. D., Schmitt, L. I., Davidson, T. J., Nakajima, M., Deisseroth, K., & Halassa, M. M. (2015). Thalamic control of sensory selection in divided attention. *Nature, 526*(7575), 705.

Yeshurun, Y., & Carrasco, M. (1999). Spatial attention improves performance in spatial resolution tasks 1. *Vision Research, 39*(2), 293–306.

Zahn–Waxler, C., Radke–Yarrow, M., Wagner, E., & Chapman, M. (1992). Development of concern for others. *Developmental Psychology, 28*, 126–136.

CHAPTER 3

······································

ATTENTION DEFICIT
HYPERACTIVITY DISORDER

······································

3.1 DIAGNOSTIC CONCEPTS

PEOPLE with attention deficit hyperactivity disorder (ADHD) show persistent patterns of inattention, hyperactivity, and impulsivity that are out of keeping with their developmental age. Most of the problems exist as a continuum in the population, and many represent immaturities. They are unified into a syndrome mostly because they tend to cluster together. Most of the research and clinical practice is based on the syndrome rather than the idea of component dimensions as set out in Chapter 2. This chapter therefore describes the diagnosis and associations of the syndrome, but with special reference to the multitude of associated problems.

Historically, the description does not stem from a single classical description but partly from its appearance in children with neurological disorders such as encephalitis, and partly from the gradual recognition of the remarkable effects of stimulant (and other) medications in reducing the core features (Taylor, 2017).

Major programmes of psychological research have shown associations between the syndrome and impairment of functions described in Chapter 2. Lack of inhibition, altered time perception, poor executive function, altered response to reward, changes in spatial and working memory, and many other impaired functions have been implicated. However, none has commanded the field or shown the high levels of predictive value required to be diagnostic tests. Accordingly, the definition remains behavioural.

Emotional over-reactiveness used to be regarded as a core feature, but this was dropped from diagnostic criteria in 1980, in keeping with a consensus that the condition then called 'minimal brain dysfunction' was grounded in neurocognitive disorder and should be called 'attention deficit'. Successive editions of the American Psychiatric Association's *Diagnostic and Statistical Manual* (now DSM-5) have maintained a tradition of description based on adding together a set of behavioural items (American Psychiatric Association, 2013). The definition applies a cut-off validated by the scores of young people who have been diagnosed with ADHD in practice. The approach has been controversial, partly because the behaviour items involved—such as 'idle, impatient and a nuisance'—can also be described in moral terms. Accordingly, a wide-ranging systematic review, consultation, and meta-analysis was undertaken by the UK guideline-making organization, NICE (National Institute for Health and Care Excellence, 2009). NICE's conclusion was clear: ADHD represented a valid disorder and should be treated by the National Health Service.

The World Health Organization's (WHO's) international classification of diseases did, for some years, take a different line from the *Diagnostic and Statistical Manual*. The tenth edition of its classification of disorders (ICD-10) called the condition 'hyperkinetic disorder', required the combination of inattention, hyperactivity, and impulsiveness all together, and had strict requirements for pervasiveness of symptoms over time and across situations (Zivetz, 1992). The result was that hyperkinetic disorder (HKD) was a subtype nested within ADHD, accounting for about a quarter of cases, and characterized by more neurodevelopmental changes in motor and language development than other forms of ADHD, a more marked short-term response to methylphenidate compared with placebo, and a greater discrepancy between a very good short-term response to medication and a weak response to behavioural treatment (Santosh et al., 2005).

HKD, however, no longer seems to be a separable condition, either genetically or in course over time. A longitudinal comparison with other forms of ADHD indicated that the outcome at age 16 was very similar between the groups: the presence of emotional disorders was a stronger predictor of poor outcome than the exact symptom pattern of inattention and impulsiveness (Arnold et al., 2018/2019).

The lack of discriminative validity for HKD has meant that the current version of ICD-11 accepts ADHD as the condition to recognize, follows the DSM-5 criteria, and mentions HKD as a severe form (WHO, 2018). It will still be a useful clinical construct as an index of severity or a "refined phenotype" (Swanson et al., 1998). ICD-11 differs from DSM-5 in not having a list of criteria to add up. Rather, it provides description of the key features and encourages clinicians to see them as a prototype to which an individual case can be referred. The difference between the schemes reflects the uses to which they will be put. Precise numbers of symptoms in DSM-5 are very desirable for research. They do not require an expensive clinical judgement; they are transparent to critical scrutiny; and they ensure that different groups of researchers are talking about similar cases. However, for clinical purposes, simply adding up criteria can miss children with very severe levels of single problems. Furthermore, the exact number is not a well-validated cut-off. Further still, the number of problems can and does fluctuate over time and is not a stable characteristic of the person.

Both DSM-5 and ICD-11 separate out two dimensions—one of inattention, and one of hyperactivity and impulsiveness. A dimensional way of thinking allows the balance of components to be assessed, and related problems brought in. Both diagnostic schemes require that the dimensions are enduring characteristics of the children and not only transient reactions to circumstances. This is made operational by expecting that problem levels have been consistent over at least 6 months and have been present in at least two kinds of situation (such as home, school, work, and extracurricular learning).

3.2 RECOGNITION AND MAKING THE DIAGNOSIS

3.2.1 Rating scales

3.2.1.1 *Informants' rating scales*

Questionnaire ratings by people who know the young person well are useful for screening purposes, triage, and monitoring interventions. Parent and teacher versions assess similar potential problems, and some of the scales also have self-report versions. Most use Likert scales, in which several items of potentially problematic behaviour are marked for their usual severity. The items rated are derived either from developmental research or from the DSM criteria described earlier.

Conners scales are widely used in the USA and UK to assess children between the ages of 6 and 18 years. They exist in several forms. They are constructed to yield T-scores, which have a mean of 50 and a standard deviation of 10. Scores above 65 are correspondingly taken to indicate potential problems. The Conners-3 (short version) was designed specifically for assessing the problems frequently associated with ADHD (Conners, 2008). Subscales include 'Inattention' (nine items) and 'Hyperactivity/Impulsivity' (nine items). There are also subscales for 'Learning problems/Executive functioning', 'Aggression' (the parents' version has eight items for oppositional, 15 for conduct), and 'Peer relations'. It is also possible to generate scores for levels of impairment, gender-specific scores, and estimates of raters' response style (positive impression, negative impression, and inconsistency). It is concise enough to be practical for repeated assessments of progress. Users, however, should beware of misinterpreting spontaneous fluctuations and regression to the mean as evidence of clinical improvement.

Some scales use similar items, but with different purposes. The SWAN (Strengths and Weaknesses of ADHD Symptoms and Normal Behaviour Rating) scale was developed with a wider range of scores for each item (including both 'far above average' and 'far below average') (Swanson et al., 2012). It will yield a more Gaussian distribution in a population survey than most other instruments and may be preferred for population genetic research. Both it and the SNAP (Swanson, Nolan, and Pelham) scale (Swanson et al., 2012) are available free from the internet (www.adhd.net).

Other scales, such as the ADHD Rating Scale (Dupaul, 1991) and the Vanderbilt ADHD Rating Scale (Bard et al., 2013), were developed directly from DSM criteria. Further useful scales aim to include ADHD features as part of a general cover of most of the common problems of psychopathology. The advantage lies in providing a systematic screen for many of the other types of psychopathology, including emotional problems. The disadvantages can be a loss of precision for ADHD features and a reduced compliance if the scale is very long.

One convenient and widely used set of general-purpose rating scales derives from the well-known Rutter scales, which were developed as the first stage of multistage epidemiological research in the general population. The Strengths and Difficulties Questionnaires (SDQ) (Goodman, 1997) have been translated into many languages and used in population surveys, so can be relevant to the needs of multicultural services. They are brief (typically being completed in around 5 minutes); appropriate for the teachers and parents of young people aged 4 to 17 years; and available free from the internet (www.sdqinfo.org). Although much shorter than the Child Behaviour Checklist (CBCL) (described below), they performed better, when judged against a semi-structured interview, in identifying inattention and impulsiveness (Goodman & Scott, 1999). Scores from the SDQ and CBCL were highly correlated and equally valuable in their primary goals of assessing mental disorder broadly: both can validly discriminate psychiatric from dental cases.

The SDQ is sometimes used to track clinical progress. It is part of a wider system of interviews and online assessments, the Development and Well-Being Assessment (DAWBA). Its extensive use in epidemiological research has allowed for estimating the expected change over 6-month periods that can be expected from non-specific influences of repeated measurement, and therefore for comparison with the effects of intervention.

The CBCL (Achenbach & Ruffle, 2000) records caregiver ratings of positive behaviours, social competence, and a wide range of common behaviour and emotion problems. There are preschool and school-age versions, and the latter includes assessment of academic functioning. There are normed scales of 'Aggressive behaviour', 'Anxious/Depressed problems', 'Attention Problems', 'Rule-breaking behaviour', 'Somatic complaints', 'Social problems', 'Thought problems', and 'Withdrawn/depressed'. These are not based on DSM diagnoses, but rather on factor analyses of problems. They are part of a wider system of assessment, the Achenbach System of Empirically Based Assessment. There is, however, an alternative system of scoring intended to parallel the concepts of DSM.

The Conners scales (mentioned earlier) also include a long version (90 minutes), called the Comprehensive Behaviour Rating Scale (CBRS), with wide coverage of an extensive range of young people's problems beyond ADHD and associated behaviours (Conners, 2008). A short version (the Conners Clinical Index) can be completed in as little as 5 minutes and is useful for tracking course.

Many of these rating scales have similar strengths and weaknesses (Burns et al., 2013). In group comparisons, they give reasonably good discrimination between people with a clinical diagnosis of ADHD and controls from the ordinary population, with an effect size of about two standard deviations, implying a substantial overlap. This discrimination is probably somewhat better for the special-purpose ADHD scales than for the general-purpose scales. Test–retest reliability is typically around 0.7; all are sensitive to the effects of medication. Agreement between teachers and parents is typically rather low, often around 0.3. All scales, used as a population screen, leave a fair number of individuals misclassified and are liable to many false positives. The rating scales are best seen as a first stage of screening, not as defining casehood.

Specificity and *sensitivity* of all the scales mentioned are moderate, around 0.8 when tested against an interview or an expert diagnosis.

3.2.1.2 *Self-rating scales*

For children aged 9 years and above, self-report is feasible using versions of the informant scales, including the CBCL and SDQ. Their validity is uncertain, and they may generate different associations from the reports of informants. For adults, a variety of self-report measures have been developed and were reviewed by Davidson (2008). The Wender Utah scales were particularly important in the early conceptualization of adult ADHD (McCann et al., 2000). The Adult ADHD Self-Report Scale (ASRS) is a symptom checklist developed for the WHO (Adler et al., 2003). It can be downloaded from: http://www.caddra.ca/pdfs/Guidelines_ENG_ChangesJuly2012.pdf

3.2.1.3 *Use of rating scales for screening*

Many rating scales, especially the parent and teacher versions of the Conners, are widely used to select cases for detailed assessment. This is frequent practice in the UK, even in spite of lack of detailed evidence for its efficiency. The problems are so frequent in the general population that some form of screening is considered essential to avoid overloading specialized services. Sensitivity and specificity therefore need to be understood. The *sensitivity* of a test is the proportion of people who test positive among all those who actually have the condition. A sensitive test helps rule out a disease when the test is negative. The *specificity* of a test is the proportion of people who test negative among all those who actually do not have that condition. A specific test helps rule in a disease when the test is positive.

Clinicians are often more concerned about *predictive value* than about specificity and sensitivity. This statistic allows clinicians to understand how likely it is that an individual actually has the condition being sought. It depends on the prevalence of the disorder being screened for. *Positive predictive value* (PPV) is the probability that, following a positive questionnaire result, the individual will truly have ADHD. As prevalence decreases, so false positives increase relative to true positives, and so the PPV falls. *Negative predictive value* (NPV) is the probability that, given a negative questionnaire result, the individual will truly not have ADHD. As prevalence decreases, NPV will increase. A rare condition will generate more true negatives for every false negative.

Screening strategies should be planned in the light of the questions being asked and the populations being examined.

3.2.2 Interviews

3.2.2.1 *Informant interview*

The most informative single method for assessing children and adolescents is a detailed interview with parents (or other main caregivers). Parents will usually have very good knowledge of attention and activity control. They do not, however, necessarily have a good knowledge about the normal range. Good clinical interviewing practice will therefore aim at descriptions of key situations such as getting ready for school, playing with toys, drawing, mealtimes, homework, and family excursions. Professional judgement can then be applied about whether those descriptions indicate abnormality of development, rather than asking informants for evaluative judgements such as 'Are they more impulsive than other children?'

Standardized interview schedules are also available. Some, such as the Diagnostic Interview Schedule for Children (DISC) (Shaffer et al., 2000), are highly structured and can be delivered by non-clinicians. Others are more interactive, can be delivered flexibly, and expect the interviewer (rather than the respondent) to be the specifier of what is rated. Examples of these 'semi-structured' instruments would be the Child and Adolescent Psychiatric Assessment (CAPA) (Angold & Costello, 2000) and the Schedule for Affective Disorders and Schizophrenia for School Age Children (K-SADS) (Ambrosini, 2000). They are time-consuming, sometimes too much so for routine clinical practice, but offer full cover of salient features.

Interviews also give information about coexistent problems, social and intellectual development, emotional life, and any physical problems. Informant interviews with teachers are often omitted for convenience. Teachers can, however, give a close and professionally informed overview of the child in the classroom. Interviewing them (e.g. by telephone) also helps to build cooperation and confidence.

3.2.2.2 *Psychiatric interview*

An interview with the child allows observation of attention and social interaction. Getting a view of the young person's understanding of their predicament usually involves speaking with them, both with and without the presence of their parents. Children, however, are not good witnesses about their own concentration and impulse control. Even affected adults are not good at describing themselves in these terms. The experience of ADHD is usually one of suffering the reactions evoked from other people, or one of repeated failure. Adults often describe an experience of whirling and interrupted thoughts (in the absence of manic features). Some children will say the same, especially if treatment has enabled them to make a comparison with another way of being.

Direct observation of the child, in a given activity or during psychometric testing, can offer a vivid idea of the nature of their problems in attending. Do they take time to appreciate what they are being asked to do? Is the tempo of their activity increased? Can they slow down when asked? Are they distracted by the setting? Do they complete tasks and play activities? Observation of play and task performance in natural settings such as classrooms can be particularly useful if informants are giving conflicting accounts.

3.2.3 Information to seek for recognition and diagnosis

The following section outlines key features of ADHD and provides notes on their recognition in the presence of other problems (as is usually the case). The verbal descriptions of key features can be misinterpreted if they are presented only as part of a checklist—especially a rating scale completed by non-professionals and interpreted by non-experts. Accordingly, each feature is elaborated here by including comments on how it can be mimicked by other conditions and how to make the necessary distinctions.

3.2.3.1 *Inattention*

The main features of inattentiveness are changes in behaviour, especially self-organization. They all need to be judged against what is expected at the individual's level of development.

3.2.3.1.1 *Failure to pay close attention*

Children, young people, and adults with ADHD often fail to give close attention to details. They often make careless mistakes in schoolwork, at work, or with other activities. Frequent mistakes can also be made for reasons other than inattentiveness. Learning difficulties can create a mismatch between a young person's competence and the demands of the task. 'Carelessness' can be a subjective and mistaken judgement about an affectation of insouciance, or a feature of people who are preoccupied. However, it is usually possible to infer it from observation of how work or schoolwork is being addressed rather than from achievement alone. Teachers are usually in a good place to know.

3.2.3.1.2 *Not maintaining attention on tasks or play activities*

The judgement of poorly sustained attention needs to be made on the basis of developmental expectations about the normative changes in sustaining focused attention (see Chapter 2, Section 2.3). The pattern in ADHD is typically that of a much younger child. Focus can be intensive for short periods but is typically fleeting. It will be important to keep in mind that the focus of attention can be maintained for much longer if the task is intrinsically exciting or pleasant. Video games, for example, often have very rapid incentives built in and can create a misleading impression of good attention that does not generalize to other activities. A much better guide will be obtained from considering activities that need a person to be self-sustaining. Building bricks, playing with toys, drawing or modelling, and reading are the kind of activities in childhood to ask about or observe.

Coexisting autism can obscure rapid shifts of attention. A favoured activity can be obsessively engaged by autistic people, leading examiners to suppose that this demonstrates good attention. When assessing the presence of ADHD-type problems in autism spectrum disorder (ASD), one should avoid rating attention on the basis of idiosyncratic preoccupations.

3.2.3.1.3 *Failure to listen*

'Often does not seem to listen when spoken to directly' should only be recognized when the examiner is clear that hearing is sufficiently intact. In many countries, hearing is a routine part of developmental assessment. Where it is not, then clinical assessment—or better, specialist audiometry when available—should be carried out. High tones carry much of the information about consonants, and selective impairment of hearing them can be missed by a casual test of the ability to hear. Intermittent hearing loss, as in recurrent episodes of otitis media, can create interfering tinnitus or a habit of ignoring sounds even at times when tested hearing is normal.

It is also possible for people in the spectrum of autism, or those with high anxiety, to be focused so intently on thoughts or activities in hand that it is hard for them to shift to another speaker.

3.2.3.1.4 *Failure to follow instructions*

'Often does not follow through on instructions' is mostly an issue in structured settings. Not finishing schoolwork, chores at home, or duties in the workplace because of becoming sidetracked is similar to 'difficulties in maintaining attention'. A distinction needs to be made from oppositional rejection of instructions. A typical presentation of ADHD would be a willing engagement to a task but premature breaking off from it.

3.2.3.1.5 *Failure to organize tasks and activities successfully*

Disorganization is a type of executive dysfunction (see Chapter 2, Section 2.5) which takes many forms. It might be seen in difficulty amassing everything that will be needed for tasks and activities, or in losing them. It may mean failing to meet deadlines for school or work. It may also reflect mind wandering interrupting the flow of activity.

It is an important part of the practical distinction between ADHD and autism spectrum conditions. Both ADHD and ASD can lead to missing an overview of the situation. However, in ADHD, the problem is in carelessness and sloppy errors; in ASD, there is an excessive focus on detail.

3.2.3.2 *Avoidance of effort*

Dislike of mental effort over a long period of time is characteristic of ADHD. Children and young people with ADHD are typically reluctant to take on tasks such as schoolwork or homework. Effort is also avoided in self-chosen activities, as well as those imposed by others. Young people with learning problems may also become highly demotivated during school tasks when they have long experience of failure. The difficulty in ADHD, however, is not confined to school or work. A distinction is also required from ASD, in which avoidance is essentially of tasks that compete with autistic preoccupations. People with ADHD typically get bored, in contrast with ASD where predictable routine tasks are seldom a problem.

3.2.3.3 *Disorganized approach to activities*

People with ADHD often lose things necessary for tasks and activities. School materials, tools, keys, paperwork, and spectacles are among the classic examples of what can easily be forgotten. Like other problems, it needs to be judged against the developmental level of the child. Forgetfulness is also a feature of intellectual disability and sometimes of preoccupying anxiety, which need to be excluded as the causes.

3.2.3.3.1 *Distractibility*

People with ADHD are consistently described as 'easily distracted'. The mere presence of irrelevant information in the outside world is seldom enough to lead to impairment of performance. Rather, the lack of orientating to a task is the key problem and is similar to the difficulties with focus described earlier. Mind wandering in ADHD can lead to distractible behaviour, rather than the latter being due only to passive capture by attractive features of the environment. This can be superficially hard to distinguish from the internal distractibility of people with high anxiety, for whom ruminations and preoccupations can be the features leading to loss of focus. It is therefore important for a diagnosis of ADHD to check that distraction is not due only to painful intrusive thoughts.

3.2.3.3.2 *Difficulties remembering*

Being forgetful in daily activities, as a feature of ADHD, is typically shown not by a defiant refusal to engage in chores but by initial engagement and only partial continuance. It is marked when several instructions have been given (e.g. 'go upstairs, clean your teeth and wash your hands') and a child presents themselves back again with a cheerful lack of recognition that all of them were to be done. For teenagers and young adults, it may be a failure to call people back on the phone, to respond to social media calls, or to be present at an expected time.

3.2.3.4 *Hyperactivity and impulsivity*

There is a wide range of activity levels in normal development. High energy and high-spirited enthusiasm should not be seen as problematic. In general, the examples of impulsive behaviour given here are intended to capture a style, of action without reflection, that can also be seen in hasty and unwise decision making, and in taking risks without considering the consequences.

- *Excessive fidgeting*. This includes movements of hands and feet and movements of the trunk while seated. It does not include stereotyped movements and tics.
- *Restless activity of the whole body*. This should be enough to take one out of the seat, and frequent enough to be clearly out of line with expectations for one's age. It should be distinguished from the situation of young or immature people who have not appreciated the nature of the expectation.
- *Running about inappropriately*. The inappropriateness in relation to context is important. The playground is not a good place in which to detect a high activity level in children. The classroom, visits to relatives, presence in church, public transport, and shopping are much more useful settings about which to enquire. As children with ADHD mature, they usually become able to modulate their gross motor activity

successfully. In adolescents and adults, the difficulty may be only that they feel very constrained in doing so.

- *Lack of quiet play or leisure activity.* This is intended to apply to young people who are unable to tone down their activity. The threshold for recognition of this as a problem should be high, to avoid false identification of ADHD in self-willed children and young people who are still able to calm down on occasion.

- *Continuous restlessness.* This should be to an extent that other people find it hard to keep up. It can be measured mechanically but needs to be distinguished from high levels of goal-directed activity that are seen in mania and hypomania. Overactivity in ADHD tends to be random and disorganized but not stereotyped.

- *Excessive talking.* Speech may well be rapid and inappropriate, but still makes sense and does not usually show the 'flight of ideas' that characterizes manic states. If autism is present, it may well be a sufficient reason in itself for any inappropriateness of language

- *Blurting out premature replies.* This is one of several ways in which a key aspect of impulsiveness—premature action before reflection—can be shown. It is not in it-self a serious problem, and it may even be linked to superior academic attainment. However, for a child with learning problems, it may be a clue to what kind of problems they are. Some clever children are bored and understimulated by the classroom en-vironment, and this should be detected in a careful assessment. Blurting out answers before the question is finished should be distinguished from the social insensitivity of some people in the spectrum of autism.

- *Failing to wait one's turn.* Typically, affected people will be aware of the conventions applying in a social situation (including joining other people's games gradually and with consent), but do not take the time and trouble required to follow them.

- *Interrupting other people's activities and conversations.* This is another way in which premature action can spoil relationships. It needs to be excessive in frequency, to dis-tinguish it from mere social gaucheness.

3.2.4 Making the diagnosis

Clinicians often wish to establish not only whether ADHD features are present, but whether they amount to an official diagnosis. Diagnosis is not the whole purpose of an assessment, but can be administratively necessary—to determine whether, for instance, a young person should have access to publicly funded services and whether medication should be prescribed (National Collaborating Centre for Mental Health (UK), 2018).

To make a formal DSM-5 diagnosis, the criteria should be followed as expressed in the manual (American Psychiatric Association, 2013). Six or more symptoms of inattention for children up to age 16, or five or more for adolescents and adults aged 17 and older need to be present. Alternatively, there should be six or more of the criteria for hyper-activity/impulsivity. They should not be wholly explicable by the presence of another psychiatric condition. DSM-5 also expects clear evidence that the symptoms interfere with social, school, or work functioning. As considered in Chapter 1, Section 1.2.8, it may be better and clearer to note such a social limitation separately from the behavioural description and include both in a diagnostic formulation.

Based on the types of symptoms, three presentations of ADHD are recognized by DSM-5: 'Predominantly inattentive', 'Predominantly hyperactive-impulsive', and 'Combined'. In practice, these 'presentations' are not very distinct, do not have validated cut-off criteria, and will often change over time. A 'predominantly inattentive' case can still have enough impulsive features to impact the course over time They should therefore not be regarded as significant subtypes. The levels of both inattentive and hyperactive-impulsive behaviours should be noted in a formulation.

No biological marker is yet very helpful in recognizing the condition. Changes, such as those in the EEG or in imaging measures of neural connectivity, suggest an immaturity in the development of the brain. They are outlined in Section 3.3 as potential risks. Nevertheless, they lack the necessary predictive value for inclusion among the diagnostic criteria. ADHD represents a pattern of behaviour, not its cause. Aetiological influences (including specific genetic conditions and severe early adversity) do need recognizing and including in a case formulation, but they should not replace the description of the condition(s). Emotional dysregulation is not part of the diagnosis but is very often present. Its status is described in Section 3.3.

3.3 DIFFICULTIES MAKING A DIAGNOSIS

Complexities in establishing the diagnosis can result from cases being close to the threshold in one way or another, symptom scores changing over time, symptoms being mimicked by other conditions, or having a varying and situation-dependent impact on function.

3.3.1 Subthreshold cases

Cases are sometimes regarded as subthreshold for a diagnosis because they show significant problems in only one of the two dimensions of inattention (IA) and hyperactivity-impulsiveness (HA-IMP). These dimensions are somewhat distinct, and either should be recognized, even on its own. HA-IMP predicts selectively to aggression, accidents, and rejection by peers; IA to poor academic function, shy and passive social behaviour in children, and lower life satisfaction in adults. The distinction is not absolute: the dimensions are correlated with each other, but they deserve separate attention in clinical assessment. *Different treatment approaches are usually needed*, especially when one dimension is present with very little evidence of the other.

The *changes in attention* (IA) dimension can exist alone. This is a purer condition than simply a 'predominantly inattentive' presentation. Clinicians should recognize that some young people who are not at all overactive or impulsive can still be seriously impaired in their concentration. Their inattentiveness carries real risks for academic achievement and for success in employment. Such children are often anxious, socially immature, and have a sluggish tempo in processing information.

The *changes in hyperactivity-impulsiveness* (HA-IMP) dimension can also exist alone. Such children can be hard to distinguish from those with oppositional-defiant disorder (ODD) only. The distinction lies in the presence in ODD of spitefulness and deliberate, wilful disobedience. Children with ADHD are often in disciplinary trouble, but it stems from silliness or hasty disregard of rules rather than being unduly headstrong. The development of oppositional or conduct disorders can be a complication (see Section 3.5.1), but most impulsive children avoid it.

The correlation between IA and HA-IMP can mostly be attributed to their having genetic influences in common. Clinicians should not be deterred from offering help to children who are severely affected in only one dimension.

Cases can also be subthreshold for the DSM-5 because the number of items does not reach the required tally. This is somewhat arbitrary. Fixed quantitative rules such as these are helpful for quality control and research, but need not drive clinical practice. The ICD-11 approach does not use them. Cases can also fall short of the diagnostic level because problems are specific to one situation (e.g. school or home). When this is the case, it should lead to more enquiry about the characteristics of the situation. For example, if problems are only at school or at work, is the regime inappropriate for the individual? Are expectations for study or achievement too high for the individual? Is there an unrecognized learning disability? Is there demotivation from long experience of failure? Is an intelligent child bored in an undemanding class? If problems are only at home, is there parental intolerance? Is school pressure leading to an upsurge of activity when children can relax at home? Are rules and expectations at home sufficiently clear and consistent?

3.3.2 Impact on function

A DSM-5 diagnosis formally requires that 'the symptoms interfere with, or reduce the quality of, social, school, or work functioning'. Chapter 1, Section 1.2.8 indicates the problems that this requirement brings for several conditions. In ADHD, it is responsible for a good deal of the international variation in prevalence. As with other types of neurodevelopmental disorder (see Chapter 4, Section 4.1.3.2.2 on diagnosis of ASD), a rich assessment will distinguish between caseness based on core features and impact on overall function. Impact will partly depend on the reactions of other people and systems.

3.3.3 Developmental appropriateness

Many of the features of ADHD would be considered normal in a younger person, and judgement is needed for each case about whether they are out of line with what is expected. Sometimes clinicians outsource this judgement to raters who know the child well. A typical rating scale will ask whether each behaviour is different from that of others of the same age. When the rater is an experienced teacher, this works well enough, but an inexperienced parent may struggle to make the judgement.

3.3.3.1 *Chronological, relative, gestational, and developmental age*

'The same age' may be an inexact description. Most classrooms in primary schools will include children whose birthdays fall between 11 months before the start of the school year and those immediately beforehand. The normal difference between the younger and older children in the class will therefore be considerable. An ability to concentrate which is less than that of the other children might therefore represent not an immaturity (as part of ADHD) but simply youth. Assessment should therefore be based on actual age, not just the usual age of the class.

A child born prematurely may well seem less mature than others simply because their age calculated from the day of birth is greater than that calculated from conception, and it is the latter that will be more relevant to their stage of brain development.

Children with generalized developmental delays in motor, cognitive, and social development are often described in terms of an overall developmental age. The way of allowing for this in assessing attention and impulse control is not obvious or universally agreed. The usual and intuitive method is for the assessor to consider what would be expected for a typically developing child whose chronological age is the same as the developmental age of the child being assessed. Conceptually, this is open to doubt. The 'developmental age' is like an average over several functions that are, in practice, often diverse. The attention and impulse control of developmentally delayed children have not been studied in sufficient detail to know whether they do in fact follow the same trajectory as that of younger children who are developing typically. For the moment, it is the preferred guide, but one can hope for better information to emerge. Clinicians experienced in developmental delays will have developed their own expectations.

3.3.4 Coexistent disorders

Coexistent disorders are the rule for people with a diagnosis of ADHD. Failure to diagnose true cases can arise from a preference for a single diagnosis and consequent overshadowing of the ADHD by another set of problems. A separate issue for diagnosticians is the need to recognize that some conditions may masquerade as ADHD by reproducing some of its features. This makes differential diagnosis necessary.

3.3.4.1 *Differential diagnosis of disruptive behaviour and emotional dysregulation*

There are plenty of reasons for disruptive behaviour apart from ADHD. *Insomnia* may produce an irritable child who is not engaging in classroom activity, but (unlike ADHD) it is accompanied by daytime sleepiness, and the problems resolve when the insomnia is relieved. *Oppositional behaviour* alone may include an appearance of not listening and refusing tasks. The distinction can be difficult. The presence or absence of inattention is a helpful guide. *Emotional dysregulation* also needs consideration. It is frequently part of an ADHD presentation, but is also a feature of bipolar disorder or can be a mood problem on its own (see Chapter 2, Section 2.9). Unlike ADHD, it is a fluctuating and episodic problem.

The problems that can masquerade as ADHD may also coexist with ADHD. The key for the diagnostician is then to discern whether the disorganized pattern of ADHD behaviour is also present, and to make the additional diagnosis (or diagnoses) as necessary.

The process of differential diagnosis is to be distinguished from the need to recognize potential causes. Brain syndromes, such as fragile-X or head injury, may well be responsible for ADHD features. Both the neurological condition and the ADHD should then be recognized. More subtly, severe neglect in early childhood is probably a cause of attention and activity abnormalities (see 'Risks', Section 3.7). If ADHD is present in such a child, it should still be diagnosed. A social worker identifying a neglect syndrome and a physician diagnosing ADHD in the same child may both be right. Good communication may be best served by a dual diagnosis.

Confusions arise in a single-diagnosis scheme, such as a national case register. Technically, this probably means coding the ADHD cluster as 'secondary neurodevelopmental syndrome', which might well lead to misunderstandings (e.g. in interpreting international statistics).

3.4 COURSE OVER TIME

Changes are sometimes described from the first year, though usually with hindsight. 'He was a very stormy baby' is too common and non-specific a temperamental difference to be a useful predictor of ADHD later. 'She never walked but ran everywhere' may well be a characteristic of high energy rather than disorganization.

During preschool years, from about the age of two, a typical presentation is of parents troubled by their child's whirlwind of activity and lack of response to themselves. The clues to this being a presentation of ADHD are probably a lack of modulation in different situations and an extreme of emotional reactiveness to frustration and disappointment. If a child is also slow to use language appropriately, it may lead to suspicions of ASD, but ADHD alone will not be accompanied by the rigidity and uncommunicativeness of autism.

Before inattentiveness can be reliably assessed, the differentiation from ODD on its own is often insecure. In any case, the intervention for both is likely to be behaviourally orientated training to help parents to a non-punitive but effective coping style. Furthermore, both ODD and ADHD can result from neurological causes, and both are influenced by the social environment. So, before the age of four, the exact form of behavioural problems does not automatically give the aetiology. Temper tantrums are very common. They are usually part of normal development. Caregivers will usually be requesting advice rather than pathological formulation.

By the age of (about) 3 or 4 years, the ADHD cluster becomes a valid way of describing problem behaviours. Longitudinal studies (e.g. Riddle et al., 2013) have shown that it is moderately stable even over periods of 6 years or more. It is even more predictive if it is accompanied by marked defiance and aggression. Chaotic family patterns, with disorganized parenting, contribute to persistence, partly because they can reflect the genetic similarity of parents with the child and heritable patterns of parenting (Mokrova et al., 2010).

As children mature and start to learn formally, inattentiveness becomes a concern and may be the reason for clinical referral. The beginning of schooling is a frequent point at which earlier concerns about a child's development are accentuated by the appearance of functional problems in relating to other children, settling into the classroom atmosphere and expectations, and learning to read and calculate. Emotional control may now be obviously problematic as storms of distress and aggression become separable from ordinary tantrums by their intensity and long duration. Falling behind in their studies, failing to be accepted by other children, and coercive struggles with parents all add to the cascade of disadvantage described in Chapter 10 as a pathway from impairment to disability.

Inattention may become more obvious and disabling as children move into more advanced classes and are expected increasingly to manage their own learning without the scaffolding provided by adults. Attention span may well have increased by the time of secondary school—for instance, from 3 to 20 minutes (Chapter 2, Section 2.3.3)—but most students of the same age will have advanced more rapidly to the higher level of persistence required for longer classroom sessions. The gap between ADHD and typically developing people does not always reduce with age. In this sense, 'inattention' can remain just as much of a problem in adolescence and young adult life, even if it has improved to the extent that diagnostic criteria are no longer met.

Impulsiveness, too, may reduce in absolute terms, but not in relative ones. Teenagers with ADHD will be less likely than their younger selves to wander around a classroom or jump on furniture at home. In relative terms, however, they may still be much more likely than their contemporaries to make hasty and unwise decisions.

Overactivity in teenagers may not necessarily appear as extreme restlessness or wearing others out with their activity, but in constant fidgeting. In young adults, it may manifest as an internal feeling of restlessness and being constrained.

Adolescence brings increasing challenges to all children for personal identity, increasing independence, risk taking, and a wider range of social and virtual relationships with other people. ADHD features can compromise all these lines of development. There is no single trajectory. In some young people, there is a changing balance of impulsive and inattentive features; in some, there is improvement in both; and in some, a progressive deviation from healthy development. There are probably some genetic influences on the course over and above those contributing to the presence of ADHD in the first place. The associated features of emotional dysregulation and conduct problems become increasingly important in influencing life course.

Emotional dysregulation strongly influences outcome, especially as an antecedent of depression. Emotional problems of anxiety and depression also tend to appear as consequences of failures, frustrations, and poor self-image. Suicidal ideation and behaviours then tend to appear more frequently than in typically developing people.

Substance misuse is also more common in those growing up with ADHD, but this is mostly accounted for by the coexistent presence of conduct problems rather than the exact level of impulsiveness and inattention. A common route is for poorly socializing young people, who have not been integrated into the lives of most of their peers, to find themselves in the company of antisocial youth and to acquire the values and customs of a deviant group, including risky use of alcohol and drugs. ADHD in itself, however, does seem to add some risk—especially to increase the likelihood of tobacco smoking, in which an element of self-medication may come into play. Cannabis use will add to the problems of inattentiveness and lack of application, especially if varieties rich in tetrahydrocannabinol happen to be used (see 'Toxins', Chapter 7, Section 7.9.11).

It may be hard to distinguish between ADHD and substance-induced impairments that affect attention, concentration, and impulsivity for the worse. Chronic marijuana use has been associated with deficits in problem solving, organization, and sustained attention that often persist even after three weeks of abstinence. When there is uncertainty, practitioners will probably give priority to treating the substance use and then reassessing for ADHD when patients are abstinent. If this is not possible, they will enquire about a period when the patient was not using toxic substances—preferably seeking contemporary evidence such as old school reports.

ADHD also adds to other kinds of risky behaviour, and accidental injuries are a specific association. If delinquency supervenes, then there is a trap into all the adverse consequences of arrest, punishment, and unemployability.

3.4.1 Developmental trajectories through adolescence

Little is currently known about the genetic and environmental factors and underlying neurobiological processes that shape these different developmental pathways. Fluctuations in the course make it hard to predict or even to fully define the varying trajectories that different people follow. Coexisting disorders can worsen the outlook; beneficial environments can reduce the impact. Sonuga–Barke and Halperin (2010) indicate the kind of research that will be needed to develop the range of preventive interventions that could reduce the variety of interacting risks that shape development.

Environmental influences on course are described in Chapter 10, for this and other neurodevelopmental disorders. For instance, parental responsiveness and tolerance, perhaps promoted by parent-focused interventions, may protect against the development of conduct problems in children with ADHD (Taylor et al., 1996). Recovery through remission and functional improvement (via the development of coping) is seen even in current practice.

3.4.2 Adult life

The transition into adult life is a turning point with many changes. Most affected people no longer meet the full diagnostic criteria for ADHD, but retain some functional impairment related to inattention and impulsiveness, albeit at lower absolute levels than those leading to a full diagnosis. Evidence of this led DSM-5 to adjust downwards the number of symptoms expected for diagnosis in adulthood.

Inattention may now be reflected in tasks being left unfinished or never started, and mind wandering becomes a major part of people's experience. Self-organization is increasingly required; for example, in budgeting, paying bills on time, remembering appointments, finding lost objects, maintaining personal appearance, and meeting deadlines. Overactivity may now be a matter of impatience or be confined to an inner feeling of restlessness. Recklessness and poor decision making can put people at risk. Emotional lability often comes to interfere with personal and business relationships. Negotiation can be impaired by hastiness and a lack of attention to long-term interests.

Many young people choose to stop taking medication as they become more able to make their own choices; for example, once they have completed school-leaving examinations. The reasons for this, and possible solutions, are described in 'Effectiveness in the long term', Chapter 9, Section 9.4.7. Whatever the resolution of this important adult decision, it will be essential to ensure that review continues, and that people have the chance of resuming medication, when and if it is appropriate.

On the one hand, there may be continuing or even increased functional impact of ADHD in adult life. On the other hand, brain maturation can bring lessening of symptoms and there may be new ways of coping. Better understanding of the condition lets many people adjust their lives for the good. They may, for instance, choose walks of life where rapid changes of activity are necessary and valued (such as sales, trading, pastoral work, publicity, and some kinds of performing arts, to name but a few). They may be able to find colleagues to take over planning duties, or routine and tedious tasks. Many will find a stable partner to take over some of the organizational tasks of everyday life.

3.4.3 First presentations in adult life

Even when it is obvious that the ADHD features were creating serious difficulties in childhood, they may well not have been recognized as such at the time. Many professional cultures have been resistant to using the label. It can still be very rewarding to treat the problems (e.g. with stimulant medication) for the first time in adult life, and many affected people find it liberating to understand the reasons for some of the difficulties they have endured. Treatment can still be helpful even when the core problems have been surrounded by cumulative disadvantages, and even when people are in prison or struggling with substance dependence.

Sometimes ADHD seems to appear for the first time in adult life. This does not necessarily mean a late onset of disorder. Inattention and impulsiveness may well have been present in childhood, but not giving rise to problems, and accordingly never been recognized as such or diagnosed. Bright children may have been able to do well in school with a 'just in time' strategy of study. Many will not have shown conduct problems, and so may well have fitted harmoniously into family life. ADHD features may only have become troublesome when adult life presents greater demands for responsibility, scheduling, and applying executive functions of self-control.

Accordingly, part of the assessment of a first presentation in adult life is a history about what patients were like in childhood. The DSM-5 diagnosis includes an expectation that the symptoms (not just functional impairment) should have started before the age of 12 years. This may be very difficult for patients to remember, or indeed to have noted at the time, so the clinician should seek information from people who knew them as children and to ask for contemporary reports from school.

Some people, however, show a late onset of ADHD features with no suggestion of their presence in childhood. Head injuries (see Chapter 6, Section 6.5) can produce a picture of secondary ADHD, and it is worth enquiring specifically about recurrent mild concussions. Chronic use of some cannabis products can produce a variety of adverse neurocognitive effects, including marked difficulties with attention, memory, and executive control. The early stages of dementing disorders include ADHD features.

There may be other causes of late presentation. Indeed, research from longitudinally studied cohorts has identified many individuals who presented ADHD features in adult life but did not show them when they were studied in their childhood (e.g. Moffitt et al., 2015). They were also less likely to have affected family members, less likely to show cognitive deficits, and more likely to have used cannabis and other drugs. It is still controversial whether or not such cases should be included as 'ADHD' or 'neurodevelopmental'. However, the problems should not be belittled and deserve recognition in a clinical formulation.

In most cases, the originating cause of ADHD problems is not exactly known and does not have pride of place in decisions about treatment. Future research on this group can be expected to clarify whether they have similar genetic, neurological, and psychological characteristics to those with typically neurodevelopmental ADHD and what interventions, if any, are appropriate.

3.5 COEXISTENT PROBLEMS OF CONDUCT, EMOTIONS, ASD, LEARNING, AND MOTOR CHANGES

Multiple mental and physical difficulties are the rule for people with ADHD, and are of several types. The presence of ADHD should be recognized even in the presence of other psychiatric conditions. This raises the further question of how to understand other types of disorder—such as ASD, oppositional/conduct problems (O/CP), intellectual disability (ID), movement problems, and anxiety—when they coexist with ADHD. They are often called 'comorbidity', but the term misleads. They are not all best seen as independent disorders. Some are developmental consequences of ADHD. Others represent the tendency of all neurodevelopmental problems to coexist because of related genetic risks (Pettersson et al., 2013). Yet others represent the beginning of adult-type disorders, such as personality disorder, for which ADHD is a risk.

In practice, multiple diagnoses are frequently made, even in International Classification of Disease (ICD) systems which discourage the practice through multiple exclusion rules. For example, Jensen and Steinhausen (2015) reported on 14,825 children and adolescents (age 4–17) diagnosed in Danish psychiatric hospitals between 1995 and 2010. Of these patients, 52.0% had at least one psychiatric disorder diagnosed in addition to ADHD; 26.2% had two or more 'comorbid' disorders. Disorders of conduct were present in 16.5% of those with ADHD; specific developmental disorders of language, learning, and motor development in 15.4%; autism spectrum disorders in 12.4%; and intellectual disability in 7.9%. These high rates need to be seen in the context of routine practice, which might have failed to detect some associated conditions. Male gender was associated with an increased risk for neuropsychiatric disorders; female gender was associated more specifically with emotional disorders. The analysis highlighted the range of problem profiles that can coexist in young people with ADHD.

3.5.1 Conduct problems and oppositionality in ADHD

Most children with ADHD are not particularly angry or aggressive. When they break rules, it is usually a matter of forgetting rules, not noticing them, or impulsively neglecting them. Conduct disorders, by contrast, are characterized by deliberate or spiteful flouting of the rules and wilful violation of the rights of other people.

Nevertheless, defiance and antisocial behaviour are very commonly present in young people with ADHD. The association is not only because of referral or selection bias. In epidemiological surveys of total populations (e.g. of 7-year-olds in a London borough by Taylor et al. (1991)), more than half of those who had high levels of pervasive HA-IMP also scored above cut-off on parent and teacher reports of O/CP. In that study, HA without O/CP was associated with cognitive, motor, and language delays. O/CP without ADHD features was not marked by those developmental difficulties; they were linked rather to social adversity and family problems. The mixed state (HA + O/CP) was marked by both types of association, but the ADHD features appeared first. O/CP in the definite absence of ADHD features is seldom a precursor of later ADHD.

Neuroimaging has not yet made it possible to differentiate reliably which children with behaviour difficulties have ADHD and which do not, or which children with ADHD are at high risk for developing conduct problems. A functional magnetic resonance study by Rubia et al. (2008) compared groups of children with ADHD but no conduct problems and a contrasting group with conduct problems but no ADHD.

They found reduced functional activation in the ventrolateral prefrontal cortex in the ADHD group, not in the group with conduct problems. Other dysfunctions, however, were shown by both groups. Both the right temporal and parietal brain regions, and the right dorsolateral prefrontal cortex showed differences from typically developing controls for conduct problems as well as for ADHD. As discussed later, we do not yet have neurological measures that can robustly differentiate ADHD from other problems of development.

3.5.1.1 *Why are conduct problems so common in ADHD?*

The combination of ADHD and conduct problems needs to be understood developmentally. Strong reliance on a single-diagnosis approach has led some clinicians to neglect one or another aspect of mixed cases. Much clinical effort can be expended in a struggle to decide 'does this person have ADHD or O/CP?' The effort may be counterproductive. In a study of international diagnosis, diagnostic overshadowing led to a low rate of diagnosis of ADHD by UK clinicians when they applied a single-diagnosis scheme, but not when they recognized as many problems as were present (Prendergast et al., 1988). In practice, ADHD should not be diagnosed by the absence of conduct problems, but by the clear presence of the core problems of inattentiveness and disorganization.

On the one hand, overfocus on the conduct problems in mixed cases risks too little use of ADHD treatments. On the other hand, overfocus on the ADHD can lead to young people with mixed problems blaming them all on the neurological problems, at the expense of developing a sense of personal agency and responsibility. It is more fruitful to take a clinical approach that recognizes complexity and seeks to analyse why a young person with ADHD should develop conduct problems as well. Several developmental trajectories are involved. They can be distinguished in individual cases.

1. As ADHD evolves, the impulsive children often come to experience the discordant family relationships that can contribute to conduct problems in any young person: abuse, poverty, parental substance abuse, and/or other mental health problems, and family conflict or violence.
2. The propensity of ADHD to develop problems of conduct could result from genes in common. Young people with aggressive behaviour have a polygenic liability score for ADHD substantially above that in the population generally (Hamshere et al., 2013).
3. Failure in school, hostile relationships with peers, counterproductive disciplinary strategies such as frequent punishment, and victimization can all result from ADHD and are all known antecedents of problems of conduct.
4. ADHD and O/CP could share environmental risks. Deprivation, for example, can be associated with both, possibly through different mechanisms. Low family income, for instance, has an association with conduct problems; a less supportive upbringing, with ADHD (Mulligan et al., 2013).
5. Other types of disorder coexisting with ADHD could be responsible for O/CP developing in some people. Emotional dysregulation is so close an association of ADHD that it used to be regarded as part of the disorder. Uncontrolled emotions

could be intensifying the anxious and aggressive reactions to the social consequences of ADHD outlined above.

The ADHD, the social consequences, and the oppositionality all need to be recognized. They predict different sorts of outcome. Inattentiveness drives academic and occupational failure. Impulsiveness creates personal problems and exacerbates oppositionality.

O/CP drive major social maladjustment, use of drugs of addiction and recreation, and the risk of prison. There are also some interactions between problems. Conduct problems in the presence of ADHD are more likely to be severe and to be accompanied by anxiety than is the case in pure presentations of antisocial disorder. ADHD in the presence of O/CP tends to accelerate the progress through the stages towards conduct disorder.

In terms of treatment, it is desirable to recognize the distinctiveness of components (see Chapter 8, Section 8.6). Antisocial problems do not necessarily respond to anti-ADHD therapies. Medications are sometimes increased or even multiplied even though they are ineffective. Impulsive/inattentive problems seldom respond to psychological treatments which have been offered in good faith because they work for coexistent behaviour difficulties.

3.5.2 Tourette disorder and tics in ADHD

Chronic tics and Tourette are frequently present as extra problems for people with ADHD. An epidemiologically based study in Melbourne compared ADHD with unaffected controls (Poh et al., 2018). The children with ADHD were four times more likely than other children to have chronic tics at the age of 7 years, and six times more likely at age 10. The presence of chronic tics in addition to ADHD was a marker to higher rates of emotional disorders and peer problems. Possible reasons for the association include misdiagnosis and effects of prescribed stimulants. They have not been shown to account for most cases of coexistence, but clinicians should bear them in mind.

High motor restlessness in Tourette may indeed represent the coexistence of ADHD but can also result directly from tics. If a child's tics are very frequent and numerous, then their repetitive and stereotyped nature may not be apparent, and they may be seen simply as restless fidgetiness. Direct observation of the pattern of overactivity is the key. When there is doubt, filming the child and subsequent slow-motion review may make repetitive patterns evident.

3.5.3 Intellectual disability (ID)

About a quarter of children and young people with ADHD will also have IQ levels low enough for an ID to be recognized. It is still useful to recognize both when they are present. It is not always easy to do so, especially when attention problems are prominent.

The presence of impulsivity and overactivity often need to be the key to diagnosing ADHD in the presence of ID, and the presence of a wide range of cognitive problems to diagnosing ID in the presence of ADHD.

Inattention needs to be disproportionate to mental age if it is to be taken as evidence for ADHD. Such a judgement is particularly difficult at lower levels of function. For those with a mental age of less than 3 years, standardized tests are usually unavailable or inadequate. It is often better to rely on the judgement of an experienced professional who has worked with both ADHD and ID.

Most of the genetic and environmental hazards described in Chapter 7 are also causes of ID. The overlap of conditions often comes about because of similar genes.

The management of ADHD is similar whether or not ID is also present. Accordingly, there may well be a case for an attempt at symptomatic treatment of ADHD (see Chapters 8 and 9) even when the distinction of which features can be attributed to ID is unclear. The results of medication in ID are similar in kind to those in uncomplicated ADHD but less successful in degree.

3.5.4 Language and specific learning problems in ADHD

Specific learning difficulties are more common in children with ADHD than in the rest of the population. The relative risk in language impairments is usually taken to be about a threefold increase in ADHD (Mueller & Tomblin, 2012). About 3–4% of the school population will show both. The risk is not very specific but applies to disorders of conduct and emotions as well as ADHD. Many children with ADHD alone show immaturities in expressive language. They need to be recognized for educational purposes. The advice of a speech and language therapist can be invaluable to ensure that communication problems are recognized and addressed.

Young people with many other impairments of learning, such as dyslexia and dyscalculia, show cognitive and behavioural evidence of attention problems. The distinction from ADHD is that the attention problems of such individuals are not confined to periods on academic tasks.

Developmental coordination disorders (DCD) are associated with ADHD, as they are with intellectual disability, dyslexia, and ASD. They are a marker to a general immaturity of brain development. In ADHD, they need to be distinguished from the unplanned and thoughtless style of motor responding that is a core part of ADHD.

3.5.5 Autism in ADHD

There is a large overlap between ADHD and ASD. About a third of those with ADHD meet criteria for ASD, too. It is desirable to recognize both when present. Medication for ADHD can still be effective when ASD is also present, though a higher rate of adverse effects will make very careful monitoring necessary. Each condition, however, can mimic the other in some respects, and complications such as challenging behaviours may derive from either or both. The combination can be confusing to families.

Studies of risk and associated biological factors give grounds for thinking that there are brain-based influences in common with both conditions. Genetic twin studies indicate both risks shared by ADHD and ASD, and other risks that are specific to one condition. The risks in common apply across a broad range of problems, even in children as young as 2 years (Ronald et al., 2010). Other twin studies have suggested a general genetic factor that influences ADHD and a broad spectrum of other neuropsychiatric conditions (Pettersson et al., 2013). Martin et al. (2014) showed that ADHD's polygenic liability predicted ASD traits in a clinical population sample.

Neuropsychologically and neurologically, ASD and ADHD seem to show some common and also some specific features (Rommelse et al., 2011). Christakou et al. (2013) reported both disorder-specific and shared functional imaging changes in ADHD and ASD. Sustained performance measures were impaired in ADHD relative to ASD boys. Underactivation of the left dorsolateral prefrontal cortex was significantly more pronounced in ADHD patients. ASD boys, by contrast, had greater cerebellar activation than either ADHD or control. Both disorder groups showed deficits in fronto–striato–parietal activation and default mode suppression. Structurally, too, some grey-matter changes are probably disorder-specific. Grey-matter reduction in the cerebellum in ADHD has been reported to be disorder-specific relative to ASD (Lim et al., 2015). In the same study, grey-matter enlargement in the right posterior cerebellum and left middle/superior temporal gyrus was a specific finding in ASD relative to ADHD.

For those wishing to decide which diagnosis—ADHD or ASD—is the primary one for each child, there are guides for considering the issue in behavioural terms (e.g. Rommelse et al., 2018). The sections in this book on recognition (3.2 and 4.1.2) give some guidance on the most specific clinical features of each. Single-category classification remains popular with parents and educators, so deserves respect. It is not, however, the best way of planning service. Clinicians will usually need to be pragmatic, and resist exclusive classification, in the interests of people with multiple impairments having their needs met. Dual or multiple diagnosis is very often more appropriate than reliance on a single label. In school, for instance, the same child may need both an autism-friendly environment and an ADHD-appropriate structuring of learning (not to mention help with communication, motor co-ordination, and so on). The combined condition is best explained as early as possible to avoid possible confusion in families faced with an apparent change of diagnosis.

3.5.6 Anxiety in people with ADHD

Anxiety is prominent in about a quarter of people referred for ADHD. The anxiety pattern is less likely to be phobic or obsessional than in anxious children without ADHD. It is often a result of prolonged failure, struggle, and victimization. Whatever the underlying causes, high anxiety can itself disrupt cognitive performance, including attention. Unfocused attention might expose children to greater recognition of more potential threats and thereby increase anxiety about the future. High anxiety in ADHD seems to be associated with reduced impulsiveness and, often, with a sluggish cognitive tempo.

Neuropsychological models for the coexistence of ADHD and anxiety states are described and reviewed by Schatz and Rostain (2006). None has yet commanded understanding. There may be some confounding with gender issues. ADHD in females needs closer study than it has received, but seems to show not only more emotional disturbance but also less impulsiveness, more cognitive inefficiency, and later referral to services than is seen in males.

3.6 Prevalence

The rates with which ADHD is diagnosed are increasing rapidly in many countries (Chapter 1, Section 1.1). Diagnostic practice is not sufficiently standardized internationally to allow for definitive estimates of geographical prevalence. The most authoritative recent figure comes from a meta-analysis by Thomas et al. (2015) which has generated an average figure of around 7.2% of schoolchildren. The adult rate is about half that of children and young people.

The figures for individual countries differ considerably, largely for reasons of methodology. The numerical estimates are given in 'Frequency and impact of neurodevelopmental disorders', Chapter 1, Section 1.1. The exact diagnostic criteria adopted, the measurement methods applied, the level of impairment required, and the sources of information used are all major influences on the estimates (Polanczyk et al., 2014). In particular, the judgement of 'clinical significance' gives rise to a good deal of the variance. It is conceivable that some of the international differences in prevalence reflect variations in risk factors (e.g. use of junk food, levels of exercise, screen use, obstetric practices) but, if so, they are dwarfed by the methodological variations.

3.6.1 What causes underdiagnosis and overdiagnosis in practice?

In the USA, influences on prevalence seem to include pressure on schools for academic results, leading to high referral rates, and managed care practices favouring diagnoses implying medication. In the UK, low rates seem to reflect underdiagnoses and cultural resistance to the concept, especially in schools.

Professional cultures also play a part in determining apparent prevalence. A comparison of diagnostic practice between USA and UK clinicians indicated that diagnostic overshadowing operated in different ways in different contexts. In mixed cases, UK clinicians diagnosed the behavioural problems, USA clinicians, the ADHD (Prendergast et al., 1988). When multiple diagnoses were encouraged, there was little difference between those diagnosing on either side of the Atlantic.

Diagnostic overshadowing and under-recognition in the UK take place at several levels. A survey in UK general practices screened for ADHD features and found that referral to a secondary service was conditioned by parental beliefs (Sayal et al., 2002). If parents had presented hyperactivity as the problem, referral to a secondary service (paediatric or mental health) was generally prompt and accurate. If they had not identified the problem, but attended because of their child's bad behaviour, uncontrollable tempers, or unhappiness, then referral was usually to community services for parent training or counselling. Those services would be appropriate to the problem presented, but not necessarily to an underlying problem of ADHD.

Under-recognition is sometimes because ASD and ID are identified at an age before that at which ADHD can be recognized. ASD or ID may thenceforward dominate subsequent management and apparent prevalence.

Under-recognition can also be encouraged by beliefs about causation. ADHD is not in fact an aetiological diagnosis, but some suppose it to be so. Such a belief can polarize professional attitudes. Those who see it as a neurological disease may be reluctant to recognize it in people without other neurological problems, or to suppose that another brain disorder rules out ADHD as a useful diagnosis. Conversely, those whose experience is with children showing the scars of neglect and abuse may suppose that a psychosocial cause of problems rules out the possibility that the form of the problems is ADHD.

3.6.2.1 *Clinical implications of influences on estimates of prevalence*

The very variable rates of recognition of ADHD imply an unmet need for reliability in clinical diagnosis.

The probable underdiagnosis in the UK argues for service improvements. Underprovision of services should be corrected. Better information for parents and teachers about ADHD could be expected to overcome stigma and create better informed referrals.

Screening in the population as a whole is not yet an evaluated way to improve outcomes: it does not necessarily make for more or more appropriate referrals, and if it did, it would risk overloading already stretched services. Nevertheless, screening within existing services of children presented for problems of behaviour or learning could well overcome the existing filters. Foreman et al. (2001) found, some years ago, that a questionnaire screen in a child mental health service enhanced the recognition of ADHD features, and subsequent diagnostic rates rose from 2% to 25% of the clinic cases.

3.7 RISKS

3.7.1 Genes and environment

Genetic and environmental influences are profoundly intertwined for ADHD, as for other types of mental dysfunction, and need to be considered jointly (Chapter 7, Section 7.5).

For ADHD specifically, strong genetic influences have been established by decades of research (Faraone & Larsson, 2019). The risk of ADHD occurring in other first-degree family members (biological parents, brothers and sisters) is raised about five-fold. Comparisons of monozygotic twins (who have the same DNA) and dizygotic twins (who share half their DNA) have suggested that heritability is quite high, at approximately 70%. Adoption studies concur in a higher rate of ADHD in biological siblings than in adoptive siblings living in the same family. Review of the genetically informative studies by Thapar et al. (2012) confirms a strong genetic influence on the syndrome.

These findings have motivated an extensive search for ADHD susceptibility genes. Variants of genes have been described that influence aspects of neurotransmission, abnormalities of structure and function in regions of the frontal lobes and basal ganglia, failures to suppress inappropriate responses, and a cascade of failures in cognitive performance and organization of behaviour.

A few known DNA changes, such as 22q11 deletion, have large effects. They also produce other consequences for mental health, and are described in Chapter 7, Section 7.4. They are rare and cannot account for most cases. Most DNA risk variants for ADHD are, individually, very small. Cumulatively, however, they explain much of the difference between people in inattention and impulsiveness. Genome-wide association studies (GWAS) have found some of them. At the time of writing, DNA variants have been reliably identified at 12 independent points along the chromosomes in people of European ancestry with ADHD (Demontis et al., 2019).

Individual genes identified include FOXP2 (at chromosome 7), which is already known to play a significant role in forming synapses and neural systems involved in learning and speech. An intron in SORCS3 on chromosome 10 encodes a transmembrane receptor believed to be important for neural development and altered in depressive disorders. The locus on chromosome 12 includes DUSP6 which is considered to influence dopamine levels in synapses.

Active research is changing understanding quickly. Frequent genetic variants are of minimal effect individually, but cumulatively they may account for much of the association between ADHD and other conditions such as depression, smoking, obesity, and low educational attainment—as well as with having children earlier and more frequently (which might help to explain its evolutionary persistence).

Polygenic risk assessment for individuals has become feasible (see Chapter 7, Section 7.4). It is now guiding major research programmes, and is increasingly being used in practice in major centres. Other parts of the inherited variance are due to copy number variants—insertion or deletion of small parts of the chromosome that are repeated a varying number of times. Individually, they are rare but can have larger effects than any of the common variants considered here. They may be especially significant if they are not inherited from typically developing parents but arise de novo in the affected person. Both common and rare genetic changes have been found, and may have independent effects (Martin et al., 2015).

Much of the heritability is still unexplained. Five of the best established genetic variants—in serotonin 1b receptor, serotonin transporter, dopamine D4 and D5 receptors, and the dopamine transporter—have been estimated to account for only 3.2% of the variance in symptoms of ADHD, and 4.2% of the heritability (Kuntsi et al., 2006). The advice given to families should still be that genetic influences are strong, but they are multiple. Nevertheless, the scientific difficulty in specifying the precise influences responsible makes genetic counselling inexact for affected families. For the moment, investigation of chromosomes and DNA for individual patients is recommended only when there are specific reasons—such as a phenotype suggesting a large gene effect (e.g. Williams syndrome), or the presence of many affected family members, or the existence of other neurodevelopmental problems (e.g. intellectual disability) that are enough in themselves to indicate genetic evaluation.

3.7.2 Environmental influences

Several, potentially harmful factors in the early environment are reliably associated with ADHD, but none is unequivocally established as a cause (Thapar et al., 2012). Toxins, allergies, and infections are covered in Chapter 7. The developmental pathways involved can be complex. Genetic factors could influence both the exposure to environmental risks (G–E correlation) and the susceptibility of the individual to them (G–E interaction). Individual environmental adversities are considered in Chapter 7.

- *Prenatal associations* include maternal smoking during pregnancy, maternal alcohol consumption and use of non-prescribed drugs of abuse, prescribed drugs such as anticonvulsants and anxiolytics, maternal stress, and maternal hypothyroidism.
- *Perinatal associations* include low birthweight, prematurity, and obstetric complications.
- *In postnatal life*, associations include an inadequate diet, iodine and vitamin B deficiencies, iron and lead poisoning, and high exposure to some artificial food colourings and preservatives. Various medical illnesses are also risks for the development of poor concentration, irritable mood, and problems of conduct. In young children, eczema and sleep problems are common reasons for the upsets, and successful treatments of these primary problems will often relieve the behavioural problems, too.
- *Screen exposure* to social media, multiple apps, and videogames are probably not responsible for modern youth having shorter attention spans and less focus in behaviour than their predecessors (see 'Encounters with the internet', Chapter 10, Section 10.10).
- *Social environment* associations of ADHD include exposure to extremely depriving institutional environments. More frequent and less severe variations in the family environment may also be implicated, probably as influences on developmental course rather than as causes of ADHD (Chapter 10).
- *Family hostility* (Chapter 10, Section 10.6) is associated with ADHD, and also with genetic influences. Lifford et al. (2009) therefore examined the causal relationships with a combination of a genetic twin study and a longitudinal analysis. For girls, genetic factors alone explained the association between parents' hostility and ADHD

symptoms. For boys, genes played a part and there was an effect of their ADHD contributing to their mothers' hostility. Even though family relationships do not seem to have much influence on the development of ADHD, parental hostility could still contribute to the transition into conduct problems.

In short, there may be several developmental pathways through which constitutional factors interact with the environment to influence ADHD. In one possible set of tracks, altered brain states lead directly to cognitive alteration, and the resulting impulsive and inattentive behaviours show direct continuity through childhood into late adolescence. In others, an understimulating environment is evoked by (and may be genetically associated with) an inattentive and cognitively impulsive style during early childhood. In yet another track, impulsiveness evokes critical expressed emotion from parents and inefficient coping strategies, which in turn contribute to the development of antisocial conduct (see 'Encounters with family problems', Chapter 10, Section 10.6). Several types of clinical formulation will therefore be needed in different presentations.

3.8 Pathophysiology

ADHD does not reflect a pathology of attention in any simple way. The functions of attention described in Chapter 2, Section 2.3 do not suggest that ADHD will reflect any one fundamental neurocognitive change. It seems more likely that ADHD, in an individual case, will prove to be associated with multiple changes in many brain circuits, associating more or less closely with multiple types of neurocognitive alteration, and with multiple types of emotional and behavioural change. Research will therefore need very large numbers of subjects and advances in the means of analysing them.

Most reviewers of neurocognitive changes in ADHD have opted to conclude that there are multiple pathways. Artificial intelligence analyses have accordingly been used to try to identify patterns of change that will give reliable guides to diagnosis, prognosis, and choice of treatment. So far there is no single consensus, in spite of good progress in developing large series with comparable measures (Castellanos & Proal, 2012).

For the moment, therefore, clinicians should avoid giving overly precise formulations to young people and their families about the neural basis of their problems. The objective tests are not necessary or sufficient to diagnose ADHD. Despite this, several commercial devices have been developed to offer objective tests to aid the diagnostic process, without solid evidence that they add significant value to the traditional approach. A randomized trial of using a computerized assessment of activity and accuracy while carrying out a continuous performance test did not find improvement in diagnostic accuracy (Hollis et al., 2018). The computerized test did, however, increase clinicians' confidence that their diagnoses were correct, and it speeded up the over-lengthy process of making and conveying the diagnosis.

For children and young people, diagnosis remains dependent on clinical interview of a parent to inquire about each symptom relative to peers of the same sex and age, detailed information from the class teacher, and a clinical judgement about whether intensity and frequency of behaviour change is extreme enough to represent impairment of function. When objective test performance is discrepant with the subjective clinical report, the latter takes priority.

The pathophysiology of ADHD remains in doubt in spite of extensive research into its neuropsychology. Many researchers proceed from a view that neurocognitive impairments are the prime ways of explaining the behaviour of children with ADHD. A vast amount of psychological experimentation has therefore contrasted children and young people at various ages (usually 8 to 14 years) who have an ADHD diagnosis or high levels of inattentiveness/impulsiveness, with unaffected children of similar ages. There are many fine reviews. Readers wanting to immerse themselves are recommended a review by Castellanos and Proal (2012). That review goes beyond the most familiar models of frontal and striatal dysfunction to implicate large-scale resting-state networks involving frontoparietal, dorsal attentional, motor, visual, and default networks (see Section 3.8.2).

3.8.1 Cognitive changes

Findings at the cognitive level are inconstant. Most of the abilities described as 'executive function' in Chapter 2, Section 2.5 have been examined (including weak inhibition of responses, working memory, and planning ahead) together with several other cognitive and motivational processes (including delay aversion, response variability, shortened delay of reward gradient, incompetent timing, and weak spatial memory). They all differentiate ADHD from controls in some studies, but do not correlate well with each other (Sonuga–Barke & Halperin, 2010).

3.8.1.1 *Findings from the experimental studies of cognition in ADHD*

- Many children with ADHD perform poorly on at least one executive function test.
- Many also show deviant function in other types of cognitive test, including high response variability, delay aversion, shortened delay of reward gradient, incompetent timing, and weak spatial memory.
- Effect sizes of ADHD on single tests—usually less than one standard deviation—are not large enough to be regarded as part of the definition.
- Somewhat larger effect sizes have been found for combinations of tests (possibly because of greater reliability when several tests have been combined).
- Poor performance is the rule, in spite of experimental control of test details. Testing is usually done in non-distracting and reasonably non-aversive circumstances, in which the nature of the task to be done is made clear. This is very different from the usual circumstances of the classroom and social life, and might limit the predictive value of

test results in the real world. It nevertheless seems that individual children have definable impairments of function and are not only the victims of adverse contexts.

- Impairments are disproportionate to IQ changes.
- No one executive function is specifically impaired. Attempts have been made to make a specific case for one abnormality (e.g. in inhibition) as primary, but none has yet clearly emerged. Maybe there are several subtypes of behaviour change in each of which there is a specific neurocognitive abnormality; maybe there are several pathways from neurocognition to ADHD. Several attempts have been made to identify a range of pathways. Many are promising (Sonuga–Barke & Halperin, 2010), none conclusive (Stevens et al., 2018).
- A considerable minority of children with ADHD have no abnormality on any of the tested functions.
- The causal direction for associations between behavioural and neurocognitive changes is not clear. Either could be responsible for the other, or they might each reflect a common cause in different ways, or the causes of each might be different but themselves be correlated.
- Treatment of one level does not necessarily improve the other, and ADHD behaviours and neurocognitive performance deficits do not, as far as we can tell at present, predict one another strongly over time. Perhaps there are many causal pathways, with some of them involving direct causation one way or the other, but none of them can emerge from the noise of considering all together as influences on a single, polythetic syndrome. Perhaps they are associated because of prior associations between neural circuits, each of which has independent actions on behaviour and cognition. Perhaps 'attention deficit' is only a good description at a behavioural (not cognitive) level and other aspects (e.g. volition?) need better understanding.

3.8.2 Neural changes

Knowledge of brain structure and function in ADHD is expanding rapidly—too rapidly for a detailed review of studies to be of any but historical interest by the time it is published in a textbook and read. It is already clear, however, that there are consistent (but sometimes quite small) differences between groups of people with ADHD and typically developing controls. The following citations are to studies, or reviews of studies, that are large enough and representative enough that the group findings are likely to be replicated.

Cortical volume is smaller in young people with ADHD than in controls, especially in the frontal lobes (Ambrosini, 2000). There are also volume differences in subcortical structures. The amygdala, accumbens, and hippocampus are all somewhat smaller in ADHD than in typically developing individuals (Hoogman et al., 2017). The differences from the usual sizes are greater for young people (up to 15 years) than for adults (21 years and over), so perhaps maturity does make for a more typical pattern. In the cerebellar white matter, those with ADHD showed slower growth in early childhood than a typically developing group, a phenomenon which had reversed by the time of late childhood (Shaw et al., 2018).

Functional imaging of patterns of connections within the brain is also generating group differences, as much in ADHD as in any psychiatric disorder (Castellanos & Aoki, 2016). There are probably multiple patterns of difference and a detailed review of pattern-recognition approaches is provided by Wolfers et al. (2015).

Functional brain imaging, especially using magnetic resonance techniques, is being widely used to test neuropsychological hypotheses. Many of the studies contrast brain activity while performing cognitive or emotional tests with activity recorded at different times. The tasks used often involve executive function and, more recently, emotional control. Rubia (2018) provides a systematic review. There is sound evidence that, as a group, both young people and adults with ADHD have alterations (usually diminished activity) in several networks that are considered to mediate cognitive control, attention, timing, and working memory. Dorsal, ventral, and medial fronto-cingulo-striato-thalamic and fronto-parieto-cerebellar networks are involved in both the right and left hemispheres. More preliminary evidence suggests abnormalities in orbital and ventro-medial prefrontal and limbic areas that mediate motivation and emotion control.

Some research has focused on brain activity when the individual is not engaged in experimental tasks. The 'default mode networks' (DMN) are revealed at rest by the appearance of spontaneous high-amplitude, very slow (<0.1 Hz) fluctuations in blood oxygenation levels in the ventrolateral and ventromedial prefrontal cortex, the posterior cingulate cortex (PCC), the cuneus, and the inferior parietal lobe. The activation reduces when other networks are engaged in mental effort (e.g. the fronto-parietal and ventral attention networks). The subjective experience during DMN activation is usually one of mind wandering or daydreaming. The suggestion from meta-analyses of neurophysiological research is that people with ADHD do not switch off the activation of DMN when engaged in a task to the same extent as other people (Cortese et al., 2012)

None of these group findings are yet good enough to guide clinicians in thinking about individuals. They have, however, helped to create a climate of understanding. ADHD is now seen as a treatable condition rather than a moral defect.

REFERENCES

Achenbach, T. M., & Ruffle, T. M. (2000). The Child Behavior Checklist and related forms for assessing behavioral/emotional problems and competencies. *Pediatrics in Review, 21*(8), 265–271.

Adler, L. A., Kessler, R. C., & Spencer, T. (2003). *Adult ADHD Self-Report Scale—v1.1 (ASRS-v1.1) Symptom Checklist.* World Health Organization.

Ambrosini, P. J. (2000). Historical development and present status of the schedule for affective disorders and schizophrenia for school-age children (K-SADS). *Journal of the American Academy of Child & Adolescent Psychiatry, 39*(1), 49–58.

American Psychiatric Association. (2013). *Diagnostic and statistical manual of mental disorders* (DSM-5).

Angold, A., & Costello, E. J. (2000). The child and adolescent psychiatric assessment (CAPA). *Journal of the American Academy of Child & Adolescent Psychiatry*, *39*(1), 39–48.

Arnold, L. E., Roy, A., Taylor, E., Hechtman, L., Sibley, M., Swanson, J. M., Mitchell, J., Molina, B. S. G., & Rohde, L. (2018/2019). Predictive utility of childhood diagnosis of ICD-10 hyperkinetic disorder: adult outcomes in the MTA and effect of comorbidity. *European Child & Adolescent Psychiatry*. https://doi.org/10.1007/s00787-018-1222-0

Bard, D. E., Wolraich, M. L., Neas, B., Doffing, M., & Beck, L. (2013). The psychometric properties of the Vanderbilt attention-deficit hyperactivity disorder diagnostic parent rating scale in a community population. *Journal of Developmental & Behavioral Pediatrics*, *34*(2), 72–82.

Burns, G. L., Walsh, J. A., Servera, M., Lorenzo–Seva, U., Cardo, E., & Rodríguez–Fornells, A. (2013). Construct validity of ADHD/ODD rating scales: recommendations for the evaluation of forthcoming DSM-V ADHD/ODD scales. *Journal of Abnormal Child Psychology*, *41*(1), 15–26.

Castellanos, F. X., & Aoki, Y. (2016). Intrinsic functional connectivity in attention-deficit/hyperactivity disorder: a science in development. *Biological Psychiatry: Cognitive Neuroscience and Neuroimaging*, *1*(3), 253–261.

Castellanos, F. X., & Proal, E. (2012). Large-scale brain systems in ADHD: beyond the prefrontal–striatal model. *Trends in Cognitive Sciences*, *16*(1), 17–26.

Christakou, A., Murphy, C. M., Chantiluke, K., Cubillo, A. I., Smith, A. B., Giampietro, V., Daly, E., Ecker, C., Robertson, D., MRC AIMS Consortium, Murphy, D. G., & Rubia, K. (2013). Disorder-specific functional abnormalities during sustained attention in youth with attention deficit hyperactivity disorder (ADHD) and with autism. *Molecular Psychiatry*, *18*(2), 236.

Conners, C. K. (2008). *Conners' rating scales* (3rd ed.). Multi Health Systems.

Cortese, S., Kelly, C., Chabernaud, C., Proal, E., Di Martino, A., Milham, M. P., & Castellanos, F. X. (2012). Toward systems neuroscience of ADHD: a meta-analysis of 55 fMRI studies. *American Journal of Psychiatry*, *169*(10), 1038–1055.

Davidson, M. A. (2008). ADHD in adults: a review of the literature. *Journal of Attention Disorders*, *11*(6), 628–641.

Demontis, D., Walters, R. K., Martin, J., Mattheisen, M., Als, T. D., Agerbo, E., . . . & Neale, B. M. (2019). Discovery of the first genome-wide significant risk loci for attention deficit/hyperactivity disorder. *Nature Genetics*, *51*(1), 63–75.

DuPaul, G. J. (1991). Parent and teacher ratings of ADHD symptoms: psychometric properties in a community-based sample. *Journal of Clinical Child and Adolescent Psychology*, *20*(3), 245–253.

Faraone, S. V., & Larsson, H. (2019). Genetics of attention deficit hyperactivity disorder. *Molecular Psychiatry*, *24*(4), 562–575.

Foreman, D. M., Foreman, D., Prendergast, M., & Minty, B. (2001). Is clinic prevalence of ICD-10 hyperkinesis underestimated? *European Child & Adolescent Psychiatry*, *10*(2), 130–134.

Goodman, R. (1997). The Strengths and Difficulties Questionnaire: a research note. *Journal of Child Psychology and Psychiatry*, *38*(5), 581–586.

Goodman, R., & Scott, S. (1999). Comparing the Strengths and Difficulties Questionnaire and the Child Behavior Checklist: is small beautiful? *Journal of Abnormal Child Psychology*, *27*, 17–24.

Hamshere, M. L., Langley, K., Martin, J., Agha, S. S., Stergiakouli, E., Anney, R. J., Buitelaar, J., Faraone, S. V., Lesch, K. P., Neale, B. M., Franke, B., Sonuga–Barke, E., Asherson, P., Merwood, A., Kuntsi, J., Medland, S. E., Ripke, S., Steinhausen, H. C., Freitag, C., . . .

& Thapar, A. (2013). High loading of polygenic risk for ADHD in children with comorbid aggression. *American Journal of Psychiatry*, *170*(8), 909–916.

Hollis, C., Hall, C. L., Guo, B., James, M., Boadu, J., Groom, M. J., Brown, N., Kaylor–Hughes, C., Moldavsky, M., Valentine, A. Z., Walker, G. M., Daley, D., Sayal, K., & Morriss, R. (2018). The impact of a computerised test of attention and activity (QbTest) on diagnostic decision-making in children and young people with suspected attention deficit hyperactivity disorder: single-blind randomised controlled trial. *Journal of Child Psychology and Psychiatry*, *59*(12), 1298–1308.

Hoogman, M., Bralten, J., Hibar, D. P., Mennes, M., Zwiers, M. P., Schweren, L. S., … & Franke, B. (2017). Subcortical brain volume differences in participants with attention deficit hyperactivity disorder in children and adults: a cross-sectional mega-analysis. *The Lancet Psychiatry*, *4*(4), 310–319.

Jensen, C. M., & Steinhausen, H. C. (2015). Comorbid mental disorders in children and adolescents with attention-deficit/hyperactivity disorder in a large nationwide study. *ADHD Attention Deficit and Hyperactivity Disorders*, *7*(1), 27–38.

Kuntsi, J., Neale, B. M., Chen, W., Faraone, S. V., & Asherson, P. (2006). The IMAGE project: methodological issues for the molecular genetic analysis of ADHD. *Behavioral Brain Function*, *2*, 27.

Lifford, K. J., Harold, G. T., & Thapar, A. (2009). Parent–child hostility and child ADHD symptoms: a genetically sensitive and longitudinal analysis. *Journal of Child Psychology and Psychiatry*, *50*(12), 1468–1476.

Lim, L., Chantiluke, K., Cubillo, A. I., Smith, A. B., Simmons, A., Mehta, M. A., & Rubia, K. (2015). Disorder-specific grey matter deficits in attention deficit hyperactivity disorder relative to autism spectrum disorder. *Psychological Medicine*, *45*(5), 965–976.

Martin, J., O'Donovan, M. C., Thapar, A., Langley, K., & Williams, N. (2015). The relative contribution of common and rare genetic variants to ADHD. *Translational Psychiatry*, *5*(2), e506.

McCann, B. S., Scheele, L., Ward, N., & Roy-Byrne, P. (2000). Discriminant validity of the Wender Utah Rating Scale for attention-deficit/hyperactivity disorder in adults. *Journal of Neuropsychiatry and Clinical Neurosciences*, *12*(2), 240–245.

Moffitt, T. E., Houts, R., Asherson, P., Belsky, D. W., Corcoran, D. L., Hammerle, M., … & Caspi, A. (2015). Is adult ADHD a childhood-onset neurodevelopmental disorder? Evidence from a four-decade longitudinal cohort study. *American Journal of Psychiatry*, *172*(10), 967–977.

Mokrova, I., O'Brien, M., Calkins, S., & Keane, S. (2010). Parental ADHD symptomology and ineffective parenting: The connecting link of home chaos. *Parenting: Science and Practice*, *10*(2), 119–135.

Mueller, K. L., & Tomblin, J. B. (2012). Examining the comorbidity of language disorders and ADHD. *Topics in Language Disorders*, *32*(3), 228.

Mulligan, A., Anney, R., Butler, L., O'Regan, M., Richardson, T., Tulewicz, E. M., Fitzgerald, M., & Gill, M. (2013). Home environment: association with hyperactivity/impulsivity in children with ADHD and their non-ADHD siblings. *Child: Care, Health and Development*, *39*(2), 202–212.

National Collaborating Centre for Mental Health (UK). (2018). *Attention deficit hyperactivity disorder: diagnosis and management of ADHD in children, young people and adults.* (NICE Guideline No. 87). British Psychological Society. https://www.ncbi.nlm.nih.gov/books/NBK493361/

National Institute for Clinical Excellence. (2009). *Attention deficit hyperactivity disorder.* British Psychological Society and The Royal College of Psychiatrists. https://www.nice.org.uk/CG72

Pettersson, E., Anckarsäter, H., Gillberg, C., & Lichtenstein, P. (2013). Different neurodevelopmental symptoms have a common genetic etiology. *Journal of Child Psychology and Psychiatry, 54*(12), 1356–1365.

Poh, W., Payne, J. M., Gulenc, A., & Efron, D. (2018). Chronic tic disorders in children with ADHD. *Archives of Disease in Childhood, 103*(9), 847–852.

Polanczyk, G. V., Willcutt, E. G., Salum, G. A., Kieling, C., & Rohde LA. (2014) ADHD prevalence estimates across three decades: an updated systematic review and meta-regression analysis. *International Journal of Epidemiology, 43*,434–442.

Prendergast, M., Taylor, E., Rapoport, J. L., Bartko, J., Donnelly, M., Zametkin, A., Ahearn, M. B., Dunn, G., & Weiselberg, H. M. (1988). The diagnosis of childhood hyperactivity: a U.S.–U.K. cross-national study of DSM-III and ICD-9. *Journal of Child Psychology & Psychiatry & Allied Disciplines, 29*, 289–300.

Riddle, M. A., Yershova, K., Lazzaretto, D., Paykina, N., Yenokyan, G., Greenhill, L., … & Posner, K. (2013). The preschool attention-deficit/hyperactivity disorder treatment study (PATS) 6-year follow-up. *Journal of the American Academy of Child & Adolescent Psychiatry, 52*(3), 264–278.

Rommelse, N. N., Geurts, H. M., Franke, B., Buitelaar, J. K., & Hartman, C. A. (2011). A review on cognitive and brain endophenotypes that may be common in autism spectrum disorder and attention-deficit/hyperactivity disorder and facilitate the search for pleiotropic genes. *Neuroscience & Biobehavioral Reviews, 35*(6), 1363–1396.

Rommelse, N., Visser, J., & Hartman, C. (2018). Differentiating between ADHD and ASD in childhood: some directions for practitioners. *European Child & Adolescent Psychiatry, 27*, 679–681.

Ronald, A., Edelson, L. R., Ahserson, P., & Saudino, K. J. (2010). Exploring the relationship between autistic-like traits and ADHD behaviors in early childhood: findings from a community twin study of 2-year olds. *Journal of Abnormal Child Psychology, 38*, 185–196.

Rubia, K., Halari, R., Smith, A. B., Mohammed, M., Scott, S., Giampietro, V., … & Brammer, M. J. (2008). Dissociated functional brain abnormalities of inhibition in boys with pure conduct disorder and in boys with pure attention deficit hyperactivity disorder. *American Journal of Psychiatry, 165*(7), 889–897.

Rubia, K. (2018). Cognitive neuroscience of attention deficit hyperactivity disorder (ADHD) and its clinical translation. *Frontiers in Human Neuroscience, 12*, 100.

Santosh, P. J., Taylor, E., Swanson, J., Wigal, T., Chuang, S., Davies, M., Greenhill, L., Newcorn, J., Arnold, L. E., Jensen, P., Vitiello, B., Elliott, G., Hinshaw, S., Hechtman, L., Abikoff, H., Pelham, W., Hoza, B., Molina, B., Wells, K., & Epstein, J. (2005). Refining the diagnoses of inattention and overactivity syndromes: a reanalysis of the multimodal treatment study of attention deficit hyperactivity disorder (ADHD) based on ICD-10 criteria for hyperkinetic disorder. *Clinical Neuroscience Research, 5*(5-6), 307–314.

Sayal, K., Taylor, E., Beecham, J., & Byrne, P. (2002). Pathways to care in children at risk of attention-deficit hyperactivity disorder. *British Journal of Psychiatry, 181*, 43–48.

Schatz, D. B., & Rostain, A. L. (2006). ADHD with comorbid anxiety: a review of the current literature. *Journal of Attention disorders, 10*(2), 141–149.

Shaffer, D., Fisher, P., Lucas, C. P., Dulcan, M. K., & Schwab–Stone, M. E. (2000). NIMH Diagnostic Interview Schedule for Children Version IV (NIMH DISC-IV): description, differences from previous versions, and reliability of some common diagnoses. *Journal of the American Academy of Child & Adolescent Psychiatry, 39*(1), 28–38.

Shaw, P., Ishii-Takahashi, A., Park, M. T., Devenyi, G. A., Zibman, C., Kasparek, S., ... & White, T. (2018). A multicohort, longitudinal study of cerebellar development in attention deficit hyperactivity disorder. *Journal of Child Psychology and Psychiatry*, *59*(10), 1114–1123.

Sonuga–Barke, E. J., & Halperin, J. M. (2010). Developmental phenotypes and causal pathways in attention deficit/hyperactivity disorder: potential targets for early intervention? *Journal of Child Psychology and Psychiatry*, *51*(4), 368–389.

Stevens, M. C., Pearlson, G. D., Calhoun, V. D., & Bessette, K. L. (2018). Functional neuroimaging evidence for distinct neurobiological pathways in attention-deficit/hyperactivity disorder. *Biological Psychiatry: Cognitive Neuroscience and Neuroimaging*, *3*(8), 675–685.

Swanson, J. M., Sergeant, J. A., Taylor, E., Sonuga–Barke, E. J. S., Jensen, P. S., & Cantwell, D. P. (1998). Attention-deficit hyperactivity disorder and hyperkinetic disorder. *Lancet*, *351*(9100), 429–433.

Swanson, J. M., Schuck, S., Porter, M. M., Carlson, C., Hartman, C. A., Sergeant, J. A., Clevenger, W., Wasdell, M., McCleary, R., Lakes, K., & Wigal, T. (2012). Categorical and dimensional definitions and evaluations of symptoms of ADHD: history of the SNAP and the SWAN rating scales. *International Journal of Educational and Psychological Assessment*, *10*(1), 51.

Taylor, E. (1994). Similarities and differences in DSM-IV and ICD-10 diagnostic criteria. *Child and Adolescent Psychiatric Clinics*, *3*(2), 209–226.

Taylor, E. (2017). Development of the concept. In T. Banaschewski, D. Coghill, & A. Zuddas (Eds.), *Oxford textbook of attention deficit hyperactivity disorder* (pp. 3–8). Oxford University Press.

Taylor, E., Chadwick, O., Heptinstall, E., & Danckaerts, M. (1996). Hyperactivity and conduct problems as risk factors for adolescent development. *Journal of the American Academy of Child & Adolescent Psychiatry*, *35*(9), 1213–26.

Taylor, E., Sandberg, S., Thorley, G., & Giles, S. (1991). *The epidemiology of childhood hyperactivity*. (Maudsley Monograph No. 33). Oxford University Press.

Thapar, A., Cooper, M., Jefferies, R., & Stergiakouli, E. (2012). What causes attention deficit hyperactivity disorder? *Archives of Disease in Childhood*, *97*(3), 260–265.

Thomas, R., Sanders, S., Doust, J., Beller, E., & Glasziou, P. (2015). Prevalence of attention-deficit/hyperactivity disorder: a systematic review and meta-analysis. *Pediatrics*, *135*(4), e994–e1001.

World Health Organization (WHO). (2018). *ICD-11 for mortality and morbidity statistics*. https://www.who.int/classifications/icd/en/

Wolfers, T., Buitelaar, J. K., Beckmann, C. F., Franke, B., & Marquand, A. F. (2015). From estimating activation locality to predicting disorder: a review of pattern recognition for neuroimaging-based psychiatric diagnostics. *Neuroscience & Biobehavioral Reviews*, *57*, 328–349.

Zivetz, L. (1992). *The ICD-10 classification of mental and behavioural disorders: clinical descriptions and diagnostic guidelines*. (Vol. 1). World Health Organization.

CHAPTER 4

....

AUTISM SPECTRUM DISORDER AND EARLY-ONSET PSYCHOSES

....

4.1 AUTISM SPECTRUM DISORDER (ASD)

4.1.1 Diagnostic concepts

AUTISM is a term to describe a pattern of reduced social communication and repetitive, restricted behaviours. They appear early in childhood and tend to persist. Alterations in social communication, sociability, language, cognitive flexibility, and repetitive motor activity are common in children with altered brains. Many, but not all children affected in this way also have problems in learning and intellectual function. Some of the features cluster together into a pattern that is now termed 'autism spectrum disorder'.

The classic description came from a paper by Leo Kanner, a paediatrician in the USA, reporting vividly on the difficulties shared by 11 children (Kanner, 1943). He was impressed by how their 'condition differs so markedly and uniquely from anything reported so far', and emphasized their 'aloneness'. Since then, experts from many countries have been impressed by the distinctiveness of the pattern. There is international consensus on the defining features. DSM-5 puts them as 'persistent deficits in social communication and social interaction' and 'restricted, repetitive patterns of behaviour, interests, or activities' (American Psychiatric Association, 2013). ICD-11 puts them in nearly identical terms as 'persistent deficits in the ability to initiate and to sustain reciprocal social interaction and social communication' and 'a range of restricted, repetitive, and inflexible patterns of behaviour and interests' (World Health Organization, 2018). Both emphasize that the deficits arise early in development, are more common in males than females, and follow a variable course of persistence into adult life. Both specify that the impairments are very much out of keeping with general developmental level.

Details vary between cultures. Nevertheless, there was an expectation that so distinctive a pattern would prove to be a disease with a specific pathophysiology and means

Box 4.1 Core features of autism spectrum disorder

- Little emotional reciprocity in social relationships
- Impairments in non-verbal communication
- Difficulties in developing and understanding relationships
- Stereotyped repetitiveness of speech and movement
- Rigid adherence to routines
- Very restricted, overfocused interests
- Over- or under-reactiveness to sensory input

Central aspects of the spectra of autism are described more fully in Section 4.1.2.1.4.

of curing it. So far, that expectation has not been realized. Genetic research, which was once considered the best hope of a biological definition, has found an extremely complex picture of multiple genes, many with very small effects and diverse consequences. Similarly, major programmes of psychological research have tried to incriminate processes such as analytic versus Gestalt processing, defective theory of mind, impaired central coherence, and many others. However, none has yet commanded the field or shown the high levels of specificity and sensitivity required to be diagnostically useful. Accordingly, the definition of autism remains behavioural.

Many clinical scientists have noted features of behaviour that are very common in identified children and not at all common outside of them. They are often called the 'core' features. The nature of this core has varied somewhat from time to time. No biological marker has been discerned to validate it. Rather, some styles of behaviour are considered central, based on clinical observations and statistical classification of behaviours.

These styles are described in the main classification schemes of psychiatry, with examples that should probably differ more between cultures than they do. Box 4.1 indicates the core features of ASD. They are widely accepted and derive from the DSM-5 (American Psychiatric Association, 2013), with which Box 4.1 is intended to be compatible. Guidance on recognition is given in Section 4.1.2. Diagnosis does not require every feature to be present, and no single feature is sufficient. The concept is polythetic; that is, of the list of commonly occurring features, no one is essential.

4.1.1.1 *Diagnosis of ASD in DSM-5*

To make a complete DSM-5 diagnosis it would be necessary to follow the full wording in the *Diagnostic and statistical manual of mental disorders* (American Psychiatric Association, 2013). There are also other requirements: early onset, evidence of limitation of function, and absence of other conditions to which the problems can better be attributed. Such distinctions should be followed to achieve standardization for projects such as administration, research, reimbursement, quality control, and distribution of resources.

4.1.1.2 *Diagnosis of ASD in ICD-11*

The eleventh edition of the World Health Organization's (WHO's) *International classification of diseases* (ICD-11) is in accepted form at the time of writing but awaits official status in most countries. It aims to be conceptually very close to the DSM-5 formulations but is written in a different way. It seeks to describe a pattern to be recognized, rather than a set of rules by which to add up signs and symptoms. It follows the DSM-5 in removing some of the features of previous formulations that have proved not to be as specific as once thought—such as pragmatic alterations of language and descriptions of altered patterns of play. Rather, it focuses more on whether children follow or impose strict rules when they play—a behaviour that can be perceived in any culture. Furthermore, it has agreed with DSM-5 in collapsing previous subdivisions of the spectrum (Asperger's, pervasive developmental disorder, disintegrative disorder) into an overall category of 'autism spectrum disorder'.

For both ICD-11 and DSM-5, the wordings can be misunderstood, and it is unwise for the diagnostician to rely totally on giving the descriptions to parents, teachers, and others who know the individual. The characteristic quality of behaviour in autism is best elicited by an experienced person directly observing it (Baird et al., 2011).

ASD can be seen either as an extreme of a continuum or a separate category. Lord and Jones (2012) argue that there may be added value in a category. As considered in Chapter 1, Section 1.2.4, both ideas have a place, for differing purposes.

4.1.2 Recognition

4.1.2.1 *Rating scales, interviews, and observations*

4.1.2.1.1 *Screening questionnaires*
Population screening is not advised for finding cases in the general population. Within at-risk populations, however, several rating scales are used, often in triage or for clarifying clinical needs. Diagnostic assessment is rather lengthy, so standardized informant ratings are often used in practice to select cases for lengthy evaluation by interview and/or observation. Rating scales are also helpful as checklists to ensure coverage of a range of potential problems. They are not, however, good ways of ruling autism either in or out. Appropriate use is reviewed by Volkmar et al. (2014) for the US context, and by NICE (National Institute for Health and Care Excellence) (2011, 2017) for the UK.

> The *Autism Behavior Checklist* (ABC) (Volkmar et al., 1988) is a wide-ranging set of 57 items and several subscales to be rated by people who know the child well.

The *Autism Screening Questionnaire* (ASQ) (Berument et al., 1999) was developed to have good discriminative validity with respect to the separation of ASD from non-ASD diagnoses at all IQ levels. It contains 40 items, with the presence of 15 performing best as a cut-off.

The *Modified Checklist for Autism in Toddlers* (M-CHAT) (Robins et al., 2001) was developed as a set of 23 items to be rated by parents, with an emphasis on detecting the features of high-functioning autism (Asperger syndrome).

The *Autism Spectrum Quotient* (AQ-Child) (Auyeung et al., 2008) was developed to detect the presence of Asperger features in children aged 4–11 years without neurological syndromes or learning disorder. It contains 50 items of parent report, scoring 0–150 with a cut-off at 76.

A review of parent-completed rating scales by Norris and Lecavalier (2010) found inadequate psychometrics of all the then available scales. The use of such measures for clinical purposes such as diagnosis is not yet advised. There are problems even with the common practice of reserving a full assessment for those with a score above a cut-off. If a screen has false negatives, it would prevent further assessment. More detailed assessment is usually required.

The spectrum of autism, in the recently developed understanding of it as a frequently occurring condition, is compatible with good general intelligence and social independence. 'High-functioning' individuals deserve both recognition and distinction from those who are also disabled or show intellectual deficit (ID). People in the spectrum, as now defined, can show ordinary language skills, social skills (including good eye contact), and affectionate contact with family members. The presence of good abilities in any one of these domains should not be a bar to referral to a team with specialist skills in the assessment of ASD.

4.1.2.1.2 *Diagnostic interviews*

Experienced clinicians will ask people with close knowledge of the person being assessed to recall their development over time. These accounts will then be used to judge the presence of the core features and associated problems. Several standardized measures have been developed to achieve reliability between different raters and to allow the use of less expert professionals in assessment.

Broad-spectrum interview methods such as the Child and Adolescent Psychiatric Assessment (CAPA) and the Kiddie Schedule for Affective Disorders and Schizophrenia (K-SADS) are cited in 'Informant interview', Chapter 3, Section 3.2. They include more information about emotional and behavioural problems than do specialized ASD measures, but less on the core problems of ASD. On their own, they are not enough for recognition of ASD. The combination of them with the specific ASD measures becomes lengthy and therefore expensive. Repeated appointments for long assessments are often perceived as impractical by families and schools in pressing need of respite. Pragmatic decisions are needed for priorities in assessment.

The autism-specific measures commonly used in UK practice are:

- The *Autism Diagnostic Interview* (ADI) (Le Couteur et al., 1989; Rutter et al., 2003)
- The *Diagnostic Interview for Social and Communication Disorders* (DISCO) (Wing et al., 2002)
- The *Asperger Syndrome Diagnostic Interview* (ASDI) (Gillberg et al., 2001)
- The *Developmental, Dimensional and Diagnostic Interview* (3di) (Skuse et al., 2004)

None is enough for a comprehensive assessment; all will miss some cases and identify some falsely. Several of these exist in both investigator-based and electronic formats. The 3di has a computer-based ASD interview for parents.

4.1.2.1.3 *Diagnostic observation*

Ideally, an assessment would draw heavily on the direct examination of the young person by a very experienced professional. The disadvantage is the scarcity of such professionals, which is responsible for long waits for full assessment. The subtlety and diversity of children's problems, and their fluctuation with time and context, has made it difficult to establish definitive tests. The best current effort is the *Autism Diagnostic Observational Schedule* (ADOS) (Lord et al., 2000). This provides different levels of assessment for young people at different ages and different levels of intellectual ability. The schedule allows the recording of the performance of young people in a range of interactive situations, including those described in Chapter 2, Section 2.5 for social understanding.

4.1.2.1.4 *Information to be sought in clinical assessment*

The combination of ADOS and ADI is often regarded as a 'gold standard' and is widely used in the UK. Even this, however, needs to be combined with an experienced clinician's evaluation (NICE, 2011). The core features to be assessed are described here, following the headings of Box 4.1 and adding considerations of the difficulties that arise from the coexisting presence of other conditions with overlapping symptoms.

Little emotional reciprocity in social relationships

There is typically a marked delay in the development of social connectedness: a lack of response to others making social overtures, or, later, of conversation in a to-and-fro style, or of sharing emotions. It may involve highly idiosyncratic styles of response.

There can be reasons for social unresponsiveness other than ASD, such as global developmental delay or deficits in hearing or facial perception, so it is important to make sure that the child has the physical capacity for understanding and response, and that their lack of complex interaction is out of keeping with developmental level. Furthermore, the key idea in autism is an inability rather than an emotionally determined withdrawal. ASD should not be confused with a generally inhibited style—and need not be if one seeks the other features of autistic interaction.

Selective mutism also needs to be distinguished from the uncommunicativeness of ASD. It also involves a marked lack of social communication—but usually not to everyone. Affected children talk little, or not at all, in complex situations involving challenge (e.g. the classroom or social groups), but typically may chatter spontaneously at home. They may also be very shy or nervous about talking with other people present. It is common for there to be an underlying difficulty with language (e.g. in situations requiring a language to which they are not native) or a coexisting language disorder.

Impairments in non-verbal communication
Eye contact may be directed away from other people rather than towards them; faces may be expressionless; gestures may not be used to communicate or be used in a way that does not square with what is being said. The usual coordination of body language, gesture, and communication may be lacking. This represents an important distinction from most disorders of communication. Expressive language disorder, for example, is accompanied by normal or even enhanced communication through gesture.

Difficulties in developing and understanding relationships
It is usually difficult for young people in the spectrum to make relationships with other people. Put baldly, it may seem to stigmatize children who are culturally distant from the other people around or have little experience with them. The lack of social under-standing is the key point (see Chapter 2, Section 2.6). In the extreme, there may be no friends or any interest in making them, or no imaginative play that involves them. In relatively mature and communicative young people, only a subtle lack of understanding may be identifiable. However, the absence or oddity of interest in others can be striking. The interest in others can be eccentric and obsessive; for instance, in the day of the week people were born or the texture of their hair.

Stereotyped repetitiveness of speech and movement
Stereotyped or repetitive motor movements, use of objects, or speech are frequent but not universal in ASD. At the extreme, these may involve endless flapping of arms or body rocking, especially in those who also show a global developmental delay. They can also be much more subtle. Play activities may show them. Toys are lined up mechanic-ally or sorted carefully by physical appearance, rather than being spontaneously used symbolically. Speech may be repeating exactly what has been said to them, but without any real intent to communicate ('echolalia').

'Insistence on sameness' has been a persistent part of the definition of autistic behaviours for many years. Young people with autism can be very distressed by change and resolute in escaping from it. The change needed to provoke an adverse reaction can be slight and hard to detect. Inflexibility can be a main cause of disability. Transitions between places and activities can be very hard to tolerate and need to be spelled out to young people in advance so that they become predictable and controllable.

Ritualistic behaviours can come about for various reasons, not all of them autistic (see 'Qualitative differences in motor development' in Chapter 2, Section 2.2.2). The lack of social understanding can present in this way as well. Greeting new people can make use of repetitive, unusual, and inappropriate questions: 'Have you an umbrella?' 'What bus did you come on?'

Autistic stereotypies need to be distinguished from the motor restlessness typical of attention deficit hyperactivity disorder (ADHD). Sometimes this is not obvious. A driven overactivity may be the result of repetitive but complex sequences. One boy had a set pattern in the classroom of standing, sitting, stretching, standing, moving to the window, tapping, and returning. This made him appear very restless, but it was a stereotyped overactivity, and lacked the disorganized quality of ADHD. (It had still led to a mistaken diagnosis of ADHD, until a failure of stimulant drug treatment resulted in prolonged observation in the classroom).

Rigid adherence to routines
Insistence on exact ways of doing things can be restricting and can exasperate other people. Strategies to acquire sameness and avoid change include seeking a high level of control over the environment. Headstrongness, however, is also characteristic of oppositional-defiant disorders, and obsessional children are often highly controlling. Headstrong insistence by itself does not mark the autism spectrum. The difference is in the nature of the challenge and the reaction to it: impatience and frustration in the case of oppositional disorders, rather than the tension, panic, and extreme avoidance of ASD.

Very restricted, overfocused interests
Highly restricted, fixated interests need to be excessive in intensity or focus if they are to be part of the recognition of ASD. At the extreme, they involve odd objects or interests not normally to be expected at all. Milder forms overlap with the everyday. Some people in the spectrum of autism develop an encyclopaedic knowledge of a small topic—such as railway timetables. Such abilities can be functional, as (in this example) when people are employed to give rail information to travellers. Even very overspecialized interests can be advantageous in the specialized niches existing in today's workplaces—for instance, in information technology.

Restrictive and fixated interests should not be confused with special interests—favourite toys, collections, imaginary friends, intense fascinations (e.g. with dinosaurs), and the like, which are not bizarre and can persist into later childhood and adolescence in many, not necessarily immature, young people. The distinguishing feature of ASD is the extent to which special interests are pursued to excess and in solitude. Preoccupations become a problem only if they crowd out more appropriate interests. In one instance, a teenager showed precocious brilliance in the languages of classical antiquity but was unable even to gain entrance into university education because of his insistence on writing about nothing except the works of one obscure Silver Latin author. (A more tolerant university might have been more accommodating.)

Oversensitivity or under-reactiveness to sensory input
Hypersensitivity and hyposensitivity to sensory changes can both occur. Oversensitivity (to pain, loud noise, bright light, and possibly to internal signals such as anxiety) has

been linked to high levels of distress and possibly to anxiety and avoidant states (South & Rodgers, 2017).

Sensory processing can be either overintense or insufficiently apprehended. All sensory modalities can be affected: sounds, sights, things, smells, tastes, or the feel of things. Indifference to pain, visual fascinations, and insistent smelling are all possible. Some of the commonest features relate to things heard—'Has trouble functioning if there is a lot of noise around or the radio is on', 'Responds badly to loud unexpected noises', and 'Covers ears with hands to protect them in the presence of noise' are all frequent descriptions, as is 'Ear plugs help.' Alternatively, they may not respond when their name is called, even though they can apparently hear well. In vision, the concerns may be that bright lights bother them, or they may cover their eyes or squint as if to protect them. Some are very attracted to moving objects and may watch them closely with peripheral vision. They may react very negatively to being touched and may have very strong preferences in clothing. Alternatively, they may seek to touch other people a great deal, for the sake of the sensation. In taste and smell, too, they may limit themselves to particular food textures or tastes or temperatures. Individuals may be avoided because of the smell of their sweat or their perfume; toileting can be difficult because of the smell of urine or faeces.

The sheer quantity of sensory information may also become very aversive and lead to 'meltdowns'—states of extreme panic. Meltdowns will usually require a quiet period with very little sensory stimulation of any kind

Apart from overall sensitivity, there can be qualitative perceptual changes. Some report that central vision is blurred but peripheral vision is experienced as quite sharp, or the opposite. Images may fragment, and it may feel much better to concentrate on detail rather than a whole object. Poor depth perception, and consequent problems with throwing and catching, can appear as clumsiness.

Sensory changes can be idiosyncratic and confusing. The same child can be both hypersensitive to ambient noise and unresponsive to pain. The changes can dominate life. Creating an autism-friendly environment often means managing these extreme reactions by appreciating and eliminating the individual sources of distress. Sound-absorbing walls and halogen lighting can help.

Less extreme patterns of reduced or increased reactiveness can also be seen in obsessive-compulsive disorder, schizophrenia, emotional dysregulation, and intellectual deficit.

4.1.3 Difficulties in current diagnoses and variant types

Several aspects of the international definitions raise diagnostic challenges for the clinician.

4.1.3.1 *Changes of definition over time*

Kanner's nuclear definition of autism was quite soon expanded as clinicians and educators became familiar with the idea. An influential paper by Wing and Gould

(1979) followed up a population survey with a recognition of the wider range of similar problems. In further work, different profiles of disturbance were described, including Asperger syndrome, pervasive developmental disorder, and pervasive refusal syndrome. Their description excluded 'full autism' and the criteria for autism itself were refined. Differentiation became problematic and it was hard to communicate satisfactorily. The DSM-5 and draft ICD-11 criteria therefore unified them into one 'autism spectrum disorder', comprising social communication and restricted/repetitive dimensions, with further distinctions based on levels of intellect and language. The criteria themselves have shifted over time—for instance, with less emphasis on specific types of language impairment. The frequencies of diagnosis have shifted correspondingly (see Section 4.1.6).

4.1.3.2 *Subthreshold cases*

Some of the core features can occur on their own. They can still be severe, and in a mixed presentation they are often referred to as 'autistic features'. It will be more precise to use phrases such as 'social communication problems' or 'features of repetitive, restrictive activity'.

Some individuals show only the features of one of the component dimensions. One component on its own—*repetitive behaviours*—can be captured, in part, by 'stereotypic movement disorder'. Another key component—*social communication changes*—can also exist alone, and DSM-5 has created a separate disorder, within a different overarching group of communication disorders, of 'social (pragmatic) communication disorder' (SCD). It expects that SCD problems are 'not attributable to low abilities in the domains of word structure and grammar'. ICD-11 uses 'pragmatic language disorder' (PLD) in the same way as SCD. PLD is described as a dimension of language disorder and could encourage an overspecialized approach.

It is not yet clear whether the new definitions of communication problems will capture all the communication deficits previously contained within 'autism spectrum'. ASD and SCD will have so much in common in their descriptions of social communication that it will probably be difficult to differentiate them:

- 'Deficits in social-emotional reciprocity' (ASD) is likely to include 'deficits in using communication for social purposes' (SCD).
- 'Failure of normal back-and-forth conversation' (ASD) reads as potentially similar to 'impairment in the ability to change communication to match context or the needs of the listener' (SCD).
- 'Deficits in nonverbal communicative behaviours used for social interaction' (ASD) will surely overlap with 'knowing how to use verbal and nonverbal signals to regulate interaction' (SCD).

Other individuals miss a diagnosis because they do not show quite enough of the required criteria. There is a spectrum of severity, as well as of types of presentation. DSM-5 expects some counting of criteria (e.g. two or more of the problem behaviours included as repetitive-restrictive). This kind of algorithmic approach is helpful for research, where replicability is a key requirement and the cut-off for the disorder needs to be simply expressed for researchers without clinical qualifications. For clinical practice, however, where individuals need to be correctly identified, it is better to think of identifying a pattern rather than adding up criteria. In any case, the diagnostician should go on to specify the range of functions on which the individual is encountering difficulties. These will be key to assessing the need for services and the response to interventions. It is likely that they will also be the route to linking changes of behaviour with neurobiological findings.

The result of specialist assessment can be that the individual is 'showing some autistic features but not the full pattern of ASD'. This should act as a call for a fuller pattern of recommendations about the local services that are best able to meet the associated needs.

4.1.3.2.1 *Developmental changes over time*

The profile of core features fluctuates over time (see Section 4.1.4). Some less severe cases may therefore go in and out of a diagnosis if criteria are applied pedantically and algorithmically. This is undesirable for care decisions, so the diagnostic assessment should include a historical perspective on how the symptoms and signs have varied over the years. Repeated specialist assessments may well be needed to review the suitability and effect of interventions.

4.1.3.2.2 *Requirement for impact*

There is an expectation in DSM-5 that the core features should not only be present but should be interfering with social function and creating a need for services. This is one way of differentiating disorder from diversity. This requirement is controversial, both for research and for practice. Reduced or inappropriate social functioning is part of the definition of the social communication dimension, creating ambiguity about what is meant by the requirement of 'poor social function'. This can be clarified by maintaining the distinction between 'dysfunction' and 'disability' (see Chapter 1, Section 1.2.8).

Some people with marked levels of the core symptoms and signs have nevertheless managed to function in age-appropriate ways in school, at home, and in work. A well-compensated person can still benefit from being regarded as autistic even though they are not disabled. A newer approach correspondingly refers to diversity rather than disorder as a key concept.

A criterion requiring impact imports uncertainty because 'disability' is not only a function of the individual but of society. Researchers seeking the genetic basis of autistic features are not likely to find them if they are muddled with the competence of people responsible for their child's upbringing. Clinicians are advised to think in terms of needs for support, and to keep that important matter separate from the clinical profile in their formulations.

Adaptation is a two-way process. It is not just a matter of the individual conforming to social rules; it is also a matter of society, families, and schools adapting their rules to the individual. *Severity* can be judged by the amount of support required.

4.1.3.2.3 Quality of information is sometimes doubtful

The diagnostic criteria are required to be present across different situations. Accordingly, the persons making the diagnosis may have to rely on imperfect accounts from people who know the child but not the condition. When in doubt, clinicians should include sources of uncertainty in their diagnostic formulations, together with the information that will need to be sought later in development. Researchers should specify the sources of uncertainty for the benefit of later meta-analyses.

4.1.3.2.4 Varying purposes of diagnosis

A diagnosis must do a lot of work in the real world. It has its own impact, independent of the individual's needs, on service provision. It may be a requirement for extra help in education or special classes. It may be a disqualifier for services that say 'we don't take autistics'—though such services are not so commonly encountered these days as they once were.

The making of a diagnosis is also an important step in a person's life (see 'Encounters with diagnosis', Chapter 10, Section 10.13). It means different things to different people, but is nearly always important for self-image and self-esteem. Psychoeducation and counselling should always follow a diagnostic assessment, whatever the decision.

4.1.3.3 Course of specialist assessment

A specialist service will begin by reviewing the referral information. Reports from family doctors and teachers will probably have much information about the history so far, the presence of language/communication problems, and the family. Routine screening tests should have identified significant early-onset medical conditions. Community health should have information about medical conditions, hearing and vision, and motor development.

Screening questionnaires (see Section 4.1.2.1.1) will be asked for if they have not been made available already. The main purpose is to develop understanding of the full range of mental health and developmental problems, which may accompany or mimic core autistic features. Core features should be assessed as described earlier. Standardized tests are not good enough in themselves for a definitive diagnosis or exclusion. The full psychiatric assessment should be accompanied by cognitive and neurological assessment, planned individually.

4.1.3.3.1 Cognitive assessment

When there is the clinical or educational suspicion of intellectual disability (ID), or a very uneven cognitive profile, standardized tests of intellect are needed (see 'Intellectual deficit', Chapter 5, Section 5.2.4.1). IQ measures need to be supplemented with an assessment of adaptive functioning, such as the Adaptive Behavior Assessment System (ABAS-3) (Harrison & Oakland, 2015) or the Vineland-3 (Sparrow et al., 2016).

4.1.3.3.2 Neurological assessment

Investigations for underlying neurological problems or genetic diseases should be carried out on an individually planned basis, not as part of a generally applicable protocol. All cases should have the benefit of enquiry about potential risk factors. A general physical examination should seek evidence of strongly associated disorders (NICE, 2011), namely:

- skin stigmata of inherited disease, including the depigmented changes of neuro-fibromatosis or tuberous sclerosis which can be detected with a Wood's (ultra-violet) lamp;
- signs of injury, for example from self-harm or maltreatment by others;
- congenital anomalies and dysmorphic features including macrocephaly or microcephaly;
- abnormalities of hearing and vision—unless these have been excluded already.

Routine genetic screening should follow the advice of the local genetics service. Fragile-X should be tested for. Evidence of specific dysmorphic features, congenital anomalies, and/or evidence of a ID will be indications for a genetic workup.

The case for extensive genetic examination as routine may well become stronger as more benefits of polygenic profiling are appreciated, and molecular tests become cheaper.

4.1.3.4 *Variant types of ASD*

Some variant types are considered to fall within the autistic spectrum. Key distinctions to make are the presence or absence of global developmental delay, the presence or absence of language delay, and the age of first appearance.

4.1.3.4.1 *Pathological demand avoidance (PDA)*

In some children, the dominating presentation is one of extreme and rigid non-compliance with everyday demands and extreme mood variability. Such inter-action styles can be very hard indeed for parents or other caregivers. They are often accompanied by other features of the autism spectrum, but sometimes without the full picture.

Newson et al. (2003) published an account of 30 children with such problems. They described it as a syndrome of 'pathological demand avoidance', and the term has proved very influential in some countries, though it has not been included in international diagnostic schemes. The children they described had much in common. In the first year, they were passive infants, and in later childhood, showed superficial sociability. They went on to resist and avoid ordinary demands of life, the strategies of avoidance being essentially forms of social manipulation. Activity always had to be on the child's terms. They needed to be very much in control, with an obsessional rigidity, and became distressed or aggressive if they failed to be in charge. They were often good at mimicry and pretend play, but idiosyncratic in games and use of language. Although these features were described as a syndrome distinct from the autism spectrum, most clinicians since have been more impressed by the similarities to ASD than the differences. Overcontrol can be an autistic type of preservation of sameness, combined with high anxiety and a lack of appreciation of other people's perspectives.

There has not been much research on PDA, but what there is has failed to show syndromic coherence or any distinction from ASD at a biological level, Nevertheless, while it is not correct to regard it as a distinct diagnosis, the pattern described has resonated with many families—especially the emphasis on controlling rigidity and social superficiality. It is usually wise and humane to work with parents' concerns and include a focus on those aspects that most concern them. There is little to be gained from arguments about terminology that risk leaving parents feeling that their concerns are unrecognized. Services that refuse treatment because the child does not meet all the ASD criteria or 'has PDA' should re-examine their priorities.

The major split in understanding relates to the implications for therapy. The therapeutic approach often recommended from the model of autism is the detailed assessment of the profile of problems and a joint plan for each of the major problems involved. This might, for instance, entail reducing the intensity of anxiety about losing control through medication or environmental modification, followed by very gradual introduction of challenges, with rewards for steps towards mastery. For many proponents of PDA, on the other hand, the core intervention is the withdrawal of challenges. Such an approach does however risk a progressive restriction of life. Sometimes it is possible to modify challenging behaviours that are motivated by escape from demands by providing an alternative way for the child to signal their need for escape (e.g. by showing a red card), allowing that escape, but introducing rewards for prolonging tolerance.

4.1.3.4.2 *Asperger syndrome*

The term 'Asperger syndrome' is seldom used nowadays and 'high-functioning autism' is preferred. Lorna Wing (1981) popularized the term to refer to an account by Johann ('Hans') Asperger (1944) which described young people who combined features of autism with typical language development and normal intelligence. Recent historical research, however, has found out so much about Asperger's relationship with National Socialism (Czech, 2018) and its programme of murder that it seems inappropriate to honour him with an eponym.

There are no behaviour changes that are not seen in other forms of ASD. Uneven development of cognitive abilities is not rare in typical ASD. Exceptional performance in memory, art, visuospatial ability, mathematics, calendar or numerical calculation, or music can coexist with intellectual deficit, and is then often called a 'savant' skill (Howlin et al., 2009). Savant skills are more frequent in autistic people than in other conditions, but are also described in brain damage, epilepsy, and in Prader–Willi, Smith–Magenis, and Williams syndromes (Treffert, 2009). Around half of people with savant abilities are in the spectrum of autism.

4.1.3.4.3 *Other disorders*

Pervasive developmental disorder was a term to describe cases in which autistic features were present but did not amount to a classic picture of autism as then defined. The concept of ASD has made it unnecessary.

Childhood disintegrative disorder (Hellers syndrome) referred to progressive loss of mental function in early life. When this process included autistic features, as it often did, it would be defined nowadays as 'regressive autism' (see Section 4.1.4.1). When it did not, but was characterized by other behavioural and cognitive changes, it would have raised the possibility of dementia, which is considered in 'Chromosomal and single gene disorders' in Chapter 7, Section 7.3.

Dementias do not cause only autistic features, but core autistic features can be part of them. In relatively late-onset diseases, such as Sanfilippo syndrome, this may mean that social communication problems are appearing for the first time after several years of typical development. The disease should be the primary diagnosis, but when, as is often the case, neurological investigation does not find an underlying disease, then childhood disintegrative disorder is still a suitable term.

4.1.4   Course over time

The course over time is variable. Typically, the signs are present by the end of the second year, and it is at about this time that most cases should be detected. Young autistic children may show little or no initiation of social action, no sharing of emotions, and no imitation of others. Language may be absent, or restricted to the immediate and concrete. The absence of joint attention is characteristic. Sometimes no abnormality is detected until after the age of 3 years. Maybe parents do not detect the signs; maybe the signs do not appear until more social expectations arise; maybe the effects of a later-onset brain disorder or disease have not yet kicked in.

During later childhood, repetitive behaviours may sometimes reduce. Restricted interests, however, tend to become even more restricted. Depth of close and specialized study can result in some people becoming extremely knowledgeable and skilled. Social interactions can be aloof and uninterested, or present but passively following others, or 'active but odd'.

During what should usually be school years, the course is strongly influenced by language development and IQ. If there is no useful language by the age of five, or there are signs of global developmental delay, then the prognosis is usually of continuing disability, but with a good deal of variability even in the core symptoms. Access to education and physical healthcare is often limited. Mortality is raised, especially when epilepsy has set in.

For the most able young people, there is even more variability. Usually, the autistic features subside somewhat but are still noticeable. Transitions (e.g. school changes, movement or reconstitution of families) can be very challenging. Adolescence can bring the onset of epilepsy. Mental health problems may appear, either from linked neurodevelopmental problems such as ADHD, or from all the disadvantages attendant upon being socially different from the norm. Death rates are still higher than in the non-autistic, even in those who were functioning reasonably well at the age of 5 years. In this high-functioning group, the major cause of death is suicide. (See also 'Encounters with illness and danger', Chapter 10, Section 10.3, for later complications.)

In a minority, perhaps 5–25%, the outcome for social function is very good and they develop increased interest in other people. Compensation happens, and social understanding benefits as some people come to calculate and learn the skills of interaction that come intuitively to most of their peers.

Vocabulary and grammar may be pretty much like anyone else's by the time they reach adolescence. Some, however, even of these high-functioning people, will still show unusual language that is stilted, or overliteral, or unresponsive to buried meanings and metaphors. The appropriate use of social language can also develop. Most are restricted but continue to adapt and compensate. There may be a high cost to pay in the effort to calculate and work out consciously what most people achieve rapidly and by intuition.

In adult life, cognition usually continues to show a diversity of strengths and weaknesses. Special cognitive abilities may have appeared. Strong attention to detail and excellent analytical powers can be advantages to set off against any problems in executive function or in missing the big picture. A meta-analysis, comparing adults with ASD and typically developing controls matched for age and IQ, is reported by Velikonja et al. (2019). It showed the greatest persisting impairments to be in social cognition: theory of mind, emotion perception, and processing. There were also problems outside the realm of social understanding: slower processing speed and poorer verbal learning and memory. No single cognitive domain was uniquely affected in ASD adults, and most of the impairments were similar in kind to those seen in schizophrenia. The authors suggested that it would therefore be worth testing cognitive enhancement techniques that have been used in other types of adult psychopathology.

The transition into adult life brings encounters with situations that create risks for other mental health problems. Many are not unique to autism. Independence from family is often difficult to achieve. Further education is often not available, though access is improving in many countries. Those who need continuing support still find it very hard to access it. Adult, intimate, and erotic relationships are increasingly challenging. Sensory hypersensitivity can make many environments intolerable. The confusing demands of workplace roles combine with stigma and prejudice to make steady paid work unavailable to most. On the other hand, the increase of jobs in information technology has motivated some employers to create more autism-friendly work environments for them. A wide range of difficulties at work is described in Chapter 10, Section 10.11.

4.1.4.1 *Regressive autism*

The clinical course is not always one of very early onset and persistence. Sometimes there is worsening, or onset after a period of ordinary development. 'Regression' occurs in several ways, differentiated by the age being considered.

In the first two or three years of life, the onset of autistic features may be after an apparently normal development. There may have been useful words and social interest, but these are lost. The onset can be gradual or sudden. A sudden onset can be accompanied by irritability. Nearly all such cases will go on to autism of the usual type. The clinical importance is in creating a false impression that there has been a different cause. A notorious example is a fraudulent claim that a triple vaccine (against measles, mumps, and rubella: MMR) caused autism. The link to MMR vaccination was in fact coincidental (see 'Infections' in Chapter 7, Section 7.6)

After school entry, fluctuations in severity are quite common but do not imply a new disease. There can indeed be regression in the sense that skills are lost. Skill loss can be at the time of onset of epilepsy, but not always—there does not seem to be a consistent relationship. The reasons remain obscure. A late onset of diagnosable ASD (after about the age of 3 years) is rare. The clinical importance is to raise the possibility of a dementing illness (see 'Single-gene disorders with progressive course', Chapter 7, Section 7.4.3).

4.1.5 Coexistent problems

The spectrum of autism overlaps with other spectra of dysfunction. When this is because the defining behaviours overlap, there is an issue of differential diagnosis, considered in Section 4.1.2. When this is because of multiple morbidity, the issues are for how to recognize and manage the other disorders in the presence of ASD.

4.1.5.1 *ADHD in ASD*

Chapter 3 on ADHD includes the issues of coexistence with ASD and separation from it. Recognizing the presence of ADHD in the presence of autism can be complicated by the effects of autism itself, which can make children appear to be inattentive because their attention is overfocused on things of special interest. Some of the flags to the simultaneous presence of ADHD should be:

- Lack of attention to details and making careless errors—which is very unlike the precision of autistic people (but is not always present in coexistent ADHD/ASD).
- Both ASD and ADHD can lead to missing the requirements of tasks and underperforming accordingly. However, the reasons are different—excessive focus in ASD, distractibility and lack of focus in ADHD.
- Clear difficulties in sustained attention are likely to be part of ADHD, especially in activities that are not part of a restricted interest.
- Struggling to engage in difficult tasks is typical of ADHD, but seldom any kind of problem for uncomplicated ASD.
- Excessive losing of things and forgetfulness in daily activities are very unlike the usual dependence on routine of people with ASD alone.
- Excessive undirected noisiness is another ADHD feature that differs from the loud insistence on specific arrangements that characterizes some ASD people.

Management of ADHD is not different because of the co-occurrence of ASD, but may be more difficult. Stimulant medication has similar positive effects, but they may be smaller and more likely to be accompanied by adverse effects.

4.1.5.2 *ID in ASD*

On average, the rate of intellectual disability (ID) in autism used to be estimated at around 70%, with only 30% of diagnosed individuals scoring in the normal range of intellectual functioning. According to Fombonne (2002), 30% scored in the mild to moderate range of ID, and 40% in the severe to profound range. The reported rate of ID in ASD, however, is falling in proportion to the increased tendency to diagnose ASD in people of average or superior intellect. This in turn is changing the perception of ASD and the needs for services of those with the condition.

Even now, a large minority of people with diagnosed ASD show some degree of ID. This is probably not an inherent part of the genetic loading for ASD. Polygenic risk scores for ASD also predict *high* scores on several cognitive tests in the general population (Clarke et al., 2016). This contrasts with the high rates of observed ID. The idea of a genetic link to superior performance has come from general population data, leaving the possibility open that a harmful influence on cognitive ability might derive from an effect of the full 'disease state' of autism.

Some medical disorders causing ID might be causally related to autism. Some are common enough to have been reported in surveys: tuberous sclerosis and Fragile X. Other rare medical conditions—such as congenital rubella, phenylketonuria, or neurofibromatosis—are sometimes reported. Overall, in 32 epidemiological surveys reviewed by Fombonne in 2002, 6.4% of subjects had an associated medical disorder of potential aetiological significance (see Chapter 6).

4.1.5.3 *Behaviour problems in autism*

Difficult-to-manage problems in typically developing children are very frequent and often linked to adversity in caregivers and temperamental differences in children. *Oppositional-defiant disorder* (ODD) is defined by a persistent pattern of irritable mood, non-compliant and defiant behaviour, and spitefulness to others. *Conduct disorder* (CD) may well include all these, but goes further to include behaviours that violate the basic rights of other people—aggression to people and animals, destruction of other people's property, truancy, stealing, and lying,

People with ASD are not immune to ODD and CD, but such problems in them are more characteristically part of a rather different pattern of *challenging behaviour* (CHB). CHB is not a recognized psychiatric syndrome and does not figure in the DSM-5. Nevertheless, it is distinctive in its pattern, associations, and therapeutic approaches (McClintock et al., 2003). Intense rages, severe aggression to others and oneself, and profound non-compliance are the key aspects. Stealing and lying, by contrast, are not typical. Unlike ODD and CD, CHB is not associated with poverty, family size, or the presence of ODD and CD in other family members. It is very much a part not only of ASD but also of chronic brain problems including ID and epilepsy (see Chapter 5, Section 5.2.4.4). Key associations for the individual are with low adaptive function, impaired communication, and physical conditions causing pain. Pain may well not be described clearly by people with communication problems and requires careful physical assessment. Other associations are with the caregiving environment rather than qualities of the person (see Chapter 5, Section 5.2.4.4). Management usually needs an individual approach rather than the well worked-out schemes of group 'parent training' that are used for CD and ODD in typically developing children and young people. Communication enhancement, avoiding precipitants, and behavioural analysis are more fruitful (see Chapter 8, Section 8.11). CHB remains a major risk for the use of psychopharmacology, family breakdown, and substitute care.

4.1.5.4 *Anxiety in autism*

Anxiety is not usually thought of as a neurodevelopmental disorder, but it has features in common and is often the most distressing aspect of ASD. High anxiety is very common in autistic people, especially the more able and the older, of whom about half will show clinically significant levels. The commonest types are simple phobia, followed by social phobia and separation anxiety disorder. Detailed empirical reviews are provided by Simonoff et al. (2008) and White et al. (2009).

In many respects, the phenomenology resembles anxiety in children and adolescents who are otherwise developing typically (Farrugia & Hudson, 2006). Subjective anxiety, negative automatic thoughts, behavioural problems, and level of life interference are all similar to those with anxiety disorders only. High physiological arousal, assessed from somatic symptoms, is high in autistic young people, as in those with anxiety disorder. Physiological changes associated with high chronic anxiety, such as reduced heart rate variability and enhanced skin sweating, are associated with anxiety in the autistic as in ordinary controls. So far as one can tell from existing research, which is limited, anxiety symptoms do not relate to supposedly fundamental core aspects of autism such as impaired central coherence. Sensory hypersensitivity, however, might indeed contribute.

There are a few specific characteristics of anxiety in autism, which may reflect pathoplastic factors rather than fundamental differences. Teacher ratings of anxiety are often higher than those made by parents, perhaps indicating that the school environment is particularly stressful for autistic people. Furthermore, autistic people's expression of anxiety may be particularly likely to involve CHB—and possibly problems in reality testing and abnormal 'psychotic' beliefs. Eliciting anxiety symptoms may be harder in the presence of communication problems.

In one study (Kleberg et al., 2017), looking away from other people's eyes (gaze avoidance) took a different form in autism and in social anxiety. They studied eye movements in 25 adolescents. High autistic traits were associated with delayed orientating *to* the eyes when presented together with distractors. By contrast, high social anxiety was associated with faster orientating *away* from the eyes, even when controlling for autistic traits.

Anxiety about gender roles is also rather characteristic. Epidemiological surveys have suggested high rates of autistic features in people with gender dysphoria (e.g. Skagerberg et al., 2015) and of gender dysphoria in ASD (e.g. Van Der Miesen et al., 2016). The reasons for an association are not known. Long experience of being 'othered' can give rise to doubts about one's identity. This uncertainty is even more marked in ASD than in related conditions. It could overflow into insecurity about gender identity specifically.

There are also a few apparent expressions of anxiety seldom seen outside autism: social discomfort that is *not* associated with a fear of negative evaluation, and compulsive behaviour that does *not* seem motivated by distress relief—but these perhaps reflect behaviours that are not anxiety-based, and need to be distinguished diagnostically (e.g. as rituals or lack of social reward mechanisms). Some autistic people present highly unusual phobias.

It is possible that subjective anxiety tends to be more aversive to autistic people than to others, and that this accounts for both the lengths to which they will go to avoid it and the extremity of behavioural changes when they cannot. That might imply greater neuroendocrine, autonomic, and central nervous system changes. However, these changes have not been demonstrated clearly in the small number of studies examining the specificity of autistic anxiety. Intolerance of anxiety could be related to intolerance of other states such as loud noise (see above, 4.1.2.1.4 "*Oversensitivity or underreactiveness to sensory input*"). In spite of these possibly specific features, the similarities to anxiety in typically developing people suggest that it is a mistake to regard anxiety symptoms, when they occur, only as an expression of core autism. It is tempting to do so, for described features of both have a lot in common. Compulsive checking, social avoidance, and avoidance of specific situations have very often been seen as expected and core aspects of autism itself. However, they can often be successfully managed by the same approaches that work in more typically developing people (see Chapter 8).

Avoidance includes social withdrawal, which can be extreme. Some autistic children are egocentric and indifferent to socializing; others are driven away from other people by phobic fears. It can be difficult to distinguish between these forms of withdrawal from the social world. It can be complicated by overinvolvement from parents—a sort of pathological kindness. An extreme form of dependence on parents is common in Japan—'hikikomori'—and is not seen only in the autistic. Psychologists in Japan recognize 'amae'—a culture-based acceptance by society of overdependent behaviours (Doi, 1977). Avoidant behaviours can also include a reluctance to engage in any challenging activity (see Section 4.1.3.4.1). Avoidance of situations eliciting anxiety does have short-term benefits in reducing overall distress. Indeed, the absence of distress can lead other people, including professionals, to suppose that anxiety does not play a part in the pathogenesis of symptoms. Far from it. It becomes evident when the strategy of avoidance fails, an unpredictable challenge appears, and a sudden and extreme level of anxiety appears in a panic, or an outburst of aggression or self-harm. It may even be that previous avoidant strategies (for instance, in removing uncertainty and unpredictability) have left the individual unprepared to cope when challenges appear. Many autism-friendly institutions succeed in dispelling uncertainty with high levels of routine and careful warning of imminent change. This can be a key to useful education. However, the combination of this with a gradual encouragement to tolerate and master the feared and hated situations of ambiguity and uncertainty requires sensitivity and skill in the caregivers.

The association between anxiety and higher IQ gives credence to the notion that a good deal of the high levels of worry are secondary to growing appreciation of one's differences from the majority and apprehension about the effects of that difference. When many aspects of the world are incomprehensible, it is natural to feel anxious and to worry. One should, however, recognize that there are many causes of anxiety besides the subjective experience of the world for those with ASD. Phobias, separation anxiety, post-traumatic stress, and social anxiety can all occur independently, and all may need recognizing and treating in their own right. Obsessions and compulsions can all be hard to distinguish from autistic rituals, except that they are often not motivated by distress and anxiety relief, but by the opportunities they provide for exerting control on an unpredictable world.

4.1.5.5 *Eating disorders in ASD*

The symptoms of anorexia and weight loss are associated with ASD (Westwood & Tchanturia, 2017). They can be life-threatening. It is not possible to give a robustly researched rate for the association. The prevalence of anorexia nervosa in ASD is uncertain because of uncertainties about the phenotypes to recognize.

For some young women with ASD, restriction of food, overexercising, and purging take an alternative form. They are not always driven by body-image problems or a phobia of fatness (though they can be). More often, they represent a way of achieving control over overwhelming feelings of anxiety. Less frequently, deliberate weight loss arises from phobias or extreme faddiness about specific foods. Sensory changes towards textures or tastes can contribute. Resistance to change can impair engagement with therapists. Neurological and genetic overlaps between causative influences on eating disorders and ASD are also conceivable (Gillberg & Råstam, 1992).

Ritual overeating and bulimia can also be driven by similarly autistic changes in ways of thinking.

4.1.5.6 *Autonomic dysfunction in ASD*

Abnormalities in pupillary light reflex, resting heart rate, heart rate response to social cognitive tasks, respiratory rhythm, and skin conductance have been found in laboratory tests (e.g. Ming et al., 2005). All suggest autonomic dysfunction in ASD. An overactive sympathetic nervous system could create a false impression of anxiety or contribute, by feedback, to the level of anxiety experienced.

Postural lightheadedness, fainting, and rapid heart rate may all need to be addressed. It is conceivable, but not demonstrated, that cardiac changes could contribute to the high rate of unexplained sudden death.

4.1.5.7 *Subjective experience*

The inner world of people with ASD can be difficult for them to describe. They may not give emotional accounts of other people in terms of situation, cause, and explanation, but describe perceptually salient elements of experiences. They may therefore possess less coherent representations of their emotional experiences. Nevertheless, one should not share the public perception that autistic people are emotionless or interested only in themselves. (The word 'autism' may be unfortunate in contributing to this misapprehension.) Their ability to describe emotions is not grossly different from that in other people (Jaedicke et al., 1994).

Subjective experience is most clearly described by adults with high levels of function. Their accounts tend to be dominated by the sense of difference from other people, the unpleasant reactions of other people to them, the experience of diagnosis—or lack of it, and sensory overload.

The sense of difference and separation from other people is often acute. Some autistic people feel frustrated and saddened by their isolation from other people. This alienation is often expressed as puzzlement at the strangeness (and sometimes the danger) of typically developing people. Others find eye contact hateful and overwhelming. Yet others want to engage and make friends, but lack the confidence or the skills (such as understanding of small talk and other conventions of social life) to do so. Some do not feel a need to engage with other people, whilst many others avoid engagement because of previous experiences of rejection and bullying. Autobiographical accounts are available and eloquent (e.g. Sinclair, 1992), although readers should remember that autistic people are a diverse lot, and should not necessarily generalize one person's experience to the entire group.

4.1.5.8 *Communication and language in ASD*

Language problems, once regarded as a central and possibly *the* central feature of autism, have retreated in importance. Research has not indicated that features of language such as pronoun reversal and delayed echolalia are in fact specific to autistic language, by comparison with other forms of impairment of language. Nevertheless, it remains true that the presence of problems in communicative language is a strong association and powerful predictor of adverse cognitive and social outcomes.

Some autistic children find it easier to acquire sign language or picture communication than spoken language. Careful and skilled examination of hearing abilities remains important.

Language development in autistic children, as a group, is not only delayed but, in some respects, follows a different path. An example comes from a study using the Macarthur Scales of parents' observations of language development (Charman et al., 2003). The study found that some patterns of language acquisition differed from those in typical development. Notably, word production was in advance of word comprehension. In the gestural domain, actions on objects were in advance of gestures involving sharing reference and direct social contact. Other patterns of association were in line with those found in typical development: the pattern of acquisition of different word categories and types was broadly similar. Further, the associations between word comprehension, and word and gesture production, were like those seen in typical development.

Social anxiety and poor communication skills influence each other. Social anxiety is often very marked in people who are impaired in social communication. Impaired communication, whatever the cause, can lead to isolation from other children, and uncertainty about what they might think and do. Anxiety about social situations can be expected to result. Conversely, social anxiety can be expected to lead to children avoiding social situations, and therefore failing to learn competence in communication. A vicious circle can therefore develop in which poor social understanding is both the cause and the result of the emotional changes of anxiety (Eisenberger & Cole, 2012). Neither needs to be considered as primary to the other.

4.1.5.9 *Movement disorders in autism*

Many autistic children have poor motor coordination. In a study by de Jong et al. (2011), 74% showed problems in posture, tone, or fine coordination (compared with 52% of children referred with other psychiatric disorders). Standardized and objective measures are available (Wilson et al., 2018). They have indicated, for instance, that children with ASD have oddities of gait including wide step width, reduced step rate, and marked variability in step length. These findings could be indicators of altered cerebellar and fronto-striatal/basal ganglia functions. The specificity to ASD is not firmly established.

For the most part, the motor problems in ASD are similar to those in developmental coordination disorder (DCD) (Caçola et al., 2017).

4.1.5.9.1 *Stereotyped movements in autism*

Most people with ASD show stereotypes, but stereotyped behaviours on their own can lead the unwary to an incorrect presumption of ASD. Avoiding this error requires a careful consideration of whether other features of autism are in fact present. There is little to distinguish the stereotyped movements in ASD from those occurring in children with ID, or indeed anyone else. They tend to be stable over time. Some of them are very similar to those of obsessive-compulsive disorder, and it can be difficult to elicit the compulsive quality in people with limited communication. Exposure with response prevention should always be considered in a treatment plan.

4.1.5.9.2 *Tics in autism*

About 22% of children with ASD have tics (Canitano & Vivanti, 2007), half of them showing the full Tourette picture. (This figure is drawn from a study of a group of autistic children referred to a neuropsychiatric unit, so could well be exaggerated by referral bias.) About half have a positive family history of tics. The phenomenology of the tics themselves does not seem to be very different from those seen in uncomplicated Tourette. The reason for the association is obscure, but both conditions have multiple genetic influences and it seems likely that some of those influences are, in some individuals, common to both.

The clinical importance is that the tics may be misinterpreted as an autistic stereotypy and not seen in their true light or treated appropriately.

4.1.6 Prevalence and epidemiology

The epidemiology of ASD has been reviewed effectively; for example, by Newschaffer et al. (2007) and Lyall et al. (2017). The diagnosed prevalence of ASD is rising (see Chapter 1, Section 1.1) and has increased dramatically in the USA and UK, from 4–5 per 10,000 up to more than 100 per 10,000 over the last 40 years. The increase in the USA has been particularly great for those with IQs in the normal range (Autism and Developmental Disorders Monitoring Network, 2012).

International estimates outside the USA and Europe are hard to compare because of major variations in case identification. It is however plain that rates of diagnosis in practice have been rising. A quantitative review by Elsabbagh et al. (2012) found that most surveys conducted since the year 2000, in different geographical regions and by different teams, gave a median estimate of 17 per 10,000 for autism and 62 per 10,000 for all 'pervasive developmental disorders' combined (the latter category being more or less equivalent to modern ASD). An exceptionally high rate of 264 per 10,000 was reported from South Korea (Kim et al., 2011), but the 2012 review by Elsabbagh et al. did not in fact find statistical evidence for systematic differences between geographical areas.

Changing definitions, better awareness, and improved diagnostic practices certainly account for a great deal of the increase. There is, however, controversy over whether these influences on recognition account for the whole of the increase, or whether something is increasing the true prevalence. The increasing age of fathers, earlier diagnosis, and increasing pollution are all potential influences that could be expected to increase true rates.

One consequence of instability in rates of diagnosis is to make it very difficult to interpret regional differences. Another consequence is that, as the rates of diagnosis increase, the distinctiveness of the condition can be expected to decrease. Public reaction might then change unpredictably—either to reduce discrimination or to trivialize the condition. Another consequence of the increase in prevalence is that adults are now presenting to services who in the past did not meet the more restrictive criteria that were then in force. They need reassessment now. It also follows that a clinician seeing a person with an existing diagnosis of ASD, or one of its variants, cannot be clear about the course of the condition from the previous diagnosis alone. Further still, clinicians need to consider the older scientific literature carefully before accepting its conclusions (e.g. on assessment and treatment), to know whether it is applicable to their current cases.

Boys are affected with ASD more frequently than are girls. The conclusion is robust across countries, but the reported male:female ratios vary greatly. The gender ratio is modified substantially by cognitive impairment; among cases without ID, the sex ratio may be more than 5:1, whereas among those who do show ID, the sex ratio may be closer to 2:1

4.1.7 Risks

Many risks identified as possible associations are probably involved in other neurodevelopmental disorders, too. Risks in relation to a general neurodevelopmental context, as discussed in Chapters 6 and 7, need to be considered, as well as the risks that have specific relevance to ASD.

4.1.7.1 Genetic risks for ASD

4.1.7.1.1 Genetics of syndromal autism

ASD is heritable, but the details of inheritance are very complex, probably involving multiple susceptibility genes in most affected people.

A large population study across five countries, based on case registers of families, has examined the risk of developing ASD as a function of the relatedness to other family members with evidence of the condition(s). This has suggested a heritability of about 80% (Bai et al., 2019). The risk of another child in the family being affected after the birth of one child with ASD is around 20%, depending on how narrowly or widely the condition is defined (Ozonoff et al., 2011).

Several studies comparing monozygotic and dizygotic twins have indicated moderate to high heritability (Posthuma & Polderman, 2013). A systematic review and meta-analysis of twin studies by Tick et al. (2016) has emphasized that ASD is mostly attributable to genetic effects. Heritability estimates in different studies ranged between 64% and 91%, in keeping with results from the family-based population study just cited.

Chapter 7 describes the genetic influences as they affect the broad range of functions involved. Many scientific studies, however, have focused on autism specifically, and their conclusions are accordingly considered here.

4.1.7.1.2 Rare genes

The effects of chromosomal abnormalities have been known for some time, and the knowledge led to an ongoing search for changes in individual genes. A few single-gene or oligogenic disorders are known to include ASD in the phenotype, but they all lead to a wider range of disabilities than simply ASD. Most of the currently defined single-gene alterations have only very small effects on ASD when considered singly. Some of the rare genetic alterations, however, have sizeable effects on the few people who carry them. Typically, they are copy number variants, arising de novo without other family members being involved.

Several genes are now identified as associations of ASD, including *NRXN1*, *SHANK1*, *SHANK3*, and *PTCHD1*. The penetrance of the underlying mutations, however, is not yet well described. By way of example, deletions in *NRXN1* are relatively common in clinically identified individuals with ASD (0.45%) and ID (0.12%), as well as in other neurodevelopmental phenotypes. In contrast, the frequency in population-based surveys is much less (around 0.02%).

Not all those with a risk gene will develop any disorder. A current estimate for penetrance of *NRXN1* mutations for all neurodevelopmental phenotypes is 33% (Woodbury–Smith & Scherer, 2018).

4.1.7.1.3 *Common gene variants*

Common gene variants are associated with ASD much more frequently than rare ones. They will typically have only very small effects, considered individually, but in aggregate account for a large part of the variance (Chapter 7, Section 7.4).

One recent genome-wide association study included 18,381 cases of ASD (and 27,969 controls). It detected five genome-wide significant signals, with a further seven loci that were associated with other traits (Grove et al., 2019).

4.1.7.1.4 *Clinical importance*

Genetic counselling is complicated but can be useful. Families can be given more precise information about the risks for their future children than simply quoting the recurrence rate.

There may be clinical aspects that suggest a detailed genetic investigation. For example, among individuals who have a head circumference greater than three standard deviations above the mean, the possibility of *PTEN* mutations should be considered: they can lead to overgrowth of the white matter in the brain. Similarly, developmental regression in a female patient should alert clinicians to the possibility of a *MeCP2* mutation (see Rett syndrome, Chapter 7, Section 7.3).

Genetic counselling sometimes makes it possible to plan treatment for a medical condition known to be associated with the genes that are altered. Mental health disorders are particularly frequent in those with 22q11 deletions, so enhanced monitoring and intervention are indicated. Those with 16p11.2 mutations have high rates of obesity, so prevention may be indicated. The chromosomal and other genetic conditions that are also associated with heart defects (e.g. 1q21.1 microdeletion) should trigger cardiovascular evaluation. Other susceptibility genes may interact with environmental exposures or be subject to epigenetic influence.

The Genetic Testing Registry (GTR) of the US National Center for Biotechnology Information (NCBI) is a useful resource for tests to use and sampling requirements. It is available at www.ncbi.nlm.nih.gov/gtr/tests/

4.1.7.2 *Non-genetic risks for ASD*

Environmental adversity plays only a minor role in generating ASD.

4.1.7.2.1 *Psychosocial adversity*

Some kinds of extreme psychological deprivation can cause problems in the spectrum of autism. Rutter et al. (1999) describe 'quasi-autistic' patterns following extreme global privation in Romanian and Eastern European orphans. These patterns were associated with the length of time during which they suffered deprivation.

4.1.7.2.2 *Immune and infective influences*

Cerebral spinal fluid and peripheral blood from older children with autism can show atypical levels of autoantibodies to neural antigens, immunoglobulins, inflammatory cytokines, and other markers that could signal dysregulation and/or dysmaturation of both adaptive and innate immune systems.

Prenatal exposure to viral agents (e.g. cytomegalovirus, rubella) has been linked to ASD, but early viral exposure is unlikely to account for many cases.

4.1.7.2.3 *Hormonal influences*

Abnormal sex hormone levels in pregnancy, especially testosterone, with its presumed effects on sexually dimorphic brain structure and behaviour, is an area of research interest. Exposure assessment, however, is challenging, and the utility of morphological markers of in utero exposure, such as digit length ratios, is unproven.

Other hormonal factors of interest have been hypothalamic/pituitary/adrenal (HPA) axis stress hormones and thyroid hormones. No consistent story has yet emerged from these case-control investigations.

4.1.7.2.4 *Toxins in pregnancy*

The multiple effects of toxins are described in Chapter 7, Section 7.9. Some studies have investigated pregnancy risks for ASD specifically. They indicate an increased risk of ASD being associated with advanced paternal age, prenatal exposure to organochlorine pesticides (e.g. dicofol, endosulfan), and air pollution related to traffic (e.g. particulate matter, nitrogen dioxide) (Rossignol et al., 2014).

Some medications carry risks for inducing brain changes. ASD is part of thalido-mide embryopathy (Strömland et al., 1994). Valproate in pregnancy is a known cause of autism. The risk does not extend to other antiepileptic drugs. In a population-wide case-register study, exposures to carbamazepine, oxcarbazepine, lamotrigine, and clonazepam monotherapy were not associated with increased risks of ASD and childhood autism; valproate was. (Christensen et al., 2013).

4.1.7.2.5 *Perinatal hazards*

Many studies have investigated associations between autism risk and maternal obstetric characteristics, labour and delivery complications, and neonatal factors. The mech-anism of association, however, appears to be that they are markers to an abnormally developing fetus rather than the causes of problems.

4.1.8 Pathophysiology

Careful empirical studies have resulted in partial support for several kinds of brain difference in ASD, but no one unifying abnormality. One enduring hypothesis has been that ASD is associated with, and therefore conceivably caused by, early brain (and there-fore head) overgrowth. The evidence for causality is absent; that for an association is not unanimous. It looks as though there may be individuals in whom changes in growth and connectivity play a part, but according to present knowledge there is no reason to think that a generalizable unifying abnormality has been found.

Surén et al. (2013), for instance, described increased *variability* in head circumference in boys at 12 months who would later be diagnosed with autism, and correspondingly there were more cases of macrocephaly. The *average* head size, however, did not differ at any age, and girls who would develop ASD later had *lower* mean head circumference than other girls at all ages. That difference, however, appeared to be largely driven by girls with genetic disorders, epilepsy, or ID rather than by any qualities of the autism.

Schumann et al. (2010) reported structural MRI changes in ASD, with widespread increases of both grey and white matter in the frontal, temporal, and cingulate cortex. More specific hypotheses of localized changes in processes of pruning cells or synapses have resulted in formulations about defined brain structures; for example, that the amygdala and hippocampus are larger in some children with autism (Schumann et al., 2004). There have been other reports to a similar effect; for example, in autistic people studied in adolescence (Groen et al., 2010). The involvement of these structures in emotional and social development makes them candidates for the putative anatomical bases of ASD. Changes in size, however, could as well be the results of the experiences of being autistic as the causes.

Neuropsychological formulations of the changes that could underlie social communication and sensory experience have invited tests that examine brain function directly. As with ADHD, they are not yet at the stage of definitive explanation or value in the diagnosis of individuals. One possible cause of difficulties in social communication would be a problem in reading facial expressions. The ability to attend to and process information from faces does in part depend on integrity of the fusiform face area and amygdala. Kleinhans et al. (2008) studied the connections from the fusiform face area with functional imaging. They found that people with ASD, by comparison with controls, had decreased connectivity to the left amygdala, posterior cingulate cortex, and thalamus. Clinical severity tended to be related to lower connectivity.

The suggestion of detailed versus global processing of information has also generated neural investigation. For instance, Herringshaw et al. (2018) found that young people with ASD were faster than others in identification of shapes (based on detailed visual processing) but less accurate in emotion identification (considered to require global- and context-sensitive processing). When identifying shapes, they showed less MRI activation in regions associated with executive control, such as the medial prefrontal cortex and middle frontal gyrus. For emotion, they showed decreased connectivity between frontal and posterior regions. However, numbers in such studies remain small and general conclusions are not yet possible.

Sensory abnormalities in ASD have attracted a separate literature of neurophysiological speculation. The focus has usually been on ideas of gain being increased or decreased, or on overfocused attention. A review by Marco and colleagues (2011) suggested that autistic adults responding to simple stimuli in a single modality show most of the changes at the late stages of physiological response, using measures such as evoked potentials. Early changes (e.g. those occurring up to 100 ms after a stimulus is presented) are inconstant. High-order processes such as selective attention therefore seem likely to be involved. Top-down cortical processes can influence the course of signals through the nervous system in autism (Dunn et al., 2008). Psychophysiological methods of studying sensory function (Green et al., 2015) have indeed indicated that high-functioning ASD youth show more activation than controls in primary sensory areas, the amygdala, and the orbitofrontal cortex when they are presented with sounds. This overactivation seems to be associated with both anxiety and sensory over-responsiveness. Difficulties with habituation suggest a neurological basis. Another association of sensory dysfunction is increased stress (indicated by cortisol secretion) during peer interactions.

4.2 EARLY-ONSET PSYCHOSES

Schizophrenia and bipolar disorder are not, strictly speaking, neurodevelopmental disorders. Their onset is most often in late adolescence and early adulthood. Nevertheless, they have a good deal in common. They are life-changing and life-threatening problems with strong genetic influences and a fluctuating course in adult life. Some forms are preceded by early-life changes in social, motor, and cognitive development. Autism was once regarded as a juvenile form of schizophrenia—but not now.

4.2.1 Diagnostic concepts: schizophrenia and related psychotic disorders

The distinction between autism and schizophrenia was a major advance for the development of neuropsychiatry (Rutter, 1972). The diagnostic criteria for schizophrenia are the same in adults and young people. They comprise:

- a cluster of 'positive symptoms' of hallucinations, delusions, and disorganized speech;
- a cluster of 'negative symptoms' such as social withdrawal, apathy, and 'avolitional' states (in which all kinds of goal-directed activity can be reduced);
- motor disorganization, such as catatonia;
- a trend for adaptive function (which is defined under 'intellectual disability' in Chapter 5, Section 5.2.4.2) to decline, and personal relationships to deteriorate.

Schizophrenia is a fairly reliable diagnosis at all ages if the DSM-5 and ICD-11 criteria are followed. It is not, however, a very predictive one. Attempts to define a key underlying change in psychological or neurological function have not been widely adopted.

Schizophrenia is a spectrum disorder, including related categories of mixed, attenuated, and brief forms. The clustering of clinical features, however, has not yet generated a robust system of subcategories or dimensions that gives a satisfactory account of course, cause(s), and response to treatment (Lawrie et al., 2016). The types described in Box 4.2 do not map closely to brain function.

> ## Box 4.2 Conditions in the spectrum of schizophrenia and psychosis
>
> - *Acute and transient psychotic disorder*: a sudden onset of positive psychotic symptoms that fluctuate rapidly in nature and intensity over a short period of time and do not last for more than 3 months.
> - *Schizo-affective disorders*: psychotic features coexist with mania, depression, or mixed symptoms *at the same time.*
> - *Psychotic disorders considered to have other causes*: for example, drug-induced psychosis, brain diseases, and post-partum psychosis.
> - *Schizotypy*: eccentric behaviour and changes in thinking and affect like those in schizophrenia, but with a static course similar to that of a personality disorder.
>
>   Many clinicians also use the idea of *attenuated psychosis* for cases in which not all the features of schizophrenia are present. In young people, however, the use of the 'not quite' diagnosis creates a risk of overdiagnosis and overtreatment.

Whether these various forms of psychosis are variations in a single spectrum or distinct conditions is obscure. Nevertheless, the traditional psychotic diagnoses of schizophrenia and bipolar disorder continue to be used and regarded as useful. They still guide practice and are regarded as acceptable by service users.

In practice, most adult psychiatrists do not closely follow the criteria of DSM-5 or ICD-11. The most frequent features in the WHO's major survey of 10 nations (Jablensky et al., 1992) were rather different from those in the current diagnostic schemes. The commonest features noted in adults were impaired insight (in about 90%), followed by suspiciousness, ideas of reference, and flat affect. Delusions and hallucinations were only present in about half of those given research diagnoses of schizophrenia. Nowadays, the ICD-11 draft guidelines refer to the following 'core symptoms', of which at least one must be present (together with other difficulties) for a diagnosis of schizophrenia:

- persistent delusion of any kind;
- distortion of self-experience (e.g. thought interference or thought withdrawal);
- passivity phenomena;
- persistent hallucinations in any modality;
- thought disorder.

ICD-11 also recommends using not only a categorical definition but also a set of specifiers and dimensions.

4.2.1.1 *Specifiers and dimensions*

A formulation should include both the core features and whether they are present with or without the following specifiers:

- acute stress
- post-partum onset

- catatonia
- high severity

A categorical diagnosis should be accompanied by the severity of the following dimensions:

- positive symptoms
- experiences of passivity and control
- negative symptoms
- depressive mood symptoms
- manic mood symptoms
- psychomotor symptoms (agitation, psychomotor retardation, catatonia)
- cognitive symptoms (e.g. deficits in speed of processing, attention/concentration, orientation, judgement, abstraction, verbal or visual learning, and working memory)

4.2.2 Bipolar disorder

Bipolar disorder (BD) is regarded as a psychosis because it often shows the 'positive' features of hallucinations and delusions. There are other similarities with schizophrenia. BD typically starts in late adolescence or early adult life (18–22 years being the most frequent age range of onset). It is accompanied by a lack of insight and has a damaging effect on the quality of life thereafter.

The major distinctions from schizophrenic disorders are in clinical presentation: the defining features are episodicity and the presence of periods of mania. The content of any delusions and hallucinations is in keeping with the changed mood state. Thought is not illogical but proceeds rapidly from one topic to another, and thereby loses coherence ('flight of ideas'). BD is seldom associated with premorbid deficits in motor and intellectual development in the same way as schizophrenia.

In young people, mania is a disputed concept. The adult features of elevated mood, overactivity, and grandiose thinking are more difficult to recognize as such in youth. Instead, irritability is the mood change most often recognized. As a result, there is a massive overlap between BD and severe emotional dysregulation (see 'Emotional regulation', Chapter 2, Section 2.9). Until the academic dispute is resolved, clinicians are advised to be sparing with the diagnosis in children and young people, and reserve it for cases in which there is clear evidence of a discrete episode of euphoria, grandiosity, and flight of ideas, as well as irritability (Leibenluft, 2011). The episode should be for 7 days to indicate bipolar I, or 4 days for bipolar II. Clear episodes of as little as 48 hours will probably raise the probability of BD later. They should indicate close follow-up.

4.2.3 Recognition of psychotic conditions

Most adult psychiatrists do not use standardized measures in routine practice but rely on their appraisal of the total situation and history. Many child psychiatrists do not have the same high level of experience and find it useful to employ the standardized measures developed for research.

4.2.3.1 *Standardized measures*

4.2.3.1.1 *Rating scales*

Five scales were compared by Kumari et al. (2017). The most widely used by researchers and clinicians is Positive and Negative Symptom Scales (PANSS) (Kay et al., 1987). It is a record of assessments by clinically qualified professionals. A 'negative symptoms' subscale assesses for blunted affect, emotional withdrawal, poor rapport, passive/apathetic social withdrawal, difficulty in abstract thinking, lack of spontaneity and flow of conversation, and stereotyped thinking. The 'positive' subscale addresses delusions, conceptual disorganization, hallucinatory behaviour, excitement, grandiosity, suspiciousness, and hostility. There is also a general psychopathology subscale addressing somatic concern, anxiety, feelings of guilt, tension, mannerisms and posturing, depression, motor retardation, uncooperativeness, unusual thought content, disorientation, poor attention, lack of judgement, and insight. The measure is rather long, but it outperforms the Brief Psychiatric Rating Scale (BPRS) (which takes about 20 minutes) in predicting clinical outcome (Obermeier et al., 2011).

A self-report questionnaire for young people, the Prodromal Questionnaire—Brief Child Version, focuses particularly on the symptoms considered to define a high-risk state for schizophrenia (Karcher et al., 2018). (The idea of a high-risk state in young people, however, should be treated with much caution, as discussed in Section 4.2.5.)

4.2.3.1.2 *Interviews*

Researchers make extensive use of structured interviews to be administered to parents or young people by lay interviewers, after short but specific training. The Diagnostic Interview Schedule for Children (DISC) (Shaffer et al., 2000) is based on lay raters, so is highly structured. The Diagnostic Interview for Children and Adolescents (DICA) can be given in both structured and semi-structured formats (Reich, 2000). The K-SADS (Kiddie Schedule for Affective Disorders and Schizophrenia) is a semi-structured interview with a similarly wide scope, designed for clinicians (Axelson et al., 2003). The Washington University K-SADS (Geller et al., 2001) extends it to give a fuller account of manic and rapid-cycling conditions. The Child and Adolescent Psychiatric Assessment (CAPA) (Angold & Costello, 2000) uses an extensively trained interviewer to provide the judgement calls in documenting the presence or absence of symptoms. The Schizophrenia Proneness Instrument: Child and Youth Version (SPI-CY) is a structured interview designed for use with young people, but with only limited data on validity at this stage (Fux et al., 2013).

4.2.3.2 *Clinical assessment of hallucinations and delusions in young people*

Assessment in the acute phase should include a detailed history of the presentation, and the earlier development of social, cognitive, and motor skills. Examination of the mental state needs to include an interview with the young person that is respectful of any difficulties in communication, fears about the situation, and the consequences of disclosing bizarre ideas. Checklist administration has the benefit of ensuring comprehensive cover but risks losing cooperation and using ideas and terminology that the young person does not understand. Young people with altered perceptions of reality (and their caregivers) often come for help because they fear madness or, more specifically, that the abnormal experiences are the beginning of schizophrenia.

The delicate but important distinction between hallucinations and misinterpretations of experience needs to be explored with sensitivity and understanding of the individual's experiences. Unpleasant thoughts can be misperceived as voices or messages from the outside world. Isolated hallucinations (i.e. those occurring in the absence of other schizophrenic features) are often confined to particular times of day such as bedtime and waking, and may be evidence of a disorder of the sleep–wake cycle.

Children with other forms of psychopathology, including consequences of psychological trauma, sometimes express previous memories, or elaborations of them, as vivid current events. The descriptions are often in more detail and loaded with more affect than in psychosis. They, or their caregivers, will usually make the connection. Hallucinatory experiences with intense emotional accompaniment—such as accusatory voices or visions of persecutors—occur in affective disorders such as major depression and bipolar depressive states.

Unsubstantiated perceptions of one's body being changed are frequent hallucinations in adolescents' presentations of schizophrenia—but are also frequent in body dysmorphic disorder (BMD). The false beliefs of BMD can be held with delusional intensity. The distinction is made from the whole picture: BMD is not characterized by the negative, cognitive, and motor symptoms of schizophrenia.

Perseverative and idiosyncratic beliefs are frequent in the spectrum of autism and can be confused with psychotic delusions if the distinction between longstanding preoccupations and recently developed suspicions is not appreciated.

4.2.4 Difficulties for diagnosis

A full picture of schizophrenia in early adolescence needs early and careful recognition. Early-onset schizophrenia (EOS), before the age of 18 years, and childhood-onset schizophrenia (COS), before 13 years, often follow a particularly adverse course. Diagnosis is therefore important, but difficult. Difficulties arise because:

- The full set of DSM-5 criteria includes persistence of problems (possibly in attenuated form) over a period of 6 months or more. Waiting for this criterion to be met could be risky.
- Problems in communication may make it hard to be clear about the severity of problems based on the individual's self-report.
- Pre-existing developmental problems may include autistic-type difficulties in communication and social interaction. These can be mistaken for negative symptoms of

schizophrenia. The distinction is between the static trajectories of the former and the recent onset of the latter. The DSM-5 criteria require that young people should show positive symptoms such as hallucinations and delusions, as well as other features, if they are to be diagnosed with schizophrenia.

- Ordinary childhood experiences, including overactive imaginations and vivid fantasies, can be misinterpreted as psychosis.
- Hallucinations and delusions are quite common in childhood and adolescence and should not be taken as pathognomonic of a psychotic illness.
- Other conditions in the spectrum of psychosis—such as affective psychoses—may be hard to rule out.
- The onset is often insidious, with early features often attenuated and therefore sub-clinical, making the timing of onset unclear.

4.2.5 Course over time, including premorbid conditions and prodromes

Even before the onset of a disorder, many people have shown identifiable problems in development. The early problems are various, including some in aspects that seem very relevant to later psychosis: reality testing, attention, social function, language, and motor control. Not all people who are eventually diagnosed show them. Most people who show the early developmental problems do not develop schizophrenia.

As an example of early risks, data were gathered on the 1946 birth cohort in the UK, during childhood and follow-up until the members were in their forties (Jones et al., 1994). Those who developed schizophrenia had, in childhood, been:

- more likely at age 4 years to have mothers whom the health visitors rated as below average in mothering skills;
- slow to reach milestones in walking and speech;
- low scorers on educational tests at ages 8, 11, and 15 years;
- happier to play on their own at ages 4 and 6 years;
- more likely to rate themselves as low in social confidence at age 13 years.

Some authorities argue that schizophrenia should be regarded as a neurodevelopmental disorder. Others see the early changes as non-specific risk factors rather than the beginning of illness.

It is agreed that:

- Many people with psychosis in adult life have no such early history.
- Neuroimaging studies in young adults suggest multiple changes in brain structure and function, going back at least to adolescence and often before.
- There are strong genetic influences on schizophrenia. We do not yet know whether these are the same influences that operate for the potentially premorbid signs.

- Changes in individual genes are many and varied. Many of those associated with schizophrenia probably exert influences primarily on prenatal and early postnatal brain development. The effects of single changes with large effect sizes (e.g. 22q11 mutations, see Chapter 7, Section 7.3) are to increase the risk for many different neurodevelopmental disorders.

The changes usually considered as prodromal are mild versions of the positive symptoms of hallucinations and delusions. They are not unique to any one adult outcome. Indeed, when studied prospectively, they may well continue, but not always as antecedents of later psychotic states, and not always specific to them (Armando et al., 2015a). For example, Garralda (1984) reported a controlled study in which 20 children, presenting with the combination of hallucinations and emotional or conduct disorders, were followed up into adulthood. (The mean follow-up time was 17 years and the mean age at follow-up was 30 years.) In childhood, the presence of hallucinations had been associated with precipitating events for the emotional disorder and a shorter duration of illness. Depressive mood changes, perceptual-cognitive dysfunction, and a family history of mood changes had been more common in those who hallucinated than those who did not. The earlier hallucinations in childhood sometimes persisted into adult life, but did not carry an increased risk for schizophrenia, depressive illness, organic brain damage, or other psychiatric disorders. They did sometimes predict continuing alterations of reality testing—including episodes of depersonalization, hallucinations, and altered awareness.

Widely-quoted evidence for continuity between psychosis-like experiences in childhood and schizophreniform conditions in adult life came from a study by Poulton et al. (2000). These investigators used data from the well-conducted Dunedin population study to relate experiences at 11 to those at 26. In their cohort of 761 11-year-old children, a structured psychiatric interview asked about psychotic experiences (mind being read by others, messages received through the radio or TV, perception of being followed, hearing non-veridical voices). The queries were answered affirmatively by 72, of whom 13 reported two or more such experiences (or gave a definite example). In the 12 children who reported two or more, and could be followed to age 26, three met criteria for a schizophreniform disorder and 70% showed at least one positive sign. Persistent anxiety problems also featured in the outcomes.

Subsequent analysis by Fisher et al. (2013) indicated that the risks conveyed for mental health at the age of 38 were not specific to schizophrenia. Very few of the children with psychotic symptoms were free of mental health problems in their adult life. Schizophrenia figured occasionally in the outcomes, but the major adult problems were post-traumatic disorders, suicidality, and substance dependence.

The concept of a high-risk state in young people based on attenuated positive symptoms is not a good way of predicting a schizophrenic illness (Garralda, 2016). The use of antipsychotic treatments does not prevent schizophrenia (Armando et al., 2015b). On the other hand, the high-risk state is a good predictor of persistently poor social functioning in adult life. In an ideal world, it would indicate measures to promote resilience and improve social adjustment and monitor course.

During adolescence, there can be real uncertainty about how seriously to take 'psychosis-like symptoms'. Merely the report of hallucinations and delusions should not be taken to indicate an early psychotic state. On the other hand, the combination of hallucinations and delusions with other potential predictors—especially, deteriorating social and cognitive function—will often be strong enough to indicate preventive treatment. The risks of antipsychotic drugs, and their limited benefit in this age group, are too great for them to be generally advised to prevent 'conversion' into frank psychosis. Psychological interventions, however, do not have the same disadvantage. Family and educational support, vocational training, and cognitive behavioural approaches to cope with distressing experiences should be considered on an individual basis.

When a full picture of schizophrenia does develop in children and young people, the outlook is not good. Hollis (2000) followed 110 consecutive patients with first-episode psychosis and child or adolescent onset (mean age at onset 14.2 years) who presented to the Maudsley Hospital in London between 1973 and 1991. They were followed up at an average of 11.5 years after first contact. Those for whom the first episode had lasted for 6 months or more had only a 15% chance of achieving full remission thereafter. The outcome is worse than for affective disorders in adolescence and first-episode psychoses in adult life. Social relationships are badly impaired.

In young adult life, the course is frequently one of a chronic and relapsing disorder with incomplete remissions. Negative symptoms and cognitive impairments often follow a course of steadily continuing impairment. Social outcomes include reduced rates of employment and financial independence, and an increased likelihood of homelessness and incarceration. An adverse course of persisting disability (Tandon et al., 2009) is predicted by:

- male gender,
- early age of onset,
- prolonged period of untreated illness,
- severity of cognitive and negative symptoms.

4.2.6 Prevalence and epidemiology

Lifetime prevalence is about 7 per 1,000 for the full picture of schizophrenia. EOS is much less prevalent than adult-onset cases. In the UK, a survey found the prevalence in people aged between 5 and 18 years to be about 4 per 1,000. It is decidedly rare before the age of 13; estimated at around 1 in 10,000. Peak incidence in most countries comes between the ages of 15 and 24 years. Males are more likely to be affected than females in youth, but there is a second peak in adult females at middle age.

The incidence varies somewhat between nations (McGrath et al., 2004). A well-known and influential study of 10 countries by the WHO (Jablensky et al., 1992) concluded otherwise, but probably lacked sufficient power, and has been replaced by systematic review. Rates are higher in migrants and probably in cities. In the UK and the

Netherlands, and probably elsewhere, there is a raised prevalence in immigrants with black skins and their offspring (Eaton & Harrison, 2000).

4.2.7 Risks

The earlier the onset of disorder, the more likely it is to be associated with a family history heavily loaded with relatives with a schizophrenia spectrum disorder. COS is rare and often preceded by impairments of academic achievement and abnormalities of language, motor, and social development (Driver et al., 2013). Indeed, some 20% of referred children with COS screened positive for autism.

BD is also highly heritable. Offspring of parents with BD show a great increase in the rates of bipolar spectrum disorder and a moderate increase in disruptive problems of behaviour (Birmaher et al., 2009). Other researchers have also found an increase in mood and anxiety disorder.

The notion of perinatal injury and illness causing adult-onset psychotic disorders has been reviewed systematically by Liu et al. (2015). Present knowledge does not support perinatal adversity as a main cause of psychosis, but the possibility is not entirely ruled out. Early deviations in neuromotor and socio-emotional development can follow obstetric problems, often reflecting earlier abnormality (see 'Birth injury', Chapter 6, Section 6.3).

Research on the neurobiology and psychosocial associations of COS is scanty, reflecting the rarity of the problem in those under the age of 13. Much of our knowledge comes from a team at the National Institute of Mental Health (NIMH) in Washington, DC. They have shown widespread anatomical changes in the brain, with progressive loss of grey matter in the prefrontal and superior temporal cortex, delayed white matter growth, and a progressive decline in cerebellar volume (Rapoport & Gogtay, 2011). This was a different pattern to that seen by the same investigators in early-onset BD in adolescents (EOS), where there was evidence for an unexpected increase in temporal grey matter on the left side and loss on the right.

Many other illnesses have a similar relationship between younger age at onset and greater genetic loading. Childs and Scriver (1986) argued that late-onset cases are more likely to have encountered a wide range of cumulative environmental adversity.

Psychosis in young people can also develop secondary to physical medical conditions including: intoxications (e.g. with recreational drugs); seizure disorders (especially complex partial epilepsy); central nervous system infections; autoimmune disorders (e.g. anti-N-methyl-D-aspartate receptor encephalitis, thyroid disease, and cerebral lupus, but rheumatoid arthritis is negatively associated); genetic syndromes (e.g. 22q11 deletion syndrome, Wilson disease, metachromatic leukodystrophy); unintended medication effects (e.g. steroids); and neoplasms. These associations are not unique to schizophrenia and are described in Chapters 6 and 7. They are mostly rare, except epilepsy and cannabis syndromes, which should always be considered. Physical assessment should be carried out in all first episodes, to seek any evidence of fever, clouding of consciousness, fluctuating mental state, localizing neurological signs, loss of language, previous medical illnesses, or exposure to toxins.

4.2.8 Pathophysiology

The pathogenesis of schizophrenic disorders in the young does not seem to differ qualitatively from that in adults. There is persuasive evidence in adults of genetic and environmental influences combining and interacting to create dysfunctional synaptic transmission, especially involving dopamine and abnormal neural connectivity (reviewed by Owen et al., 2016). Other brain circuits are probably involved as well. Studies of structural and functional connection between brain structures in adults continue to suggest complex patterns that may be linked to schizophrenia, but there is not yet a clear consensus about either their causal significance or their development before the clinical onset (see Zhou et al., 2018). The exact details are not yet known.

4.2.9 Management of suspected schizophrenia in young people

The diagnosis is important to establish. Very careful assessment is required because of the possibilities of both underdiagnosis and overdiagnosis, and the strong therapeutic implications. Once the diagnosis is agreed and other problems are addressed, treatment planning should include vigorous use of psychopharmacological, psychotherapeutic, and psychosocial interventions as described in Chapters 8 to 10. The treatment plan should be drawn up with, and carefully conveyed to, the young person and their family.

The severity of COS and EOS is likely to present challenges to child and adolescent mental health services. Indeed, in many areas, they are dealt with by adult services or by highly specialized teams. Antipsychotic medication is required (see Chapter 9, Section 9.6), but often has only a small effect in these severe and unusual cases. Clozapine, however, has an effect like that in adults with refractory psychosis, and is often resorted to. Even when carefully managed, the outcome is usually a worse social adjustment than is the case for onsets in adult life (see Section 4.2.5).

A combination of medical and psychological interventions has been recommended (e.g. by NICE), even in the absence of a satisfactory evidence base (National Collaborating Centre, 2013a and b). A more recent systematic review by Armando et al. (2015) found tentative support for psychosocial interventions. Approaches to remediation by cognitive and behavioural methods are considered in Chapter 8, Section 8.12 and by McGurk et al. (2009) and (McClellan (2018). Psychoeducational, supportive, vocational, and family interventions are usually needed. Services for substance abuse and suicidality may also need to be called on. Some young people need specialized educational programmes and/or vocational training programmes to address the cognitive and functional deficits associated with the illness.

4.2.10 Catatonia

Catatonia is mentioned in Chapter 2, Section 2.2.2 as a pathology of volition rather than motor control. *Stupor* is a sustained state of immobility and/or mutism. There may also be marked and unusual motor changes:

- Posturing for long periods
- Waxy flexibility (flexibilitas cerea) describes the sustained maintenance of a posture into which the examiner has placed the person
- Negativism (Gegenhalten) is an exaggerated resistance to the examiner moving their limbs
- Automatic obedience and echoing of examiners' movements or speech
- Ambitendency: an alternation between negativism and echoing
- Speech abnormalities, including 'verbigeration'—rapid, irrelevant, and monotonous utterances
- Autonomic instability (e.g. sweating, pallor, blood pressure change)

If these are present in addition to other motor signs, clinicians should look for fever and clouding of consciousness: it could be the onset of *malignant catatonia*, or a warning that prescription of antipsychotics could increase the risk of *neuroleptic malignant syndrome*. Both these complications are dangers to life and medical emergencies.

Rating scales are available (e.g. Bush et al., 1996) and their systematic use has led to an appreciation that the features are not rare. In adults, the features are usually treated with benzodiazepines—which can be a diagnostic test—and with electroconvulsive therapy (ECT).

Catatonia was originally described in the nineteenth century as a type of schizophrenia, but it has since become clear that it can be seen in several other conditions: other than schizophrenia, BD with mania and psychotic depression are probably the commonest. Other associations in adults include metabolic disorders, encephalopathies, epilepsy (for instance, in temporal lobe epilepsy or as a part of non-convulsive status epilepticus), toxic effects of cocaine, and antipsychotics or antipsychotic withdrawal.

Children and young people can develop catatonia, but research is scanty and mostly confined to single case reports (summarized by Takaoka & Takata, 2003). Most stress one or the other of increased slowness in movement and speech responses, difficulty in initiating actions or completing them, rigid posturing, and dependence on cueing by others to start and continue movements. All these can lead to confusion with juvenile Parkinsonism, in which the same problems are often described. Wing and Shah (2000) drew attention to the appearance of catatonic features in autistic people, especially in adolescence. Even when they present as part of a wider pattern of autism spectrum, they are worth separate notice because of the need to consider neurological referral and/or benzodiazepines and ECT.

REFERENCES

American Psychiatric Association (2013). *Diagnostic and statistical manual of mental disorders* (DSM-5).

Angold, A., & Costello, E. J. (2000). The child and adolescent psychiatric assessment (CAPA). *Journal of the American Academy of Child & Adolescent Psychiatry*, *39*(1), 39–48

Armando, M., Pontillo, M., De Crescenzo, F., Mazzone, L., Monducci, E., Cascio, N. L., Santonastaso, O., Pucciarini, M. L., Vicari, S., Schimmelmann, B. G., & Schultze-Lutter, F. (2015a). Twelve-month psychosis-predictive value of the ultra-high risk criteria in children and adolescents. *Schizophrenia Research*, *169*(1–3), 186–192.

Armando, M., Pontillo, M., & Vicari, S. (2015b). Psychosocial interventions for very early and early-onset schizophrenia: a review of treatment efficacy. *Current Opinion in Psychiatry*, *28*(4), 312–323.

Asperger, H. (1944) Die 'autistischen psychopathen' im kindesalter. *Archiv für Psychiatrie und Nervenkrankheiten*, 117, 76–136.

Auyeung, B., Baron–Cohen, S., Wheelwright, S., & Allison, C. (2008). The Aautism Spectrum Quotient: Children's Version (AQ-Child). *Journal of Autism and Developmental Disorders*, *38*(7), 1230–1240.

Axelson, D., Birmaher, B. J., Brent, D., Wassick, S., Hoover, C., Bridge, J., & Ryan, N. (2003). A preliminary study of the Kiddie Schedule for Affective Disorders and Schizophrenia for School-Age Children mania rating scale for children and adolescents. *Journal of Child and Adolescent Psychopharmacology*, *13*(4), 463–470. https://doi.org/10.1089/104454603322724850

Autism and Developmental Disabilities Monitoring Network Surveillance Year 2008 Principal Investigators, & Centers for Disease Control and Prevention. (2012). Prevalence of autism spectrum disorders. *MMWR Surveillance Summary*, *61*(3), 1–19.

Bai, D., Yip, B. H. K., Windham, G. C., Sourander, A., Francis, R., Yoffe, R., Glasson, E., Mahjani B., Suominen, A., Leonard, H., Gissler, M., Buxbaum, J. D., Wong, K., Schendel, D., Kodesh, A., Breshnahan, M., Levine, S. Z., Parner, E. T., Hansen, S. N., . . . & Gissler, M. (2019). Association of genetic and environmental factors with autism in a 5-country cohort. *Journal of the American Medical Association Psychiatry*, *76*(10), 1035–1043.

Baird, G., Douglas, H. R., & Murphy, M. S. (2011). Recognising and diagnosing autism in children and young people: summary of NICE guidance. *British Medical Journal*, *343*(d6360). https://doi.org/10.1136/bmj.d6360.

Berument, S. K., Rutter, M., Lord, C., Pickles, A., & Bailey, A. (1999). Autism screening questionnaire: diagnostic validity. *British Journal of Psychiatry*, *175*(5), 444–451.

Birmaher, B., Axelson, D., Monk, K., Kalas, C., Goldstein, B., Hickey, M. B., Obreja, M., Ehman, M., Iyengar, S., Shamseddeen, W., Kupfer, D., & Brent, D. (2009). Lifetime psychiatric disorders in school-aged offspring of parents with bipolar disorder: the Pittsburgh Bipolar Offspring study. *Archives of General Psychiatry*, *66*(3), 287–296.

Booth, R., & Happé, F. (2010). 'Hunting with a knife and… fork': examining central coherence in autism, attention deficit/hyperactivity disorder, and typical development with a linguistic task. *Journal of Experimental Child Psychology*, *107*(4), 377–393.

Bush, G., Fink, M., Petrides, G., Dowling, F., & Francis, A. (1996). Catatonia. I. Rating scale and standardized examination. *Acta Psychiatrica Scandinavica*, *93*, 129–136.

Caçola, P., Miller, H. L., & Williamson, P. O. (2017). Behavioral comparisons in autism spectrum disorder and developmental coordination disorder: a systematic literature review. *Research in Autism Spectrum Disorders*, *38*, 6–18.

Canitano, R., & Vivanti, G. (2007). Tics and Tourette syndrome in autism spectrum disorders. *Autism*, *11*(1), 19–28.

Charman, T., Drew, A., Baird, C., & Baird, G. (2003). Measuring early language development in preschool children with autism spectrum disorder using the MacArthur Communicative Development Inventory (Infant Form). *Journal of Child Language*, *30*(1), 213–236.

Childs, B., & Scriver, C. R. (1986). Age at onset and causes of disease. *Perspectives in Biology and Medicine*, *29*(3), 437–460.

Christensen, J., Grønborg, T. K., Sørensen, M. J., Schendel, D., Parner, E. T., Pedersen, L. H., & Vestergaard, M. (2013). Prenatal valproate exposure and risk of autism spectrum disorders and childhood autism. *Journal of the American Medical Association*, *309*(16), 1696–1703.

Clarke, T. K., Lupton, M. K., Fernandez–Pujals, A. M., Starr, J., Davies, G., Cox, S., Pattie, A., Liewald, D. C., Hall, L. S., MacIntyre, D. J., Smith, B. H., Hocking, L. J., Padmanabhan, S., Thomson, P. A., Hayward, C., Hansell, N. K., Montgomery, G. W., Medland, S. E., Martin, N. G., . . . & McIntosh, A. M. (2016). Common polygenic risk for autism spectrum disorder (ASD) is associated with cognitive ability in the general population. *Molecular Psychiatry*, *21*(3), 419.

Czech, H. (2018). Hans Asperger, national socialism, and 'race hygiene' in Nazi-era Vienna. *Molecular Autism*, *9*(1), 29.

De Jong, M., Punt, M., De Groot, E., Minderaa, R. B., & Hadders–Algra, M. (2011). Minor neurological dysfunction in children with autism spectrum disorder. *Developmental Medicine & Child Neurology*, *53*(7), 641–646.

Doi, T. (1977). *The anatomy of dependence*. Kodansha America.

Driver, D. I., Gogtay, N., & Rapoport, J. L. (2013). Childhood onset schizophrenia and early onset schizophrenia spectrum disorders. *Child and Adolescent Psychiatric Clinics*, *22*(4), 539–555.

Dunn, M. A., Gomes, H., & Gravel, J. (2008). Mismatch negativity in children with autism and typical development. *Journal of Autism and Developmental Disorders*, *38*, 52–71.

Eaton, W., & Harrison, G. (2000). Ethnic disadvantage and schizophrenia. *Acta Psychiatrica Scandinavica*, *102*, 38–43.

Eisenberger, N. I., & Cole, S. W. (2012). Social neuroscience and health: neurophysiological mechanisms linking social ties with physical health. *Nature Neuroscience*, *15*(5), 669.

Elsabbagh, M., Divan, G., Koh, Y. J., Kim, Y. S., Kauchali, S., Marcín, C., Montiel–Nava, C., Patel, C. S., Wang, C., Yasamy, M. T., & Fombonne E. (2012). Global prevalence of autism and other pervasive developmental disorders. *Autism Research*, *5*(3), 160–179.

Farrugia, S., & Hudson, J. (2006). Anxiety in adolescents with Asperger syndrome: negative thoughts, behavioral problems, and life interference. *Focus on Autism and Other Developmental Disabilities*, *21*(1), 25–35.

Fisher, H. L., Caspi, A., Poulton, R., Meier, M. H., Houts, R., Harrington, H., Arseneault, L., & Moffitt, T. E. (2013). Specificity of childhood psychotic symptoms for predicting schizophrenia by 38 years of age: a birth cohort study. *Psychological Medicine*, *43*(10), 2077–2086. https://doi.org/10.1017/S0033291712003091

Fombonne, E. (2002). Epidemiological trends in rates of autism. *Molecular Psychiatry*, *7*(S2), S4.

Fux, L., Walger, P., Schimmelmann, B. G., & Schultze-Lutter, F. (2013). The Schizophrenia Proneness Instrument, Child and Youth Version (SPI-CY): practicability and discriminative validity. *Schizophrenia Research*, 146(1-3), 69–78.

Garralda, M. E. (1984). Psychotic children with hallucinations. *The British Journal of Psychiatry*, 145(1), 74–77.

Garralda, M. E. (2016). Research into hallucinations and psychotic-like symptoms in children: implications for child psychiatric practice. *The British Journal of Psychiatry*, 208(1), 4–6.

Geller, B., Zimerman, B., Williams, M., Bolhofner, K., Craney, J. L., DelBello, M. P., & Soutullo, C. (2001). Reliability of the Washington University in St Louis Kiddie Schedule for Affective Disorders and Schizophrenia (WASH-U-KSADS) mania and rapid cycling sections. *Journal of the American Academy of Child & Adolescent Psychiatry*, 40(4), 450–455.

Gillberg, C., Gillberg, C., Råstam, M., & Wentz, E. (2001). The Asperger Syndrome (and high-functioning autism) Diagnostic Interview (ASDI): a preliminary study of a new structured clinical interview. *Autism*, 5(1), 57–66.

Gillberg, C., & Råstam, M. (1992). Do some cases of anorexia nervosa reflect underlying autistic-like conditions?. *Behavioural Neurology*, 5(1), 27–32.

Green, S. A., Hernandez, L., Tottenham, N., Krasileva, K., Bookheimer, S. Y., & Dapretto, M. (2015). Neurobiology of sensory overresponsivity in youth with autism spectrum disorders. *JAMA Psychiatry*, 72(8), 778–786.

Groen, W., Teluij, M., Buitelaar, J., & Tendolkar, I. (2010). Amygdala and hippocampus enlargement during adolescence in autism. *Journal of the American Academy of Child & Adolescent Psychiatry*, 49(6), 552–560.

Grove, J., Ripke, S., Als, T. D., Mattheisen, M., Walters, R., Won, H., Pallesen, J., Agerbo, E., Andreassen, O. A., Anney, R., Awashti, S. Belliveau, R., Bettella, F., Buxbaum, J. D., Bybjerg–Grauholm, J., Baekvad–Hansen, M., Cerrato, F., Chambert, K., Christensen, J. H., … & the 23 and Me Research Team. (2019). Identification of common risk variants for autism spectrum disorder. *Nature Genetics*, 51(3), 431–444.

Harrison, P., & Oakland, T. (2015). *Adaptive Behavior Assessment System* (3rd ed.). Pearson.

Herringshaw, A. J., Kumar, S. L., Rody, K. N., & Kana, R. K. (2018). Neural correlates of social perception in children with autism: local versus global preferences. *Neuroscience*, 395, 49–59.

Hollis, C. (2000). Adult outcomes of child- and adolescent-onset schizophrenia: diagnostic stability and predictive validity. *American Journal of Psychiatry*, 157(10), 1652–1659.

Howlin, P., Goode, S., Hutton, J., & Rutter, M. (2009). Savant skills in autism: psychometric approaches and parental reports. *Philosophical Transactions of the Royal Society B: Biological Sciences*, 364(1522), 1359–1367.

Jablensky, A., Sartorius, N., Ernberg, G., Anker, M., Korten, A., Cooper, J. E., Day, R., & Bertelsen, A. (1992). Schizophrenia: manifestations, incidence and course in different cultures. A World Health Organization ten-country study. *Psychological Medicine Monograph Supplement*, 20, 1–97.

Jaedicke, S., Storoschuk, S., & Lord, C. (1994). Subjective experience and causes of affect in high-functioning children and adolescents with autism. *Development and Psychopathology*, 6(2), 273–284.

Jones, P., Murray, R., Rodgers, B., & Marmot, M. (1994). Child developmental risk factors for adult schizophrenia in the British 1946 birth cohort. *Lancet*, 344(8934), 1398–1402.

Kanner, L. (1943). Autistic disturbances of affective contact. *Nervous Child*, 2(3), 217–250.

Karcher, N. R., Barch, D. M., Avenevoli, S., Savill, M., Huber, R. S., Simon, T. J., Leckliter, I., Sher, J. J., & Loewy, R. L. (2018). Assessment of the Prodromal Questionnaire–Brief Child

Version for measurement of self-reported psychoticlike experiences in childhood. *Journal of the American Medical Association Psychiatry*, *75*(8), 853–861.

Kay, S. R., Fiszbein, A., & Opler, L. A. (1987). The positive and negative syndrome scale (PANSS) for schizophrenia. *Schizophrenia Bulletin*, *13*(2), 261–276.

Kim, Y. S., Leventhal, B. L., Koh, Y. J., Fombonne, E., Laska, E., Lim, E. C., Cheon, K. A., Kim, S. J., Kim, Y. K., Lee, H., Song, D. H., & Grinker, R. R. (2011). Prevalence of autism spectrum disorders in a total population sample. *American Journal of Psychiatry*, *168*, 904–912.

Kleberg, J. L., Högström, J., Nord, M., Bölte, S., Serlachius, E., & Falck-Ytter, T. (2017). Autistic traits and symptoms of social anxiety are differentially related to attention to others' eyes in social anxiety disorder. *Journal of Autism and Developmental Disorders*, *47*(12), 3814–3821. https://doi.org/10.1007/s10803-016-2978-z

Kleinhans, N. M., Richards, T., Sterling, L., Stegbauer, K. C., Mahurin, R., Johnson, L. C., Greenson, J., Dawson, G., & Aylward, E. (2008). Abnormal functional connectivity in autism spectrum disorders during face processing. *Brain*, *131*(4), 1000–1012.

Kumari, S., Malik, M., Florival, C., Manalai, P., & Sonje, S. (2017). An assessment of five (PANSS, SAPS, SANS, NSA-16, CGI-SCH) commonly used symptoms rating scales in schizophrenia and comparison to newer scales (CAINS, BNSS). *Journal of Addiction Research & Therapy*, *8*(3), 324–340.

Lawrie, S. M., O'Donovan, M. C., Saks, E., Burns, T., & Lieberman, J. A. (2016). Improving classification of psychoses. *Lancet Psychiatry*, *3*(4), 367–374.

Le Couteur, A., Rutter, M., Lord, C., Rios, P., Robertson, S., Holdgrafer, M., & McLennan, J. (1989) Autism diagnostic interview: a standardized investigator-based instrument. *Journal of Autism and Developmental Disorders*, *19*, 363–387.

Leibenluft, E. (2011). Severe mood dysregulation, irritability, and the diagnostic boundaries of bipolar disorder in youths. *American Journal of Psychiatry*, *168*(2), 129–142.

Liu, C. H., Keshavan, M. S., Tronick, E., & Seidman, L. J. (2015). Perinatal risks and childhood premorbid indicators of later psychosis: next steps for early psychosocial interventions. *Schizophrenia Bulletin*, *41*(4), 801–816.

Lord, C., Risi, S., Lambrecht, L., Cook, E. H. Jr, Leventhal, B. L., DiLavore, P. C., Pickles, A., & Rutter, M. (2000). The autism diagnostic observation schedule-generic: a standard measure of social and communication deficits associated with the spectrum of autism. *Journal of Autism and Developmental Disorders*, *30*, 205–223.

Lord, C., & Jones, R. M. (2012). Annual Research Review: Re-thinking the classification of autism spectrum disorders. *Journal of Child Psychology and Psychiatry*, *53*(5), 490–509.

Lyall, K., Croen, L., Daniels, J., Fallin, M. D., Ladd-Acosta, C., Lee, B. K., Park, B. Y., Snyder, N. W., Schendel, D., Volk, H., Windham, G. C., & Newschaffer, C. (2017). The changing epidemiology of autism spectrum disorders. *Annual Review of Public Health*, *38*, 81–102.

Marco, E. J., Hinkley, L. B., Hill, S. S., & Nagarajan, S. S. (2011). Sensory processing in autism: a review of neurophysiologic findings. *Pediatric Research*, *69*(5 Pt 2), 48R–54R

McClellan, J. (2018). Psychosis in children and adolescents. *Journal of the American Academy of Child & Adolescent Psychiatry*, *57* (5), 308–312.

McClintock, K., Hall, S., & Oliver, C. (2003). Risk markers associated with challenging behaviours in people with intellectual disabilities: a meta-analytic study. *Journal of Intellectual Disability Research*, *47*(6), 405–416.

McGrath, J., Saha, S., Welham, J., El Saadi, O., MacCauley, C., & Chant, D. (2004). A systematic review of the incidence of schizophrenia: the distribution of rates and the influence of sex, urbanicity, migrant status and methodology. *BMC Medicine*, *2*(1), 13.

McGurk, S. R., Mueser, K. T., DeRosa, T. J., & Wolfe, R. (2009). Work, recovery, and comorbidity in schizophrenia: a randomized controlled trial of cognitive remediation. *Schizophrenia Bulletin, 35,* 319–35.

Ming, X., Julu, P., Brimacombe, M., Connor, S., & Daniels, M. (2005). Reduced cardiac parasympathetic activity in children with autism. *Brain Development, 27,* 509–516.

National Collaborating Centre for Mental Health (UK). (2013a). *Psychosis and schizophrenia in children and young people: recognition and management* (No. 155). Royal College of Psychiatrists.

National Collaborating Centre for Mental Health (UK). (2013b). *Autism: the management and support of children and young people on the Autism Spectrum* (NICE Clinical Guidelines, No. 170). British Psychological Society & Royal College of Psychiatrists. https://www.ncbi.nlm.nih.gov/books/NBK299062/

National Institute for Health and Care Excellence. (2011 & 2017). *Autism spectrum disorder in under 19s: recognition, referral and diagnosis* (Clinical Guidelines, No. 128). Royal College of Psychiatrists.

Newschaffer, C. J., Croen, L. A., Daniels, J., Giarelli, E., Grether, J. K., Levy, S. E., Mandell, D. S., Miller, L. A., Pinto-Martin, J., Reaven, J., Reynolds, A. M., Rice, C. E., Schendel, D., Windham, G. C. (2007). The epidemiology of autism spectrum disorders. *Annual Review of Public Health, 28,* 235–258.

Newson, E., Le Marechal, K., & David, C. (2003). Pathological demand avoidance syndrome: a necessary distinction within the pervasive developmental disorders. *Archives of Disease in Childhood, 88,* 595–600.

Norris, M., & Lecavalier, L. (2010). Screening accuracy of level 2 autism spectrum disorder rating scales: a review of selected instruments. *Autism, 14*(4), 263–284.

Obermeier, M., Schennach-Wolff, R., Meyer, S., Möller, H. J., Riedel, M., Krause, D., & Seemüller, F. (2011). Is the PANSS used correctly? a systematic review. *BMC Psychiatry, 11*(1), 1–5.

Owen, M. J., Sawa, A., & Mortensen, P. B. (2016). Schizophrenia. *Lancet, 388,* 86–97.

Ozonoff, S., Young, G. S., Carter, A., Messinger, D., Yirmiya, N., Zwaigenbaum, L., Bryson, S., Carver, L. J., Constantino, J. N., Dobkins, K., Hutman, T., Iverson, J. M., Landa, R., Rogers, S. J., Sigman, M., & Stone, W. L. (2011). Recurrence risk for autism spectrum disorders: a Baby Siblings Research Consortium study. *Pediatrics, 128*(3), e488–e495.

Posthuma, D., & Polderman, T. J. C. (2013) What we have learned from recent twin studies about the etiology of neurodevelopmental disorders? *Current Opinion in Neurology, 26*(2), 111–121.

Poulton, R., Caspi, A., Moffitt, T. E., Cannon, M., Murray, R., & Harrington, H. (2000). Children's self-reported psychotic symptoms and adult schizophreniform disorder: a 15-year longitudinal study. *Archives of General Psychiatry, 57*(11), 1053–1058.

Rapoport, J. L., & Gogtay, N. (2011). Childhood onset schizophrenia: support for a progressive neurodevelopmental disorder. *International Journal of Developmental Neuroscience, 29*(3), 251–258.

Reich, W. (2000). Diagnostic interview for children and adolescents (DICA). *Journal of the American Academy of Child & Adolescent Psychiatry, 39*(1), 59–66.

Robins, D. L., Fein, D., Barton, M. L., & Green, J. A. (2001). The Modified Checklist for Autism in Toddlers: an initial study investigating the early detection of autism and pervasive developmental disorders. *Journal of Autism and Developmental Disorders, 31*(2), 131–144.

Rossignol, D. A., Genuis, S. J., & Frye, R. E. (2014). Environmental toxicants and autism spectrum disorders: a systematic review. *Translational Psychiatry, 4*(2), e360.

Rutter, M. (1972). Childhood schizophrenia reconsidered. *Journal of Autism and Childhood Schizophrenia*, 2(3), 315–337.

Rutter, M. (1999). Autism: two-way interplay between research and clinical work. *Journal of Child Psychology and Psychiatry and Allied Disciplines*, 40(2), 169–188.

Rutter, M., Andersen–Wood, L., Beckett, C., Bredenkamp, D., Castle, J., Groothues, C., Kreppner, J., Keaveney, L., Lord, C., & O'Connor, T. G. (1999). Quasi-autistic patterns following severe early global privation. *Journal of Child Psychology and Psychiatry and Allied Disciplines*, 40(4), 537–549.

Rutter, M., Le Couteur, A., & Lord, C. (2003). Autism Diagnostic Interview—Revised. *Western Psychological Services*.

Schumann, C. M., Hamstra, J., Goodlin–Jones, B. L., Lotspeich, L. J., Kwon, H., Buonocore, M. H., Lammers, C. R., Reiss, A. L., & Amaral, D. G. (2004). The amygdala is enlarged in children but not adolescents with autism; the hippocampus is enlarged at all ages. *Journal of Neuroscience*, 24(28), 6392–6401.

Schumann, C. M., Bloss, C. S., Barnes, C. C., Wideman, G. M., Carper, R. A., Akshoomoff, N., Pierce, K., Hagler, D., Schork, N., Lord, C., & Courchesne, E. (2010). Longitudinal magnetic resonance imaging study of cortical development through early childhood in autism. *Journal of Neuroscience*, 30(12), 4419–4427.

Shaffer, D., Fisher, P., Lucas, C. P., Dulcan, M. K., & Schwab–Stone, M. E. (2000). NIMH Diagnostic Interview Schedule for Children Version IV (NIMH DISC-IV): description, differences from previous versions, and reliability of some common diagnoses. *Journal of the American Academy of Child & Adolescent Psychiatry*, 39(1), 28–38.

Simonoff, E., Pickles, A., Charman, T., Chandler, S., Loucas, T., & Baird, G. (2008). Psychiatric disorders in children with autism spectrum disorders: prevalence, comorbidity, and associated factors in a population-derived sample. *Journal of the American Academy of Child & Adolescent Psychiatry*, 47, 921–929.

Sinclair, J. (1992). Bridging the gaps: an inside out view of autism (or, do you know what I don't know?) In E. Schopler & G. B., Mesibov (Eds.), *Individuals with autism* (pp. 294–302). Plenum Press.

Skagerberg, E., Di Ceglie, D., & Carmichael, P. (2015). Brief report: Autistic features in children and adolescents with gender dysphoria. *Journal of Autism and Developmental Disorders*, 45(8), 2628–2632.

Skuse, D., Warrington, R., Bishop, D., Chowdhury, U., Lau, J., Mandy, W., & Place, M. (2004). The developmental, dimensional and diagnostic interview (3di): a novel computerized assessment for autism spectrum disorders. *Journal of the American Academy of Child & Adolescent Psychiatry*, 43(5), 548–558.

South, M., & Rodgers, J. (2017). Sensory, emotional and cognitive contributions to anxiety in autism spectrum disorders. *Frontiers in Human Neuroscience*, 11, 20.

Sparrow, S. S., Cicchetti, D. V., & Saulnier, C. A. (2016). *Vineland adaptive behavior scales (Vineland-3)* (3rd ed.). Pearson.

Strömland, K., Nordin, V., Miller, M., Akerström, B., & Gillberg, C. (1994). Autism in thalidomide embryopathy: a population study. *Developmental Medicine & Child Neurology*, 36(4), 351–356.

Surén, P., Stoltenberg, C., Bresnahan, M., Hirtz, D., Lie, K. K., Lipkin, W. I., Magnus, P., Reichborn–Kjennerud, T., Schjolberg, S., Susser, E., Øyen, A. S., Li, L., & Hornig, M. (2013). Early growth patterns in children with autism. *Epidemiology*, 24(5), 660.

Takaoka, K., & Takata, T. (2003). Catatonia in childhood and adolescence. *Psychiatry and Clinical Neurosciences*, 57(2), 129–137.

Tandon, R., Nasrallah, H. A., & Keshavan, M. S. (2009). Schizophrenia, 'just the facts' 4. Clinical features and conceptualization. *Schizophrenia Research*, 110(1–3), 1–23.

Tick, B., Bolton, P., Happé, F., Rutter, M., & Rijsdijk, F. (2016). Heritability of autism spectrum disorders: a meta-analysis of twin studies. *Journal of Child Psychology and Psychiatry*, 57(5), 585–595.

Treffert, D. A. (2009). The savant syndrome: an extraordinary condition. A synopsis: past, present, future. *Philosophical Transactions of the Royal Society B: Biological Sciences*, 364(1522), 1351–1357.

Van Der Miesen, A. I., Hurley, H., & De Vries, A. L. (2016). Gender dysphoria and autism spectrum disorder: a narrative review. *International Review of Psychiatry*, 28(1), 70–80.

Velikonja, T., Fett, A. K., & Velthorst, E. (2019). Patterns of nonsocial and social cognitive functioning in adults with autism spectrum disorder: a systematic review and meta-analysis. *Journal of the American Medical Association Psychiatry*, 76(2), 135–151.

Volkmar, F., Siegel, M., Woodbury–Smith, M., King, B., McCracken, J., & State, M. (2014). Practice parameter for the assessment and treatment of children and adolescents with autism spectrum disorder. *Journal of the American Academy of Child & Adolescent Psychiatry*, 53(2), 237–257.

Volkmar, F. R., Cicchetti, D. V., Dykens, E., Sparrow, S. S., Leckman, J. F., & Cohen, D. J. (1988). An evaluation of the autism behavior checklist. *Journal of Autism and Developmental Disorders*, 18(1), 81–97.

Westwood, H., & Tchanturia, K. (2017). Autism spectrum disorder in anorexia nervosa: an updated literature review. *Current Psychiatry Reports*, 19(7), 41.

White, S. W., Oswald, D., Ollendick, T., & Scahill, L. (2009). Anxiety in children and adolescents with autism spectrum disorders. *Clinical Psychology Review*, 29(3), 216–229. https://doi.org/10.1016/j.cpr.2009.01.003

Wilson, R. B., McCracken, J. T., Rinehart, N. J., & Jeste, S. S. (2018). What's missing in autism spectrum disorder motor assessments? *Journal of Neurodevelopmental Disorders*, 10(1), 33.

Wing, L. (1981). Asperger's syndrome: a clinical account. *Psychological Medicine*, 11(1), 115–129.

Wing, L., & Gould, J. (1979). Severe impairments of social interaction and associated abnormalities in children: epidemiology and classification. *Journal of Autism and Developmental Disorders*, 9(1), 11–29.

Wing, L., Leekam, S. R., Libby, S. J., Gould, J., & Larcombe, M. (2002). The diagnostic interview for social and communication disorders: background, inter-rater reliability and clinical use. *Journal of Child Psychology and Psychiatry*, 43(3), 307–325.

Wing, L., & Shah, A. (2000). Catatonia in autistic spectrum disorders. *British Journal of Psychiatry*, 176 (4), 357–62. https://doi.org/10.1192/bjp.176.4.357

Woodbury–Smith, M., & Scherer, S. W. (2018). Progress in the genetics of autism spectrum disorder. *Developmental Medicine & Child Neurology*, 60(5), 445–451.

World Health Organization. (2018). *ICD-11 for mortality and morbidity statistics*. https://www.who.int/classifications/icd/en/

Zhou, Y., Zeidman, P., Wu, S., Razi, A., Chen, C., Yang, L., Zou, J., Wang, G., Wang, H., & Friston, K. J. (2018). Altered intrinsic and extrinsic connectivity in schizophrenia. *NeuroImage: Clinical*, 17, 704–716.

CHAPTER 5

TOURETTE AND LEARNING IMPAIRMENTS

5.1 CHRONIC TICS AND TOURETTE

5.1.1 Diagnostic concepts

TICS are defined and distinguished from other disorders of movement in Chapter 2, Section 2.1. They are brief, sudden, stereotyped, involuntary or semi-voluntary acts.

DSM-5 and ICD-11 both include chronic tics and Tourette as neurodevelopmental disorders (American Psychiatric Association, 2013; WHO, 2018). Neurology and psychiatry both claim them, and they are often accompanied by problems of mental health. They are visible and audible problems, and quite easy to recognize. Because of this clarity, it has long been plain that there is a continuum from single, transient tics that are not necessarily noticed by anyone, to life-altering conditions of multiple tics affecting speech as well as movements. The psychopathological definitions are therefore based wholly on their extent and persistence.

Persistent motor or vocal tic disorder is defined by the tics themselves, which must have lasted for a year or more, and be limited to *either* motor *or* vocal, and have started before the age of 18 years. *Tourette disorder* describes the presence of *both* multiple motor *and* one or more vocal tics (not necessarily all at the same time).

5.1.2 Recognition

Marked fluctuations of severity and frequency of tics are the rule. Clinicians assessing should not form their judgements solely on a single period of observations. Standard rating scales are available. The Yale Global Tic Severity Scale (YGTSS) (Leckman et al., 1989) is widely used and is recommended. It includes clinical ratings of the varieties of tics and their severity, frequency, interference with life, and overall impairment. Clinical severity of coexistent obsessions can be rated with the Children's Yale–Brown Obsessive-Compulsive Scale (CY-BOCS) (Scahill et al., 1997), of which there are also self-report and parent versions and a form designed for those with coexistent autism spectrum disorder (ASD). Attention deficit hyperactivity disorder (ADHD) scales are widely available (Chapter 3, Section 3.2).

The premonitory urges outlined in Chapter 2, Section 2.2.3.4 can be described and monitored with a short self-report measure: the Premonitory Urge for Tics Scale (PUTS) (Woods et al., 2005).

5.1.3 Prevalence

There is a continuum of severity, so estimates of rates in the population vary with the level of severity chosen to define a disorder. Prevalence has been examined with a meta-analysis (Knight et al., 2012). This summary of 17 studies indicated that Tourette disorder is diagnosed in about 1% of boys and 0.25% of girls. The diagnosis of 'transient tics' affects around 4% of boys and 3% of girls. Rates in adults are lower. These figures are possibly an underestimation of current rates. They are based on an earlier DSM-IV definition which required 'experiencing significant disability attributable to their condition'. This criterion has been dropped from subsequent versions and DSM-5 defines as given in Section 5.1.1. In other disorders, such as ADHD, a requirement for disability has set a significant limit on rates.

5.1.4 Course over time

The frequency and intensity of bursts of tics often follow a trajectory of increasing through later childhood, peaking at 13 to 15 years, and declining thereafter. An optimistic approach to counselling is therefore reasonable. However, one should not promise that all will be well by the time they are grown up. To do so is to invite disappointment and distrust if it turns out not to be the case. Adverse pointers to outcome probably include an early onset before the age of 6 years, high anxiety levels, low IQ, and possibly a lack of appropriate support. Medical treatment (see Chapter 7, Section 7.3) can indeed suppress tics, but there is no evidence that I know of to suggest that the natural history is modified by treatment. There is still much to be done by education and by helping the individual to cope (Chapter 8, Section 8.4).

At the extreme, tics can develop into a picture memorably described by Gilles de la Tourette in 1885. The vocal tics turn into foul utterances (coprolalia), the movements into obscene or violent gestures, and there may be an uncontrolled sudden repetition of what another person has just said or done. Sudden interruptions of speech can be mistaken for stammering. So extreme a picture is rare, but its dramatic quality has led to depiction in plays and films that can be very worrying and stigmatizing to affected people. The term 'Tourette syndrome' has found a place in popular discourse and in professional classification schemes. It no longer necessarily refers to the full picture originally described, but just to the combination of multiple motor and vocal tics (Robertson et al., 2009).

Extremely intense tics can be dangerous, both through self-injury and through sudden violent movements to others. Their semi-voluntary nature allows for children and adolescents both to be blamed unfairly and also (less commonly) for them to use the diagnosis as an excuse for misbehaviour. Most cases, however, are mild and need not have a major impact on quality of life. Much of their impact is cosmetic, together with the effects on self-image and social relationships that result from the reactions of other people.

Associated problems of mental health are usually the most severe aspects. Coexistent disorders are very frequent, especially obsessional-compulsive disorder (OCD), ADHD, and anxiety. The reasons are not entirely known.

5.1.5 Coexistent obsessions and ADHD

OCD in the presence of chronic tics is different in several ways from other types of OCD. It is more likely to be associated with early onset of tics, male gender, and a poor response to anti-obsessional medication. The pattern of obsessions is also different from those in simple OCD. They are marked particularly by preoccupations with symmetry, counting, and rituals about repeating and arranging. Perhaps tic-related OCD needs to be thought of as a distinct neurodevelopmental condition, but the genetic and longitudinal evidence is equivocal and decisions about therapy in the condition are not (yet) specific. Pauls (2008) argued for genetic overlap between Tourette and OCD, and the point is generally accepted. It has, however, been difficult to tie down precisely. Genome-wide association studies (G-WAS) have been applied in both conditions, but without a statistically significant finding, so far, of common genes (Yang et al., 2019). Studies with large enough numbers of cases to detect overlap are awaited.

ADHD features are present in about half of children with Tourette. The full reasons are not clear. Sometimes the Tourette only comes to light because the ADHD has created a prior need for assessment. Sometimes (as described in Chapter 3, Section 3.5), the assessment has falsely described multiple tics as restlessness and therefore made an artefactual link with ADHD. Both conditions have genetic and prenatal risks, but the evidence at present is contradictory about whether those risks are shared between the conditions. The combined condition does have a worse outlook for social adjustment than Tourette alone, but the enhanced risks are essentially those of ADHD. Treating one does not necessarily help the other. Indeed, stimulant drug treatment of ADHD carries a (small) risk of worsening tics.

5.1.6 Risks for chronic tics

Genetic risk factors are surely involved. Concordance between twins is higher for the monozygotic (around 77%) than for the dizygotic (around 30%) twin (Price et al., 1985).

Some individual genes have been identified: for example, *IMMP2* (which codes for inner mitochondrial membrane peptidase 2), *CNTNAP2* (coding for contactin-associated protein-like 2, *SLITRK 1* (coding for SLIT and NTRK-like 1), *NLGN4X* (neuroligin-4, X-linked), and *HDC* (histidine decarboxylase) (see Deng et al., 2012). A recent large study by Yu et al. (2019) carried out a meta-analysis of G-WAS and constructed a polygenic risk score. The score identified nearly all the heritable influences and correlated well with the worst-ever tic severity. It could well prove clinically useful in predicting the likelihood of progression to severe impairment in individuals, and in clarifying the reasons for associations with other heritable conditions.

Environmental factors are often invoked, especially infective and immune conditions (see Chapter 7), and perinatal adversity. The causal roles are not clearly established. Increases in severity are often triggered by impactful life events.

Brain changes, studied with neuroimaging, are not totally consistent. They have given some support to frontal and striatal changes in children with Tourette disorder. White matter deep to the orbital and medial prefrontal cortex has been reported to be reduced, and grey matter to be increased in the thalamus and hypothalamus (Greene et al., 2017)

5.2 LEARNING IMPAIRMENTS

Several persisting problems in development can be conceptualized as difficulties in learning of various kinds. Motor skills, spoken language (and signing in the deaf), written language, and calculation are considered here. They have in common a continuum of ability, and most of them have a definition of impairment referenced by age norms rather than effect on social function. Impairments of the complex sets of skills comprising intellectual capacity will be considered separately.

5.2.1 Developmental coordination disorder (DCD)

Problems of muscular coordination can be rather persistent and should be recognized whether they are present with other neurodevelopmental conditions (which is usually the case) or as an isolated difficulty. They represent an immaturity of motor development, in which the individual is behaving like a younger person in showing poor coordination and overflow movements. Combining simple movements into integrated and purposive actions is impaired. Balance and spatial awareness are often poor. Clumsiness in large-scale movements of limbs can amount to knocking into other people or things and to ineptness in games and physical pursuits. Abilities to catch objects and to ride a bicycle are achieved later than for other children. Fine movements can be uncontrolled to the point of inability to manage dressing oneself or to control writing and drawing. Motor milestones have often been delayed.

The aforementioned features can be present in any of the neurodevelopmental disorders and are sometimes called 'soft neurological signs'. No specific patterns have been found with specific implications for causes or psychological concomitants. Other kinds of developmental problems, such as specific language and computational difficulties, are often present, but only inconsistently so. The effects of persisting clumsiness (Chapter 2, Section 2.2) include restriction of peer relationships and self-image, with anxiety often prominent.

5.2.1.1 *Diagnosis and terminology*

The diagnosis of developmental coordination disorder (DCD) is not based only on the aforementioned neurological features. In common with many other neurodevelopmental conditions, there also needs to be evidence that the features are severe enough to cause problems in everyday life and are not attributable to cerebral palsy, a muscular dystrophy, global developmental delay, or the other movement disorders outlined in Box 1.1. Furthermore, there needs to be evidence that the onset of symptoms is in the early developmental period. The detailed criteria are set out in DSM-5 (American Psychiatric Association, 2013; p. 74).

The diagnostic terminology is disputed, but DCD is generally preferred. 'Developmental dyspraxia' is often used as a partial synonym or alternative for DCD, but this can be confusing. It invites confusion with adult dyspraxia, which usually refers to an acquired condition in association with brain damage. 'Dyspraxia' is also sometimes used to describe the association of DCD with problems of executive dysfunction. The two often go together. It is not always clear in the individual case whether clumsiness or impulsiveness is primary. Certainly, a lack of motor coordination is frequently present at the same time as difficulties in remembering instructions, organizing one's time, respecting deadlines, and carrying out complex tasks involving several steps in sequence.

Not surprisingly, therefore, ADHD is a common 'comorbidity'—in large part because it simply reflects the way that the criteria for the two conditions overlap. It is also possible for the impulsiveness of ADHD to mimic a problem in motor control. Children who appear clumsy because they are hasty and uncontrolled in everything they do need to be distinguished from those who are uncoordinated even when they are giving themselves sufficient time to carry out motor tasks competently.

The term 'DAMP'—Disorder of Attention, Motor Control, and Perception—is often used to highlight the similarity and frequent coexistence of conditions. The linked concept of 'ESSENCE'—Early Symptomatic Syndromes Eliciting Neurodevelopmental Clinical Examinations—is not a diagnosis but an umbrella term conveying the same idea of multiple, related, and often coexisting difficulties (Gillberg et al., 2013). Whether the clinician should use such a general term or a specific diagnosis will depend on the purpose and the context. The umbrella term should not be seen as an effective description of an individual child, but as an indicator of the need for investigating a range of possible problems and reassessing as the young people develop and change.

Assessment of very clumsy children should include a neurological examination to detect any of the medical disorders listed as causes of clumsiness in Table 1.1. Measurement of creatinine kinase levels in serum can help to exclude Duchenne muscular dystrophy. Asymmetry and progression of motor signs are not part of DCD and should trigger specialist neurological evaluation and DNA testing.

5.2.2 Developmental language disorder (or delay) (DLD)

The section on the development and pathology of communication (Chapter 2, Section 2.8) has indicated a variety of ways in which children's language may be delayed. There are also various possible causes. Language delay in young children may be secondary to limited exposure (e.g. where the home language is not the main one of the culture); to medical conditions (e.g. acquired epileptic aphasia); to other brain abnormalities (e.g. auditory processing deficit); to sensory impairments (e.g. deafness); or to motor impairments of the organs of speech (e.g. cerebral palsies, verbal dyspraxia). All these should be considered in the early stages of evaluating why a child is not communicating as well as their peers.

The concept of developmental language disorder (DLD) arose to describe impairments that were not wholly secondary to defined causes such as those just mentioned. It used to imply more—that it was 'disproportionate to' general intelligence—but this restriction has largely lost its importance because of evidence that language develops in similar ways whatever the exact level of IQ (Bishop, 2003). If specific language impairment (SLI) were considered to require assistance only if defined relative to IQ, the need for services could be underestimated. SLI is nowadays usually used to mean DLD in the absence of intellectual disability.

DLD is characterized by persistent deficits in understanding or production of language or both. All the aspects of language delineated can be slow to develop. The mean length of utterance (usual number of morphemes) is a simple guide to overall level. Uneven development of cognitive skills is very common and does not justify a scientific distinction between 'delay' and 'disorder'. Knowledge and use of words are immature; problems with grammar lead to an oversimplified sentence structure. There can also be problems in discourse, for instance in building sentences to form a coherent narrative or to keep up connected conversation.

Evidence should preferably come from standardized tests showing a significant discrepancy from the level of language expected for the age. Such tests are available for many spoken languages. The *Clinical evaluation of language fundamentals* (fifth edition) (CELF-5) (Wiig et al., 2013) is probably the most widely applied. It is well standardized, but mostly on children in the USA. A review by Dockrell and Marshall (2015) explains many limitations of the tests. They need to be appreciated by clinicians seeking to interpret them as evidence for a developmental problem. A language is not unitary, but includes a variety of language systems, some amounting to dialects. Children and young people are often being tested on Standard English when they are, in fact, acquiring English in a local form or as a second language.

A formal diagnosis adds that the difficulties arise in early development, are not the result of a medical condition, and cannot be attributed solely to intellectual disability (American Psychiatric Association, 2013).

Signed language can also be affected by identifiable forms of pathology. Some children brought up in signing environments can show analogous linguistic problems to those using speech. One may recognize hesitant and effortful signed production, single-sign utterances, absence of syntactical markings, and disordered grammar such as errors in spatialized markings and problems in sentence comprehension (Mason et al., 2010). Problems analogous to stuttering can also be recognized from the hesitations and repetitions of hand and finger movements, or from jerky signs, involuntary interjections, and extra movements.

Children and young people with SLI have above-expected rates of DCD and low achievement on cognitive tests, including those of attention and executive function.

5.2.2.1 *Prevalence*

Most official estimates of the prevalence of DLD indicate some 6–8% of young schoolchildren to be affected. Surveys have been variable and dependent on the exact measures chosen. A survey of kindergarten children in the Midwest USA indicated a rate of 7.4% (8% for boys, 6% for girls) for those having language delays that were not attributable to sensory problems or to low IQ (Tomblin et al., 1997).

5.2.2.2 *Course over time*

Language difficulties in preschool and elementary schoolchildren tend to persist. As a group, they consistently lag behind their peers, not only in early development but, to a similar extent, during later childhood and adolescence (Conti–Ramsden et al., 2012). Predicting the course for individuals is much harder, but those with severe or long-lasting delays, literacy problems, and/or low non-verbal IQ are particularly at risk. In adult life, employment opportunities are restricted. Consequences in later adolescence and adult life include hindered communication, social participation, and academic achievement. Even those whose language difficulties do not persist can encounter these problems. Many find fulfilling training in vocational rather than academic further education, and many succeed in creative professions.

Mental health is often compromised (Yew and O'Kearney, 2013). Oppositional disorders and conduct problems are particularly common when the expression of language is delayed. Very often, the mechanism is the frustration and anger involved in being unable to express oneself, and the irritated reaction of other children and adults in having to concentrate to understand. Promotion of resilience and coping skills is likely to help. Assisted communication may be needed in severe cases—even signs to convey immediate needs and feelings. Inner language is also one of the ways in which children learn to instruct themselves in aspects of self-control and the regulation of emotions. Accordingly, language delays may not only increase the likelihood of miscommunication and conflict with others, but also increase the intensity of emotional reactions to them.

The risk for ADHD is nearly doubled, and some of this increase in risk may be attributable to similarities in the brain circuits involved in language and in attention impulse control. ASD is also closely associated with language difficulties.

Problems in understanding other people's language also raise the risks of mental health difficulties—in this case, especially of social problems and depression. By adolescence, there is a particular risk for developing psychosis-like symptoms (Sullivan et al., 2016).

These behavioural and emotional changes in language disorders are so common that they are often the reason for referral to mental health services, even when the language difficulties have not been recognized. Clinicians involved in mental health therefore need to be vigilant for these (as other) developmental delays.

5.2.2.3 *Associated disorders*

Other conditions affecting language include autism, ADHD, Landau–Kleffner syndrome, selective mutism, and social communication disorder (a DSM-5 diagnosis, described in Chapter 4, Section 4.1.3.2, and overlapping strongly with pragmatic language disorder in ICD-11).

5.2.2.3.1 *Pragmatic language disorder*

Pragmatic language disorder can be a serious barrier to communication, even when vocabulary and grammar are intact. Children with the condition have problems with the meaning behind what other people say. They tend to have difficulty understanding messages that involve abstract ideas, such as idioms, metaphors, and irony. They may struggle to produce messages that are socially appropriate for a given listener or context. They can be verbose and may come to appear uninterested in communicating with others. The resulting social difficulties are so marked that they can produce an impression of ASD. In ASD, however, the repetitiveness and rigidity extend beyond communication in speech. Pragmatic language difficulties can coexist with other language problems, but typically do not.

5.2.2.3.2 *Selective mutism*

Selective mutism involves a failure to speak in some social situations but not in others. Typically, children will speak at home but be mute outside, or communicate only in whispers or with a few selected adults. The condition is not common but is more frequent in children for whom the language at home is different from that of the neighbourhood. Social anxiety is often present as well, and the later outcome carries substantial risks for anxiety and depression (Steinhausen et al., 2006).

Treatment usually involves methods of reducing anxiety, including desensitization, and anti-anxiety medication may have a small part to play. Accordingly, selective mutism is usually classified with the anxiety disorders rather than those of language.

Nevertheless, many affected children do show abnormalities of language even in situations where they speak freely. It is likely that any disorder of speech or language can generate embarrassment and anxiety about speaking, with consequent avoidance. Language problems should be considered from the outset and monitored over time.

Acquired epileptic aphasia (Landau–Kleffner syndrome) is described in Chapter 6, Section 6.2.

5.2.2.3.3 *Prevalence*

There is so much variability in published rates of language disorder that no overall prevalence figure can be given to guide the provision of services. Many authorities quote rates of around 5% of preschool and elementary schoolchildren. 'Rates of disorder' will naturally depend on how severe a problem has to be in order to count as a 'disorder'. Two or more standard deviations below the mean on a valid norm-referenced test would nearly always imply a substantial problem for development, but smaller deviations from the expected may still imply a need for help. (Indeed, need for help, as indexed by referral, may be more heritable and more predictive than scores on standardized tests.) Validated norm-referenced tests, furthermore, may not be available for children from cultural and linguistic minorities. Low scores can reflect different problems, such as poor vision, poor hearing, fatigue, or emotional state at the time of testing. Also, such tests may not pick up difficulties that appear only in demanding contexts such as rapid conversation in distracting circumstances. Test scores will usually need to be supplemented by a knowledgeable person's observation of the individual's language function.

5.2.2.4 *Risks*

5.2.2.4.1 *Genetic inheritance*

Language problems tend to run in families, and genetic inheritance plays a part. Heritability estimates from comparisons of monozygotic and dizygotic twins give varying results. Most indicate heritability of 0.5 or more, but the age of the children studied and the methods of ascertainment influenced the results considerably (Bishop & Hayiou–Thomas, 2008). A few rare mutations with large effect have been discovered in investigations of people with specific language impairment. FOXP2 is the best known. This is a regulatory gene on chromosome 17 that encodes a transcription factor regulating the expression of many other genes in many parts of the body, including the brain, lungs, and oesophagus. It is expressed widely within the brain, including in parts of the cortex, striatum, and cerebellum. Its role in language problems was discovered in one family in which a three-generation pedigree (and one unrelated individual) showed an unusual form of verbal dyspraxia and proved to have other linguistic and cognitive problems (Lai et al., 2001). According to current knowledge, it probably plays little part in generating common forms of language difficulty, and its effects are by no means confined to the development of language.

Other genes associated with language problems include *CNTNAP2* on chromosome 7. It codes for the protein CASPR2, a member of the neurexin family which is involved in the attachment of presynaptic neuronal membranes to postsynaptic ones. *CNTNAP2* has been implicated in many different neurodevelopmental disorders (Newbury et al., 2010). *ATP2C2* (coding for a calcium-transporting ATPase) and *CMIP* (coding for *c*MAF-inducing protein) are both on chromosome 16. Their association is essentially with performance on tests of memory for non-words rather than any particular pattern of language disorder.

It seems that the most important genetic contribution to language impairment is, like that in similar conditions, the product of a highly complex set of many genes interacting with each other and with the environment.

5.2.2.4.2 *Environmental risks*

Environmental risks exist, but are unlikely to be sufficient to cause lasting impairment in the child unless there is also deprivation in the rest of their environment. Restricted language at home may well be associated with restricted vocabulary in young children, and with oversimplified grammar, but the interpretation of this is complicated by the likelihood that both parents' and children's language are affected by the same genetic variations.

5.2.2.4.3 *Brain changes*

Verbal short-term memory has often been linked to language function, but children with DLD tend to show a rather widespread set of impairments of executive function rather than one specific problem (Henry & Botting, 2017). Language, attention, and memory are all considered to be functions of large-scale neurocognitive networks and distributed processing (Mesulam, 1990). Their dysfunctions tend to cluster together. Attempts to discover which circuits are primary in disorders of language have not yet led to a clear taxonomy on the basis of neuropsychological deviations, or to useful prescriptive education.

Groups of children with DLD show a wide variety of neurological and neuroimaging deviations from typical development (Trauner et al., 2000). A developmental delay in left-sided frontal and parietal regions is probably the commonest finding.

Neuroimaging techniques have been applied to individual diagnosis. The most robust predictions, however, have derived from machine-based learning techniques (e.g. support vector machine) and need more evidence of generalizability. They are, nevertheless, improving all the time. Their predictive value does not depend on showing localization of lesions and could, in the near future, become sufficiently predictive to acquire a role in routine investigation.

5.2.3   Specific learning difficulty (disorder) (SLD)

By contrast with developmental language and motor problems, some problems are only apparent in subjects to be learned at school.

5.2.3.1 *Reading and writing problems*

'Dyslexia' and 'dysgraphia' are contested terms—people use them in different ways, and care is needed in their use. Poor literacy can arise for several reasons that need to be assessed:

- Lack of opportunity (e.g. non-attendance at school)
- Lack of instruction (e.g. impoverished education)
- Unfamiliar language
- Sensory impairments (e.g. low visual acuity)
- Motor problems (e.g. clumsiness or poor posture affecting writing)
- Low motivation (e.g. poor self-esteem)
- Spoken language impairment (e.g. in production and comprehension)
- Cognitive disabilities (e.g. intellectual deficit)

All these should be considered in an assessment of a child who is not reading as expected. The aspect that is most argued over is whether a diagnosis such as developmental dyslexia (or, in DSM-5, 'specific learning disorder with impairment in reading') should only be entertained if IQ is within the normal range. Scientifically, there is little to justify the practice. Specific dyslexia is not stable over time (Wright et al., 1996) and does not predict underlying psychological changes better than simple inability to read (Bishop, 2015). Nevertheless, many clinicians and educators still use the restrictive concept and it governs much biological research. The term 'reading backwardness' is used when the reading age is substantially less than the chronological age (e.g. by two or more standard deviations). 'Reading retardation' or specific reading impairment (SRI) implies that the reading age is substantially less than the chronological age *and* the measured mental age or IQ (Conti-Ramsden et al., 2012).

Some authorities have restricted SRI to those with supposedly distinctive symptoms such as reversing letters when writing or right–left disorientation. Research, however, has largely discredited the notion that these 'distinctive' features cluster into a syndrome or that they are different from the kinds of mistake that are made by typically developing children in the early stages of learning or by those with the broader problems of reading backwardness. Problems in perceiving and remembering sounds in words characterize poor readers as a class, not a neurologically defined subgroup within them (Stanovich, 1994). Indeed, many education authorities, in recent years, have rejected the validity of distinguishing SRI or dyslexia from poor reading altogether. This argument is strongest when it points out the undesirability of making good general intelligence a condition for receiving remedial instruction. It can also be unrealistic for expensive, standardized measures to be a prerequisite for the recognition of problems and access to extra help in education. There are many parts of the world where educational psychology is available only to the privileged. Even so, many education systems do require the approval of an educational psychologist for access to special help. Clinicians may then find themselves acting as advocates for their patients in negotiating with school systems.

5.2.3.1.1 *Prevalence*

Reported rates vary, not only between countries but also between males and females, and deprived inner-city areas and more privileged areas. Severe decoding difficulties (i.e. more than two standard deviations below the mean on a test of single-word reading) affected about 4% of schoolchildren in England (Snowling et al., 2009)

5.2.3.1.2 *Risks*

Family, twin, multiple regression, and adoption studies have concurred in establishing a strong role for genetic inheritance (Gayan & Olson, 1999). Twin studies, for instance, have suggested that about 60–70% of the variability between people in reading words can be attributed to genetic influences, with possibly 30% attributable to the environment that both twins share (including some of the effects of schooling), and the remaining 10% to individual factors (including chance) (e.g. Harlaar et al., 2014).

The hope for research has therefore been to find genes of large and specific influence that could illuminate the operation of neurological and psychological risk and be useful predictors of reading disability. So far, however, there has been little sign of anything of the sort emerging. Indeed, the general finding for neurodevelopmental conditions— that nearly all the genetic influences, considered singly, are of small effect—applies to written language, too. Linkage analyses have already generated findings in chromosome regions 1p34–p36, 6p21–p22, 15q21, and 18q11. They have been known for several years (Schumacher et al., 2007), and some are linked to neuronal migration. There is, however, little evidence for distinct associations with neurocognitive alterations (Bishop et al., 2015).

In summary, genetic analyses have not added to the credibility of a syndrome of dyslexia. They do support the idea that some children who are slow in learning to read have inherited risks. Affected children can usually be recognized with a simple test of nonword repetition, and they also often have difficulties in the development of spoken as well as written language.

Theories of the neurocognitive bases abound. They have included lack of phonetic awareness, deficient phonological short-term memory, visual problems in recognition of alphabetic characters, deficits in naming speed, limitations in speed of auditory processing, problems in automatizing processes such as visual–phonetic integration, poor directional sense, right–left discrimination problems, poor finger recognition, and a changing pattern of any one of these being salient, depending on developmental stage. All of these have received some support in a large literature. Many of them have proved to be associated with poor reading. None of the single-process formulations, however, has led to an uncontested place in the pathogenesis or to a robust system of subtypes (Fletcher & Morris, 2014). The strongest support has come for problems in matching phonemes (i.e. the sounds of a spoken word) to graphemes (i.e. the smallest functional units of a writing system) (Snowling, 1980). It is also reasonable to suppose a variety of different underlying impairments.

Anomalous patterns of cerebral dominance have long been invoked as brain causes of reading difficulties. On the basis of hand preference and coordination, both left- and mixed-handedness are more common in reading disabilities—but so is extreme right-handedness (Annett, 1998).

Some workers in educational psychology still make considerable use of right-brain versus left-brain explanations of educational difficulties. This is full of traps. The two sides of the brain are specialized, not hierarchical. It is usually mistaken to classify an individual as a 'left-brain' or 'right-brain' type. Even if an individual has greatly superior visuospatial skills and is backward in language, they will still be using the left hemisphere for the comprehension of syntax and production of speech (see 'Localized structural lesions', Chapter 6, Section 6.6). The concept of a right-brain type might be useful in specific circumstances, for instance for someone using a right-brain type of cognitive strategy, in preference to a left-brain type, for tasks that could be accomplished in either way. This is seldom what is meant in practice. It is nevertheless possible that it applies to a few individuals (e.g. those with 'deep dyslexia') who may rely on right-hemisphere processing (Coltheart, 2000).

Many neuroimaging studies have compared patterns of brain activation in good and poor readers. In skilled readers, there is no centre for reading. There is no reason that evolution should have developed one in brains: reading is acquired culturally and has only been around for about 5,000 years. It seems that a range of predominantly left-sided brain areas are activated during reading the English language, including the inferior frontal gyrus, temporoparietal cortex, and occipitotemporal regions (Price, 2012). In poor readers of English, there tends to be less activation in those areas, and rather more in areas more typically associated with visual recognition or articulation of speech (Martin et al., 2015).

Correspondingly, no single neuropsychological intervention has been proved to add much to practice and encouragement in reading. Children with reading difficulties have, for many years, been subjected to training programmes involving non-linguistic activities such as greater use of the less favoured hand or foot, catching bean bags, breathing through masks, solving jigsaws, or doing somersaults. They have not helped much (Burns et al., 2016). This does not mean that 'dyslexia is a myth'. It remains important to understand that a variety of inherited and acquired influences on brain development can affect an individual's literacy separately from the quality of instruction and stimulation that they receive.

The neuropsychological evidence on letter–sound (graphene–phoneme) correspondence has been influential in guiding educators towards phonic techniques in early reading (Kearns et al., 2019). It is often advised that if little progress is being made, a shift to practice in visual recognition of words is in order. It is, however, not yet empirically clear that this recommendation is any better than an enhanced focus on encouragement and practical support to read material in which the individual is interested.

5.2.3.1.3 *Management*

Effective programmes for pupils with impaired reading are characterised by being structured, sequential, cumulative and thorough. Pupils also benefit from phonetics teaching, overlearning and a multi-sensory approach that makes the link between sound, symbol and written form. Classroom interventions can be effectively reinforced by home visits and summer schools.

5.2.3.1.4 *Associated problems*

Many young people will be referred for specialist help (not usually to psychiatry) because of unexplained difficulties in learning. Mental health services also need to be able to detect learning difficulties not already recognized. These difficulties can have strong influences for the worse by generating emotional and behavioural problems.

Reading difficulties are often accompanied by disruptive behaviour. The association continues into adult life, when the association largely derives from environmental influences; notably through low self-esteem and consequent antisocial and criminal behaviour, and poor economic prospects (Trzesniewski et al., 2006). The consequences for emotional life are just as strong (review by Livingston et al., 2018). Low self-esteem, anxiety and depression become more marked through adolescence and mark a low quality of adult life. Early identification of problems is helpful to many. Many say that a diagnosis of 'dyslexia' has been valuable to them. Notwithstanding the reservations expressed above about the scientific validity of the concept, it can be a welcome relief to many young people and their families, by lightening the burden of stigma and the inferences of stupidity or laziness. It can also be a trigger to sensible management. Electronic presentation of written material, audiobooks and readers can all help mastery. Recognition and valuing of other skills are keys to a more positive self-image.

5.2.3.2 *Difficulties with handwriting and calculating*

Problems such as visual-spatial deficit, dyscalculia, dysgraphia, spatial disorientation, and dyspraxia are frequent, and disruptive to emotional development because of the academic problems that they entail. They are sometimes regarded together as 'non-verbal learning disability (NVLD)'. The category, however, is very heterogeneous and has not been included in DSM or ICD lists of disorders.

5.2.3.2.1 *Handwriting problems*

Handwriting problems can result from many causes:

- Abnormalities of grip and posture may need correcting.
- ADHD failures of organization and persistence may be responsible for messy presentation of written work.
- Poor visuospatial skills may give rise not only to a low quality of spontaneous writing but also to marked problems in drawing, copying from text, and letter reversals.
- Poor spelling and drawing are often due to DCD (Missiuna et al., 2008).
- Difficulties in the attachment of phonemes to graphemes may be a particular problem for writing as well as for their contribution to reading problems.

Once recognized, skilled teaching can help both with particular problems and with explanation to the child of the nature of the problem. Use of keyboards can help; spellcheckers may be indicated; and some young people may need extra time for written tests or even an amanuensis.

5.2.3.2.2 *Difficulties with use of numbers and calculating*

Like literacy problems, poor performance for age level is a continuously distributed variable, usually defined as a discrepancy from age on standardized tests. In the absence of standardized scales, an experienced teacher's judgement will also be used. Inability to perform at age level is not the same as 'maths anxiety', in which a fear of failure dissuades some young people from attempting maths problems.

There is a variety of possible causes of inability, that can coexist:

- Lack of motivation and persistence
- Disorganized written presentation
- Poor short-term memory, restricting ability to keep track of computations
- Limitations of executive function such as planning and working memory

It is also conceivable that some cognitive functions specific to manipulating numbers can be involved. These have been less studied than the cognitive/linguistic processes in language impairments. They could include difficulties in estimating magnitudes, counting, remembering the rules of addition and other arithmetical processes, and linking numbers to other ordered phenomena such as lists and succession of events. None is established as a cause (see 'Risks' below).

Prevalence

Rates of specific numeracy deficits are dependent on the criteria of severity that are applied. A rate of 3.6% was described in children aged 9–10 years in the UK, of whom more than half also showed literacy problems (Lewis et al., 1994).

Risks

Genetic influences accounted for about 65% of the variance in teacher-reported mathematics ability in a large twin study in the UK (Oliver et al., 2004). The estimate was very similar for the child population as a whole and for those defined by low performance. Sometimes traumatic brain damage is followed by enough problems with attention and working memory to make trains of thought and calculation impossible. ADHD can have a similar effect.

More specific neurological impairments of magnitude estimation, mental computation, maths fluency, and quantitative reasoning have been formulated. Some adults seem to have a problem in mapping an array of objects to the symbol that denotes their number, and this could be linked to functioning around the right intraparietal sulcus (Price et al., 2007). No evidence establishes this or any other neurological dysfunction as a root cause of dyscalculia. It seems more likely that several dysfunctions will prove to be involved, in different combinations for different people.

5.2.4 Intellectual disability (ID); generalized learning disability (GLD)

Intellectual disability (ID), generalized learning disability/difficulty (GLD), and intellectual developmental disorder (IDD) are different names for the combination of cognitive impairment with poor adaptive function. It involves poor performance in the abilities needed to understand information, to reason, learn, and plan in an age-appropriate way, and to cope with everyday life. It begins in childhood.

Earlier terms such as 'mental retardation' have dropped out of use because they are perceived as stigmatizing, and because not all difficulties can be conceptualized as representing the level of achievement that would be attained by a typically developing child of a younger chronological age. Rather, the standard for cognitive impairment is a comparison with other children of the same age. IQ is the score on tests that have been given to large numbers of youngsters. Many IQ tests are constructed to have a normal distribution with a mean of 100 and a standard difference of 15. They yield difference scores whose meaning will depend upon the population for which they were standardized. Scales have to be restandardized from time to time because the population average itself is increasing (the Flynn effect). An IQ of less than 70 (approximating to two standard deviations below the population mean) is a cut-off for the cognitive part of the definition of ID.

5.2.4.1 *Psychological testing of intelligence*

There is no single psychological test of cognitive function, any more than there is a precise meaning for 'intellect'. Rather, IQ tests are developed as an average of many cognitive abilities, including language, executive function, memory, and spatial reasoning. They are unlikely all to be at exactly the same level, but the average of them is a useful guide for several purposes. Individually administered scales for IQ require a skilled examiner. Such a person can record and allow for non-intellectual difficulties in performance.

Wechsler intelligence scales provide a measure of IQ. Current versions are: for adults, the WAIS-IV (Wechsler Adult Intelligence Scale); and for children, the WISC-V (Wechsler Intelligence Scale for Children) (suitable for ages 6 to 16 years). The child version provides separate scores for verbal comprehension, visual-spatial ability, fluid reasoning, working memory, and processing speed (Canivez et al., 2017). The version for preschool children is the WPPSI (Wechsler Preschool and Primary Scale of Intelligence), which can be administered to children from the age of 30 months to 7 years (Wechsler, 2012).

The full *Kaufman Assessment Battery for Children* (KABC-II NU) is a measure of cognitive ability that claims to be culturally fair and is based on psychological theory

(Kaufman & Kaufman, 2018). It is designed for young people from the ages of 3 to 18 years and has the advantage of not requiring detailed verbal instructions. The *Leiter performance scales* (Roid et al., 2013) dispense with verbal instructions entirely and are particularly suitable for children with problems in communication.

Some tests are designed to be appropriate for the testing of young children in the first three years of life (e.g. Bayley, 2006). Their predictive validity to later childhood and adolescence is not as high as that of tests given after infancy.

There are also some brief tests available, such as the Kaufman Brief Intelligence Test (KBIT 2), which can be administered by a wide range of professionals and forms a useful screen for problems of intellectual level (Kaufman, 2004). It yields indices of crystallized (verbal) ability and fluid (non-verbal matrices) ability.

Group tests are also available, which can be administered to a large number of individuals at the same time. Scoring can be automated. They can be valuable for educational purposes, such as considering whether the educational achievement of a school is accounted for by the ability of the pupils. They are not, however, sufficient for assessment of an individual. Individual testing allows a skilled examiner to interpret IQ scores in the light of other influences on performance, such as anxiety, fatigue, and application to the test.

5.2.4.2 *Significance of test results*

Marked differences between the various subtests are a useful guide for thinking about education. When the differences are great, they may lead to the individual being considered as showing a specific learning difficulty. Specific difficulties in learning should be recognized whether or not there is also a generalized difficulty.

IQ scores are not sufficient in themselves as a guide to diagnosis. In modern classifications, they must be combined with judgements about adaptive function—the ability of the individual to cope with the demands of the world in daily living. These expectations vary with age. They include:

- Achieving milestones in motor skills and use of language
- Self-help and self-care skills
- Planning and problem solving (e.g. in adjusting to new situations)
- Keeping up with other children in school
- Social maturity

Both low IQ and poor adaptive function are required for a diagnosis. This is comparable to practice in neurodevelopmental disorders (e.g. ASD, ADHD), for which the international diagnostic schemes expect defined symptoms to be combined with disability in the form of restricted opportunities for activity and participation. IQ is associated with adaptive function, but they are not identical and should not be used to define each other. Sometimes the grades of IQ deviation are overused to set rigid expectations about daily life. Measures for adaptive function include the third edition of the *Adaptive behavior assessment* (Harrison & Oakland, 2015) and the third edition of the *Vineland adaptive behavior scales* (Sparrow et al., 2016).

Children with mild cognitive difficulties will, by definition, have an IQ of 50–69. Most will not have difficulties recognized until they start at school. Thereafter, they can be expected to learn reading and mathematics skills, self-care such as dressing and washing, cooking, and going safely about their neighbourhood. They may well be slower than most to learn such skills, and need more assistance than most, but the range is great, and most affected people will lead independent adult lives and get gainful employment. Care should be taken in assessment of children from cultural backgrounds that vary markedly from those of the locally dominant culture. Many skills may have been learned (e.g. weaving, fishing, animal care) that are not reflected in current IQ scales but are highly adaptive in cultures of origin.

Moderate ID (35–49), severe ID (20–34), and profound ID (19 or below) entail progressively more need for support in everyday living. Severe and profound levels are said to be present when individuals are unable to care for themselves independently and will probably need a caregiver throughout their adult lives.

5.2.4.3 *Risks*

At mild levels of ID, the causes are usually the same interplay of genetic and environmental influences that determine IQ in the general population. A minority will have specific causes such as identifiable chromosomal or genetic conditions, brain damage and disease, or very adverse environments. In moderate and severe cases, more than half will show syndromic causes, and most will have structural abnormalities of the brain.

Medical causes of ID should be sought. Chromosomal and genetic testing is now practical for the diagnosis of many conditions such as Down syndrome and fragile-X (Chapter 7, Section 7.3). The management of learning disorders is a key concern for education. Health professionals should seek family consent to share their evaluations with schoolteachers.

5.2.4.4 *Coexistent psychiatric problems*

Neuropsychiatric disorders, and other behavioural and emotional problems, are frequent complications of ID. In mild ID, oppositional and anxiety-based problems often appear when academic progress is slow and/or parents are demanding. The recognition of ID can then clarify the true predicament. Standardized testing of IQ is crucial, and best done by a qualified psychologist. Behaviourally defined conditions such as ADHD and ASD are not only more frequent in ID than in typically developing young people, but they also make up a higher proportion of all psychological disturbance. Low IQ worsens their outlook.

Behavioural problems can be intense, frequent, and severe, at which point they are then often called 'challenging'. Behaviour that challenges is not a diagnosis but is a frequent complication of ID as well as ASD. It is described further in Chapter 4, Section 4.1.5.3. The 'challenge' is to services, family members, or caregivers. For the person showing it, it may well be serving a useful purpose. It may be attracting attention, creating sensory stimulation, avoiding demands, making a protest, or getting help. It should al-ways be considered in the context of the suitability of the care environment to the person.

Is challenging behaviour the result of painful conditions (e.g. sore throats, toothache, earache) which are not recognized? Is there a lack of occupation? Are there unpleasant conditions, such as smell or excessive noise (remembering that some people may be highly sensitive to noise levels that would be unremarkable for most)? Is the person suffering neglect or abuse? (See also 'Substitute care and accommodation', Chapter 10, Section 10.7 and 'Interventions to aid communication and language', Chapter 8, Section 8.9.)

5.2.4.5 *Management*

It is not usually possible to increase IQ with medical treatment unless it is secondary to a remediable medical illness (e.g. phenylketonuria, which can be treated with special diets from infancy) or to harmful environmental exposure (see 'Toxins', Chapter 7, Section 7.8).

Adaptive function, however, can be helped by education and family support. They are key concerns for special education. In societies making much use of residential systems for care, clinicians have been instrumental in ending oppressive care (see Chapter 10, Section 10.7). Clinicians are also involved in assessing progress and delivering interventions—not only for treating psychiatric complications, but also through speech and language therapy, occupational therapy, family counselling, physical therapy, and diet.

Families can be helpfully advised to encourage their child's independence and trying new things. Involvement in group activities and community groups will help social skills. Overcoming obstacles to social involvement (e.g. stigma) is still a struggle in some societies. Other families encountering similar struggles can be a great resource.

References

American Psychiatric Association. (2013). *Diagnostic and statistical manual of mental disorders* (DSM-5).

Annett, M. (1998). Handedness and cerebral dominance: the right shift theory. *The Journal of Neuropsychiatry and Clinical Neurosciences, 10*(4), 459–469.

Bayley, N. (2006). *Bayley scales of infant and toddler development.* PsychCorp, Pearson.

Bishop, D. V. (2003). Specific language impairment: diagnostic dilemmas. In L. Verhoeven & H.v. Balkom, (Eds.), *Classification of developmental language disorders: theoretical issues and clinical implications* (pp. 309–326). Lawrence Erlbaum.

Bishop, D. V. (2015). The interface between genetics and psychology: lessons from developmental dyslexia. *Proceedings of the Royal Society B: Biological Sciences, 282*(1806), 20143139.

Bishop, D. V. M., & Hayiou–Thomas, M. E. (2008). Heritability of specific language impairment depends on diagnostic criteria. *Genes, Brain and Behavior, 7*(3), 365–372.

Burns, M. K., Petersen–Brown, S., Haegele, K., Rodriguez, M., Schmitt, B., Cooper, M., Clayton, K., Hutcheson, S., Conner, C., Hosp, J., & VanDerHeyden, A. M. (2016). Meta-analysis of academic interventions derived from neuropsychological data. *School Psychology Quarterly, 31*(1), 28.

Canivez, G. L., Watkins, M. W., & Dombrowski, S. C. (2017). Structural validity of the Wechsler Intelligence Scale for Children–Fifth Edition: confirmatory factor analyses with the 16 primary and secondary subtests. *Psychological Assessment, 29*(4), 458.

Coltheart, M. (2000). Deep dyslexia is right-hemisphere reading. *Brain and Language, 71*(2), 299–309.

Conti–Ramsden, G., St Clair, M. C., Pickles, A., & Durkin, K. (2012). Developmental trajectories of verbal and nonverbal skills in individuals with a history of specific language impairment: from childhood to adolescence. *Journal of Speech, Language, and Hearing Research, 55*(6), 1716–1735.

Deng, H., Gao, K., & Jankovic, J. (2012). The genetics of Tourette syndrome. *Nature Reviews Neurology, 8*(4), 203.

Dockrell, J. E., & Marshall, C. R. (2015). Measurement issues: assessing language skills in young children. *Child and Adolescent Mental Health, 20*(2), 116–125.

Fletcher, J. M., & Morris, R. D. (2014). Reading, laterality, and the brain: early contributions on reading disabilities by Sara S. Sparrow. *Journal of Autism and Developmental Disorders, 44*(2), 250–255.

Gayan, J., & Olson, R. K. (1999). Reading disability: evidence for a genetic etiology. *European Child & Adolescent Psychiatry, 8*(3), S52.

Gillberg, C., Fernell, E., & Minnis, H. (2013). Early symptomatic syndromes eliciting neurodevelopmental clinical examinations.

Gilles de la Tourette, G. (1885). Etude sur une affection nerveuse caracterisee par de l'incoordination automat accompagnee d'echolalie et de coprolalie. *Archives in Neurology, 9*, 158–200.

Greene, D. J., Williams III, A. C., Koller, J. M., Schlaggar, B. L., & Black, K. J. (2017). Brain structure in pediatric Tourette syndrome. *Molecular Psychiatry, 22*(7), 972.

Harlaar, N., Trzaskowski, M., Dale, P. S., & Plomin, R. (2014). Word reading fluency: role of genome-wide single-nucleotide polymorphisms in developmental stability and correlations with print exposure. *Child Development, 85*(3), 1190–1205.

Harrison P, Oakland T. (2015). *Adaptive Behavior Assessment (ABAS-3)* (3rd ed.) Pearson.

Henry, L. A., & Botting, N. (2017). Working memory and developmental language impairments. *Child Language Teaching and Therapy, 33*(1), 19–32.

Kaufman, A. S. (2004). *Kaufman Brief Intelligence Test* (2nd ed.) (KBIT-2). *American Guidance Service.*

Kaufman, A. S., & Kaufman, N. L. (2018). *Kaufman Assessment Battery for Children* (2nd ed.), normative update. Pearson.

Kearns, D. M., Hancock, R., Hoeft, F., Pugh, K. R., & Frost, S. J. (2019). The neurobiology of dyslexia. *TEACHING Exceptional Children, 51*(3), 175–188.

Knight, T., Steeves, T., Day, L., Lowerison, M., Jette, N., & Pringsheim, T. (2012). Prevalence of tic disorders: a systematic review and meta-analysis. *Pediatric Neurology, 47*(2), 77–90.

Lai, C. S., Fisher, S. E., Hurst, J. A., Vargha–Khadem, F., & Monaco, A. P. (2001). A forkhead-domain gene is mutated in a severe speech and language disorder. *Nature,* 413, 519–523. https://doi.org/10.1038/35097076

Leckman, J. F., Riddle, M. A., Hardin, M. T., Ort, S. I., Swartz, K. L., Stevenson, J. O. H. N., & Cohen, D. J. (1989). The Yale Global Tic Severity Scale: initial testing of a clinician-rated scale of tic severity. *Journal of the American Academy of Child & Adolescent Psychiatry, 28*(4), 566–573.

Lewis, C., Hitch, G. J., & Walker, P. (1994). The prevalence of specific arithmetic difficulties and specific reading difficulties in 9- to 10-year-old boys and girls. *Journal of Child Psychology and Psychiatry, 35*(2), 283–292.

Livingston, E. M., Siegel, L. S., & Ribary, U. (2018). Developmental dyslexia: emotional impact and consequences. *Australian Journal of Learning Difficulties, 23*(2), 107–135.

Martin, A., Schurz, M., Kronbichler, M., & Richlan, F. (2015). Reading in the brain of children and adults: a meta-analysis of 40 functional magnetic resonance imaging studies. *Human Brain Mapping, 36*(5), 1963–1981.

Mason, K., Rowley, K., Marshall, C. R., Atkinson, J. R., Herman, R., Woll, B., & Morgan, G. (2010). Identifying specific language impairment in deaf children acquiring British Sign Language: implications for theory and practice. *British Journal of Developmental Psychology, 28*(1), 33–49.

Mesulam, M. M. (1990). Large-scale neurocognitive networks and distributed processing for attention, language, and memory. *Annals of Neurology, 28*(5), 597–613.

Missiuna, C., Pollock, N., Egan, M., DeLaat, D., Gaines, R., & Soucie, H. (2008). Enabling occupation through facilitating the diagnosis of developmental coordination disorder. *Canadian Journal of Occupational Therapy, 75*(1), 26–34.

National Institute for Health and Care Excellence (NICE). (2015). *Challenging behaviour and learning disabilities: prevention and interventions for people with learning disabilities whose behaviour challenges.* NICE guideline. [NG11] https://www.nice.org.uk/guidance/ng11

Newbury, D. F., Fisher, S. E., & Monaco, A. P. (2010). Recent advances in the genetics of language impairment. *Genome Medicine, 2*(1), 6.

Oliver, B., Harlaar, N., Hayiou Thomas, M. E., Kovas, Y., Walker, S. O., Petrill, S. A., Spinath, F. M., Dale, P. S., & Plomin, R. (2004). A twin study of teacher-reported mathematics performance and low performance in 7-year-olds. *Journal of Educational Psychology, 96*(3), 504.

Pauls, D. L. (2008). The genetics of obsessive compulsive disorder: a review of the evidence. *American Journal of Medical Genetics Part C: Seminars in Medical Genetics, 148*(2), 133–139.

Price, C. J. (2012). A review and synthesis of the first 20 years of PET and fMRI studies of heard speech, spoken language and reading. *Neuroimage, 62*(2), 816–847.

Price, G. R., Holloway, I., Räsänen, P., Vesterinen, M., & Ansari, D. (2007). Impaired parietal magnitude processing in developmental dyscalculia. *Current Biology, 17*(24), R1042–R1043.

Price, R. A., Kidd, K. K., Cohen, D. J., Pauls, D. L., & Leckman, J. F. (1985). A twin study of Tourette syndrome. *Archives of General Psychiatry, 42*(8), 815–820.

Robertson, M. M., Eapen, V., & Cavanna, A. E. (2009). The international prevalence, epidemiology, and clinical phenomenology of Tourette syndrome: a cross-cultural perspective. *Journal of Psychosomatic Research, 67*(6), 475–483.

Roid, G. H., Miller, L. J., & Koch, C. (2013). *Leiter international performance scale.* Stoelting.

Scahill, L., Riddle, M. A., McSwiggin-Hardin, M., Ort, S. I., King, R. A., Goodman, W. K., Cicchetti, D., & Leckman, J. F. (1997). Children's Yale–Brown obsessive compulsive scale: reliability and validity. *Journal of the American Academy of Child & Adolescent Psychiatry, 36*(6), 844–852.

Schumacher, J., Hoffmann, P., Schmäl, C., Schulte-Körne, G., & Nöthen, M. M. (2007). Genetics of dyslexia: the evolving landscape. *Journal of Medical Genetics, 44*(5), 289–297.

Snowling, M. J. (1980). The development of grapheme–phoneme correspondence in normal and dyslexic readers. *Journal of Experimental Child Psychology, 29*(2), 294–305.

Snowling, M. J., Stothard, S. E., Clarke, P., Bowyer-Crane, C., Harrington, A., Truelove, E., & Nation, K. (2009). *York Assessment of Reading for Comprehension (YARC).* GL Assessment.

Sparrow, S. S., Cicchetti, D. V., & Saulnier, C. A. (2016). *Vineland adaptive behavior scales* (Vineland-3) (3rd ed.). Pearson.

Stanovich, K. E. (1994). Annotation: Does dyslexia exist?. *Journal of child psychology and psychiatry, 35*(4), 579–595.

Steinhausen, H. C., Wachter, M., Laimböck, K., & Metzke, C. W. (2006). A long-term outcome study of selective mutism in childhood. *Journal of Child Psychology and Psychiatry*, 47(7), 751–756.

Sullivan, S. A., Hollen, L., Wren, Y., Thompson, A. D., Lewis, G., & Zammit, S. (2016). A longitudinal investigation of childhood communication ability and adolescent psychotic experiences in a community sample. *Schizophrenia Research*, 173(1–2), 54–61.

Tomblin, J. B., Records, N. L., Buckwalter, P., Zhang, X., Smith, E., & O'Brien, M. (1997). Prevalence of specific language impairment in kindergarten children. *Journal of Speech, Language, and Hearing Research*, 40(6), 1245–1260.

Trauner, D., Wulfeck, B., Tallal, P., & Hesselink, J. (2000). Neurological and MRI profiles of children with developmental language impairment. *Developmental Medicine and Child Neurology*, 42(7), 470–475.

Trzesniewski, K. H., Donnellan, M. B., Moffitt, T. E., Robins, R. W., Poulton, R., & Caspi, A. (2006). Low self-esteem during adolescence predicts poor health, criminal behavior, and limited economic prospects during adulthood. *Developmental Psychology*, 42(2), 381.

Wechsler, D. (2012). *Wechsler preschool and primary scale of intelligence* (4th ed.). Psychological Corporation.

Wiig, E. H., Semel, E., & Secord, W. A. (2013). *The clinical evaluation of language fundamentals* (5th ed.) (CELF-5). Pearson.

Woods, D. W., Piacentini, J., Himle, M. B., & Chang, S. (2005). Premonitory Urge for Tics Scale (PUTS): initial psychometric results and examination of the premonitory urge phenomenon in youths with Tic disorders. *Journal of Developmental & Behavioral Pediatrics*, 26(6), 397–403.

World Health Organization (WHO). (2018). *ICD-11 for mortality and morbidity statistics.* https://www.who.int/classifications/icd/en/

Wright, S. F., Fields, H., & Newman, S. P. (1996). Dyslexia: stability of definition over a five year period. *Journal of Research in Reading*, 19(1), 46–60.

Yang, Z., Wu, H., Lee, P. H., Tsetsos, F., Davis, L. K., Yu, D., … & Paschou, P. (2019). Cross-disorder GWAS meta-analysis for attention deficit/hyperactivity disorder, autism spectrum disorder, obsessive compulsive disorder, and Tourette syndrome. *bioRxiv*, 770222.

Yew, S. G. K., & O'Kearney, R. (2013). Emotional and behavioural outcomes later in childhood and adolescence for children with specific language impairments: meta-analyses of controlled prospective studies. *Journal of Child Psychology and Psychiatry*, 54(5), 516–524.

Yu, D., Sul, J. H., Tsetsos, F., Nawaz, M. S., Huang, A. Y., Zelaya, I., Illmann, C., Osiecki, L., Darrow, S. M., Hirschtritt, M. E., Greenberg, E., Muller–Vahl, K. R., Stuhrmann, M., Dion, Y., Rouleau, G., Aschauer, H., Stamenkovic, M., Schlögelhofer, M., Sandor, P., & the Psychiatric Genomics Consortium Tourette Syndrome Working Group. (2019). Interrogating the genetic determinants of Tourette's syndrome and other tic disorders through genome-wide association studies. *American Journal of Psychiatry*, 176(3), 217–227.

CHAPTER 6

....

PSYCHIATRIC CONSEQUENCES OF BRAIN SYNDROMES

....

6.1 BRAIN DAMAGE AND DISEASE

THIS chapter outlines the nature of common and notable brain disorders that have psychiatric consequences for children and young people.

Epilepsy can itself be seen as a common neurodevelopmental disorder, albeit its origins are not always in very early life. The effects on psychosocial adjustment are often the most disabling parts of the disorder. Management often falls in the gap between neurology and psychiatry. *Cerebral palsy* and *hydrocephalus* arise very early in life and have major impacts on the development of mental function. *Acquired traumatic injury* has a somewhat later origin and is equally the concern of neurological and psychiatric habilitation. *Localized structural brain illness* is important for its frequency and for giving clues about brain–behaviour relationships. *Diseases with diffuse brain involvement* affecting mental function include endocrine disorders and sickle cell disease. *Infective and immune encephalopathies* are considered in Chapter 7, Sections 7.6 and 7.8 in relation to environmental hazards. *Functional neurological disorders* present problems usually taken to be caused by brain disorders, but without evidence for brain involvement. They are often considered to be psychogenic conditions, but 'unexplained' would be more accurate, and they are described here.

These all have strong psychiatric and psychological consequences and need contributions from mental health professionals. The consequences of each condition are sometimes severe and usually diffuse, but none of the physical disorders individually is common enough to make them major causes of the syndromes defined at a behavioural level that were described in previous chapters. Those potentially causative influences will be taken up in the next chapter on genetic and early environmental influences on the main neurodevelopmental impairments, and considered transdiagnostically. Where there are risks specific to an individual syndrome, they will have been considered in the chapter on that disorder.

6.2 Epilepsy

Epilepsy is a tendency to have seizures—which are transient episodes of signs and/or symptoms associated with abnormal (excessive or synchronous) neural activity in the brain. It is said to be present when an individual has had two (or more) unprovoked seizures occurring at least 24 hours apart. It is therefore a recurring condition—but should not be seen as a diagnosis for life. It is 'resolved' after 10 seizure-free years, with five of them off medication. In childhood-limited conditions, a shorter period may suffice.

Epilepsy is a chronic neurological condition in children and young people. It very often begins in childhood. It is also a social position, with unique aspects of rejection and exclusion. Indeed, for most people in most countries, the worst things about epilepsy are stigma and restriction of life. Their importance through the life span was emphasized by an analysis of factors contributing to overall quality of life in adult patients (Suurmeijer et al., 2001). Psychosocial variables such as distress, coping and adjustment, and perceived stigma accounted for twice the amount of variance in quality-of-life scores than did clinical variables such as seizure frequency and adverse effects of antiepileptic drugs.

Mental health professionals make important contributions to the diagnosis, by helping to distinguish seizures from 'psychogenic' conditions. In many countries, they are the key professionals coordinating management. In most countries, they are closely involved in treatment by describing and addressing the behavioural, cognitive, emotional, and social complications which often constitute the major problems for adjustment and quality of life.

6.2.1 Types of seizure

Seizures can have many causes and can be of various types. They are usually divided into those of focal, generalized, or unknown onset. Each category is further classified into motor and non-motor, with focal seizures divided into those with retained or impaired awareness (Fisher et al., 2017). Older, anatomical classifications have proved to be of limited value for epilepsies in children. Their epilepsies are usually network conditions, rather than deriving from clearly localized lesions.

6.2.1.1 *Focal seizures*

Focal seizures in full awareness can take many forms, depending on the parts of the brain that are involved. They are all short-lived episodes and can be remembered afterwards, even if there has been apparent unresponsiveness at the time. Altered perceptions can amount to hallucinations, to involuntary muscular movements, to apparent stereotypies or compulsions. Deja vu experiences, an unusual smell or taste, and a sudden intense feeling of fear or joy are all frequent. Sometimes, the experience is indescribable and spoken of only as a 'strangeness'.

Emotion-related behaviours, such as laughing and crying, can sometimes be produced by a focus, and give a false impression of emotional dysregulation. One clearly localized form is the epilepsy resulting from a congenital malformation of the hypothalamus. The seizures begin with a brief attack of laughing (gelastic) or crying (dacrystic). The subjective experience, however, is not one of the appropriate emotions. There may be a feeling of dread, and young children may suddenly seek reassurance from their parent.

Focal seizures with altered awareness ('complex partial seizures') may begin with an aura and can proceed to motor changes such as lip smacking and complex hand movements. They can last for up to a couple of minutes and are often followed by a period of confusion. Hallucinations can be present in any sensory field. EEG may be quite normal between seizures or may show localizing changes. They used to be regarded as certainly indicating a focus in the temporal lobe, but can also be associated with evidence of other sites of EEG abnormality (e.g. a frontal lobe focus) or with none.

One common form of focal lesion, however, does derive from a localized lesion: hippocampal sclerosis. This is probably both a cause of focal seizures (if the initial discharge spreads enough) and a result of previous prolonged seizures. One series, following more than 200 children who had febrile status epilepticus, found later evidence from magnetic resonance imaging of either medial temporal sclerosis or reduced hippocampal volume, at a much higher rate than children who had suffered a febrile convulsion that was not prolonged (Lewis et al., 2014).

6.2.1.2 *Generalized seizures*

Absence seizures ('petit mal') are frequent, often several times a day, and brief, lasting not more than 30 seconds. Minor motor changes during the seizures are common—indeed, episodes characterized only by vacant staring and with no other motor change are quite unusual. There is often an automatism or a fluttering of the eyelids, but this can be missed by teachers and parents. Mental activity is suddenly interrupted during the episode. The EEG signature is 3 c.p.s. symmetrical spike or spike-and-wave complexes. Hyperventilation usually induces an absence and is helpful diagnostically (e.g. in differentiating from a focal seizure with interruption of awareness).

Seizures involving motor changes can be:

- *Clonic:* muscles develop rhythmic spasms for a few minutes.
- *Tonic:* sudden stiffening of muscles, often for less than a minute, often in sleep.
- *Tonic–clonic:* classic 'grand mal' episodes, usually starting with limbs contracting, perhaps a scream, and a fall, evolving into rhythmic shaking; often accompanied by loss of bladder and bowel control, and followed by a period of unresponsiveness, confusion, drowsiness, and headache.
- *Myoclonic:* sudden jerking.

- *Atonic:* sudden limpness—only for a few seconds, but often leading to a fall and potential injury.

Most seizures last for only a few minutes at most. Status epilepticus, however, occurs when there is continuous seizure activity, or repetitive activity without recovery between episodes. It is dangerous, and needs treating urgently if a seizure has gone on for longer than 5 minutes of tonic–clonic convulsion, or 10 minutes of absence status. After 30 minutes of tonic–clonic status, or 60 minutes of focal status with reduced conscious level, there is real danger of neuronal damage, and it needs treating as a medical emergency. Buccal midazolam is widely used—and should be made readily available for people at risk. (The exact length of a seizure, before urgent anti-seizure medication should be considered, varies between authorities; the figures above are taken from recommendations by the International League Against Epilepsy (Trinka et al., 2015)).

Non-convulsive status can be hard to recognize if consciousness is retained: the EEG is crucial. It should be considered as a possibility in people with epilepsy who develop a change in personality or worsening cognitive performance.

Recurrent epilepsy should be distinguished from single and provoked seizures. Even grand mal episodes are not necessarily a sign of epilepsy. There are many causes, and they are not always likely to recur. They may be provoked by, for example, very low blood sugar, a head injury, or a high fever.

Febrile seizures are common in childhood. They are not epilepsy but can occur in people with epilepsy. If prolonged, however, they canf cause damage to the brain—including a risk of epilepsy. In a first presentation, examination of the cerebrospinal fluid is important, to detect or rule out infections. An EEG is not necessarily required. Continuous seizures lasting for more than 30 minutes, without recovery of consciousness, are called 'febrile status' and need to be treated as a medical emergency. Status can damage the brain in itself and can reflect underlying brain pathology.

6.2.2   Discrimination from non-epileptic seizures

Dissociative convulsions ('pseudoseizures', 'psychogenic non-epileptic seizures') are a 'functional neurological' condition (as described here). They can sometimes be distinguished, by observation, from those with an organic cause. There are characteristic features—but any one of them can be misleading. Mistakes can be made both ways.

Any convulsive movements typically comprise histrionic shaking or flailing around, rather than the rhythmic clonus of grand mal. Injury after a fall during a non-epileptic attack is rare, and painful events are avoided. Typically, a non-epileptic convulsion, unlike grand mal, will have a gradual onset and a sudden recovery, with no post-ictal confusion or abnormal reflexes. 'Typical', however, is not 'universal'. All these features of non-epileptic seizures can be absent. There will often be an emotional trigger or a functional purpose (e.g. in escaping punishment or disgrace). Note, however, that there can also be emotional triggers for epileptic attacks. Dissociative episodes tend not to occur in the absence of witnesses (but this can, by definition, be hard to establish).

Dissociative episodes are very often experienced by people who also have epilepsy. The EEG is not usually helpful unless it can be recorded during an episode—but combined video and EEG can be very illuminating in uncertain cases. Indeed, the absence of change in the EEG during a witnessed seizure is as close to a gold standard as one can get. Even then, however, one should take other features of the episodes into consideration. Occasionally, a deep-seated epileptic focus is not detectable from a surface EEG.

Young people presenting with non-epileptic seizures can be affronted by the label 'psychogenic'. Their parents may embark on a course of further opinions, and there is a risk of continuing exposure to the adverse effects of antiepileptic drugs. 'Medically un-explained' might be a more accurate term. Many of the young people do show emotional problems, and other somatizing symptoms are a frequent feature—but the same can be said about those with proven epilepsy. Coexistent psychological problems, therefore, do not help in the differential diagnosis.

Dissociative seizures often, but not always, disappear after empathic explanation. In a recent long-term study of adults and young people with the diagnosis, telephone en-quiry elicited that nearly half of those with a definite non-epileptic diagnosis from a spe-cialist unit had continued to have seizures (Asadi–Pooya et al., 2019). (Note, however, that this series may well have been formed of severe cases, and there was no psycho-logical intervention, so it may give an over-gloomy picture).

Periods of unresponsiveness, of blank staring, can represent epileptic absences, but there are other causes, too. *Daydreaming* lasts for minutes and can usually be interrupted. The subjective experience is complex and dreamlike rather than an aura. An EEG seldom shows changes. *Mind wandering*, as in attention deficit hyperactivity disorder (ASD), lasts for seconds and occurs frequently. The subjective experience tends to be of thoughts disappearing. An EEG might show intrusion of default mode (Chapter 3, Section 3.8). *Sensory overload*, as in people with autism spectrum disorder (ASD), may lead to a brief withdrawal and apparent lack of registration of events.

The distinction between epileptic and non-epileptic disturbances of consciousness is not absolute; individuals can show both. They can usually be distinguished by descrip-tion or observation during an attack. Good questions to ask include: Was there any motor change or arrest? Could the episodes be terminated by touching or questioning? For how long did they last? Was there any recall later of events that happened during the episode?

6.2.3 Recurrent episodes of sudden transient behaviour change

There are also many non-epileptic conditions that can present with episodic alterations of behaviour and therefore act as a diagnostic challenge in which psychiatrists or psychologists may be involved.

Sleep-related disorders are common but also include rare conditions such as Smith–Magenis syndrome (Chapter 7, Section 7.3). Frequent problems, such as the parasomnias described here, usually just need recognition for what they are and a calm reaction from parents.

Night terrors occur in the transition out of deep sleep. Children give signs of panic, such as screaming and thrashing around. Eyes may be open, and children may appear conscious, but the episodes are lost to memory next day. Benzodiazepine drugs will usually prevent them by reducing deep stages of sleep, but are seldom needed. They have usually disappeared by the time children are 8 years old.

Sleepwalking (somnambulism) also occurs during deep non-REM (rapid eye movement) sleep and is not remembered next day. There are occasionally complex behaviours. Sometimes it can even be dangerous, and if so it may be necessary to ensure safety and wake the sufferers before the expected time of onset.

Nightmares are associated with strong feelings of anxiety and even terror. They often occur during REM sleep and are associated with bizarre and dream-like ideation. Children have usually grown out of them by about 7 years. Recurrent nightmares can be a feature of post-traumatic disorders and may call for counselling.

Sleep paralysis is also associated with REM sleep. When people wake, they have the distressing, but usually short-lived experience of inability to move their limbs.

Kleine–Levin syndrome is a rare condition of unknown cause, affecting perhaps one in a million, many of them adolescents. It is characterized by episodes lasting between a week and several months. Between episodes there are no problems. During episodes there is extreme sleepiness, and sometimes overeating and apathy. No consistent EEG changes are reported, and treatment with antiepileptic medication does not affect it. There are a few reports of successful therapy with lithium, but antidepressants have no evidence base for their use.

Panic attacks and *tantrums* in the daytime can have many causes. Sometimes the precipitants are not recognized. In ASD, the precipitant may be an apparently trivial change of routine. Phobic states are sometimes not recognized if the feared objects are unusual and not described. Tantrums can be misperceived as seizures because the children appear out of control and the tantrums are sometimes not remembered. Only rarely do they result from fits (see Section 6.2.5).

Laughing spells resulting from drugs such as cannabis can be confused with those resulting from focal epilepsy.

Severe emotional dysregulation, *bulbar palsy*, and *intermittent explosive disorder* all include brief outbursts of irritability. Outbursts often arise from little or no provocation, include uncontrolled rage after minimal provocation, last for an hour or so, and are followed by exhaustion. They can all be misperceived as epilepsy and wrongly treated as such. Episodes of proneness to anger are also a recognized feature of Tourette disorder (Budman et al., 2003).

Narcolepsy (NC) presents excessive daytime sleepiness, cataplexy, and sleep paralysis with hypnagogic or hypnopompic hallucinations. Estimated prevalence is about

1 in 2,000. This, however, is not a scientifically based rate and is almost certainly an underestimation. Onset is usually between the ages of 7 and 25 years. Daytime sleepiness takes the unusual form of sudden, brief, episodic attacks. The individual wakes in full consciousness and maintains full alertness unless and until they suffer the rapid onset of an overwhelming need for sleep. After a short period—a few minutes at most—they awake, again into full consciousness. During the sleep, they sometimes continue the previous activity but in a distorted form. Sleep at night can also be fragmented.

Cataplexy is frequently part of narcolepsy, seen in about 70% of cases. It is a sudden loss of tone in muscles without loss of consciousness. Severity varies, from a collapse with total loss of power to a subtle variation of posture or expression. It is like the loss of tone that occurs during normal REM sleep. Hallucinations and paralysis are also comparable to dreaming in REM sleep. Hallucinations are vivid and frightening.

NC may often go undiagnosed or be mistaken for seizures. There is, however, no epileptic activity in the EEG. Nevertheless, the EEG is still useful diagnostically. In combination with recording muscle activity, breathing, and eye movements (polysomnography), it can be good evidence of narcolepsy. Furthermore, altered sleep architecture is often evident in an unduly swift onset of REM sleep. The multiple sleep latency test, often carried out on the day after polysomnography, detects over-rapid sleep onset and onset of REM.

Furthermore, human leukocyte antigen (HLA) levels can give a diagnostic clue. The family of genes determining HLAs are considered to play a role in distinguishing one's own proteins from external ones and, therefore, to contributing to autoimmune disorders. Several genes in this system are associated with the presence and severity of narcolepsy. Most people with the 'risk' genes do not develop NC.

Cataplexy, in particular, is associated with extremely low levels of the naturally occurring chemical hypocretin in the cerebrospinal fluid. The causes of low hypocretin levels appear to involve destruction of the cells producing it. Autoimmune factors could be responsible.

Treatment is usually with lifestyle changes to reduce the disruptiveness of uncontrollable sleep. Safety precautions similar to those for epilepsy may be required. Schools and employers may need to be persuaded to allow rescheduling of activities and tolerance of episodic non-involvement. There may also be a lifelong need for medication, usually with modafinil, antidepressants, or stimulants that reduce the need for sleep. More recently, sodium oxybate (a metabolite of gamma hydroxy butyrate, GHB) is being prescribed in resistant and disruptive cases, with close monitoring and control.

Alternating hemiplegia of childhood is shown in recurrent brief episodes of paralysis that can affect varying parts of the body. Onset is typically before the age of 18 months. Episodes last from a few minutes to a few days. They are not epileptic but can coexist with seizures. Episodes are typically relieved by sleep but recur on waking. They can be genetic (mutations in *ATP1A3*) but are usually not inherited.

6.2.4 Prevalence of epilepsy

The exact prevalence of epilepsy does vary somewhat between countries, but it is an international problem. Fiest et al. (2017) provided a meta-analysis of 63 population studies. The pooled point prevalence of *active* epilepsy (meaning either a seizure in the last year or continuing prescription of an antiepileptic drug) was 6.38 per 1,000 persons. The rate was broadly similar at different ages, rising to its highest level during adolescence and early adulthood, and roughly equal between males and females. Higher rates have been reported from low- and middle-income countries—especially children in tropical countries, where head injuries and premature births are disproportionately frequent.

6.2.5 Mental health problems in epilepsy

The prevalence of all psychiatric disorders is markedly raised in young people with epilepsy. A classic epidemiological study by Rutter et al. (1970) found higher rates than in children with non-neurological physical illnesses or even with other neurological conditions below the brain stem. There were disproportionately high rates of heavily neurologically influenced psychiatric diagnoses that were then considered to be rare in children without brain diseases (such as autism and hyperkinetic disorder).

Subsequent research has been in line with this general picture of mental vulnerability from neurological compromise. As an example, a study from California examined 114 children, aged 5 to 16 years, with epilepsy but an average IQ and an absence of underlying neurological disease, recruited from clinical and community sources (Ott et al., 2003). They were, accordingly, an advantaged group by comparison with many children with epilepsy. They all had either 'complex partial seizures' (focal with loss of awareness) or 'petit mal' (primary generalized seizures with absence). There was little difference between these two diagnostic groups in terms of mental health problems (in contradiction to earlier clinical accounts). Even so, some 60% had a DSM-5 psychiatric diagnosis. Strikingly, however, the great majority of those affected received no mental healthcare. More recently, a community-based study in schools in Sussex, UK (the CHESS study) surveyed all the children aged 5 to 15 years who were known to have active epilepsy and reported high rates for neurodevelopmental diagnoses: ADHD in 33%, ASD in 21%, developmental coordination disorder in 18% (Reilly et al., 2014).

The mental effects are generally not constant to the pathological type of epilepsy but depend more upon the severity of any underlying brain disease, the presence of intellectual impairment, and impact on everyday life. Antiepileptic drugs, especially polypharmacy, can also create problems (see Chapter 9). The mental changes that are often noted in people with epilepsy can conveniently be described according to their relationship in time with the seizures.

6.2.5.1 *Pre-ictal mental changes*

Pre-ictal changes are seen in the few hours or days leading up to a seizure. Children and young people sometimes become irritable and even aggressive; sometimes more anxious. The eventual seizure will often clear the air and be followed by relief of the emotional tension.

6.2.5.2 *Ictal mental changes*

Ictal changes coincide with the seizure, so are recognized from their sudden appearance and usual disappearance after no more than a few minutes. The first to appear is an *aura* of subjective experience. This may be a hallucination, in any of the senses. There can be a strong emotional component—most frequently, of anxiety, fear, and dread. Children can lash out at these times. Anger, however, is not a common aura—even though it is very frequently suspected and even investigated, because of the similarity of description of 'epileptic rages' to the much commoner problem of non-epileptic tantrums. Indeed, children can often appear oblivious to the outside world in an ordinary tantrum, thus magnifying the similarity to a seizure (see Chapter 2, Section 2.9). Feelings of depression, guilt, and hopelessness can also accompany a seizure. Brief, ecstatic experiences are also sometimes described. Some children find their seizure experiences to be delightful and even seek to induce them (e.g. with flashing lights).

Focal motor seizures are sometimes very similar to a purposive activity such as searching for a (nonexistent) object. Occasionally, they have been responsible for injury to oneself or others, but without awareness at the time or memory for them afterwards. Sometimes, the only behaviour change is an interruption of mental activity. Automatisms are complex and seemingly purposive acts carried out without intention and without recollection.

Brief cognitive impairment (BCI) can masquerade as poor attention, especially if the episodes are frequent. Subtle behaviour changes during seizures may need combined video and EEG changes to detect their nature. If they are being observed without recording equipment, it can help for the observer to say an unusual word while the change is happening, in order to ask for recall afterwards and note any absence of registration.

6.2.5.3 *Post-ictal mental changes*

Confusion and amnesia are the rule after a grand mal seizure and can also follow less obvious episodes. They may continue for hours (or even days) and be responsible for aggression, overactivity, and/or disinhibited conduct. Depression and anxiety can also be part of these post-ictal changes; psychotic-type distortions of reality are also possible.

6.2.5.4 *Inter-ictal*

Inter-ictal disturbances can be hard to recognize as related to epilepsy because of their lack of a direct temporal association. Surveys have made it clear that young people with epilepsy have unusually high rates both of chronic mental health diagnoses and high scores on dimensions of mental health problems. For instance, Dunn et al. (2009) found ADHD, disruptive behaviour disorder, and anxiety disorder each to be present in about 20–30% of their sample of 173 children aged 9 to 14 years who had been affected by epilepsy for at least 6 months. Approximately one child in ten had evidence of a mood disorder.

6.2.6 Causes of psychiatric disorders in epilepsy

It is possible for individual cases to arise as a direct consequence of epilepsy:

- As a result of brain damage during a seizure (hippocampal sclerosis).
- As one part of the progress of one of the described but unexplained epilepsy syndromes considered here, or one of the increasing number of reported single-gene mutations, such as those responsible for autosomal dominant nocturnal frontal lobe epilepsy, genetic epilepsy with febrile seizures plus, or severe myoclonic epilepsy of childhood (Shorvon, 2011).
- As an encephalopathy or a set of receptor changes resulting from kindling or multiple seizures. Early onset in the first 2 years seems to predict autism and intellectual disability later.
- As a result of partial status or frequent seizures in sleep. Disruption of synaptic function in early life could be responsible.
- As a result of the psychological effects of frequent seizures. Hallucinations and delusions are frequent ictal events in temporal lobe epilepsy, and they can become incorporated into paranoid inter-ictal thinking about the world.

For most young people with epilepsy, however, the coexistence of mental health problems is not strongly linked to epilepsy variables, such as frequency and type of seizures. It is unlikely that most of the psychiatric syndromes in young people are the direct result of having seizures. Pericall and Taylor (2017) described factors leading to major mental health problems in children and young people with epilepsy. Early onset, and severity as indexed by seizure frequency, were not strong predictors. Family dysfunction and mental health difficulties before the epilepsy did predict higher rates of disorder. Females with epilepsy were only a little less likely than males with epilepsy to show ASD and/or ADHD—but the gender ratio was much more equal than in people without epilepsy.

For some people with epilepsy, the discontinuation of seizures may be a trigger for psychiatric disorder (forced normalization).

6.2.6.1 *ADHD and attention problems in epilepsy*

There are multiple possible causes for impaired attention in young people with epilepsy, including coexistent presence of ADHD or intellectual disability, the immediate effects of current seizures, effects of chronic seizures on cognitive functioning, and adverse effects of antiepileptic drugs (AEDs). In clinical practice, all these mechanisms can be encountered and often coexist.

There is no consistent evidence for a close relationship between ADHD severity and epilepsy variables, such as type or even frequency of seizures within the usual range of severity. Children with seizures are more than twice as likely as those without to have showed ADHD symptoms (especially inattention) *before* their first recognized seizure (Hesdorffer et al., 2004). Austin et al. (2001) found similar results for behaviour problems generally in 224 children aged 4 to 14 years whose mothers were interviewed shortly after the first recognized seizure. There was a clear story of ADHD being present before the epilepsy. To complicate the picture, they also found that those who had shown possible but unrecognized seizure events in the 6 months before the first recognized seizure were at even higher risk of behaviour problems than those with no such history.

By contrast, coexistent problems such as low IQ and underlying brain disease are consistently reflected in higher ADHD rates. In most respects, including presence of coexistent conditions, ADHD in epilepsy seems to be comparable with that in people without epilepsy—except that girls are nearly as likely as boys to be affected. In particular, stimulant medication is comparable in efficacy whether or not the person has epilepsy too (see Chapter 9, Section 9.4).

Some severe forms of epilepsy, such as partial status epilepticus, can reproduce many of the features of ADHD. Reduced awareness of the environment as a result of seizures can include apparent failures of concentration, memory, and learning. The distinction from usual ADHD is important. The key to improving function may well be a determined use of anti-epileptic drugs to control the seizures. An EEG is therefore a key measure and is recommended especially for children whose learning and social function are deteriorating.

6.2.6.2 *ASD and epilepsy*

Autistic people have been known for some time to be prone to developing seizures: 22% of those enrolled in a longitudinal study were so (Bolton et al., 2011). One review reported a sevenfold increased risk of epilepsy in individuals with ASD relative to the general population (Thomas et al., 2017). A key reported risk factor is the presence of intellectual disability, which increases epilepsy risk in ASD by three to five times over that in people with epilepsy but ordinary levels of IQ. There is also an increased risk of epilepsy in intellectually able people with ASD, but that risk is rather smaller than in those with low IQ.

More recently, population data have shown that people with epilepsy are at increased risk of showing ASD. A meta-analysis by Strasser et al. (2018) focused on 19 studies: there was a wide range of estimates—overall, a pooled ASD prevalence of 6.3% in individuals with childhood-onset epilepsy. Risk factors reported in the studies included the presence of intellectual disability. Male gender, however, was not a risk, unlike the situation in neurotypical people.

A Swedish clinical database found 85,201 individuals with epilepsy (Sundelin et al., 2016). A clinical diagnosis of autism had been recorded in 1.6%—a tenfold increase in the hazard ratio when compared with non-epileptic controls at that time. There was also an increased rate of autism in the siblings, mothers, and offspring of people with epilepsy, so perhaps genetic factors contribute to the association. The offspring of epileptic mothers were more likely to show autism than the offspring of affected fathers, raising the possibility of uterine influences such as antiepileptic medication.

6.2.6.3 *Psychosis in epilepsy*

A systematic review by Clancy et al. (2014) gathered together several surveys of clinical populations. The prevalence of psychosis in children and adolescents with epilepsy was given as 5.4% (like the rate in adults, which is 5.6%). The rate in temporal lobe epilepsy (TLE) was only somewhat (and not statistically significantly) higher at 7%.

No specific type of seizure characterizes young people with both epilepsy and psychosis (Pericall & Taylor, 2010). A long-standing clinical belief implicates TLE specifically, but this has not been empirically established. Perhaps TLE must be present for a long period before it generates psychosis. Perhaps the profile of psychotic features in TLE is so untypical that it is not recognized as such. The presentation of schizophrenia-like symptoms in TLE is often distinctive. It is dominated by command hallucinations, third-person auditory hallucinations, and other 'first-rank' symptoms. Personality and affect tend to be well preserved, and maintenance of social interest and warmth is the rule.

Both in children and in adults, the associated psychiatric presentations often do not represent the crystallized textbook diagnostic syndromes. Rather, they show partial forms of mixed conditions. Existing classifications of major mental health problems do not do justice to the clinical realities (Krishnamoorthy et al., 2007).

6.2.6.4 *Common mental health problems*

The most frequent forms of mental health disturbance in childhood—anxiety, misery, and oppositional problems—are also more frequent in people with epilepsy, and not only because of the coincident presence of ADHD or ASD. Stigmatization, cognitive and linguistic problems, social adversity, the burden of care in families, and bullying all play a role for children with epilepsy, and psychopathology occurs in 37–77% of them (Plioplys et al., 2007).

Children and young people who encounter environmental adversity will often develop emotional and behavioural reactions to the vulnerability, disempowerment, and discrimination associated with having seizures. A systematic review of international qualitative studies identified frequent themes relating to stigma: loss of body control, loss of privacy, feelings of inferiority and futility, therapeutic burden, and navigating healthcare (Chong et al., 2016).

6.2.6.5 *Iatrogenic problems*

Many of the AEDs carry risks for inducing problems of irritability, aggression, sedation, and mood disturbance. These must be set against the beneficial effects of reducing or preventing seizures. Some AEDs are particularly prone to negative effects on mental health. Phenobarbitone, phenytoin, topiramate, valproex sodium, and probably gabapentin have earned particularly bad reputations among clinicians. Comparative trials find several of them more likely than other AEDs to impair cognitive performance

(Burns et al., 2018). Carbamazepine, levetiracetam, and lamotrigine are not implicated in the same way. Interactions between antiepileptic and psychotropic medications can be troublesome, and require either a single prescriber or careful communication between teams (see also "strategic planning" in Chapter 9, section 9.3.2.4).

6.2.6.6 *Epilepsy syndromes*

Some of the many syndromes recognized by the International League Against Epilepsy have strong implications for cognitive and behavioural outcomes. The severity of some of them calls attention to a need for psychiatric assessment, but scientific evaluation is too scanty to allow for syndrome-specific recommendations for psychiatric intervention.

The frequent syndromes of *early-onset childhood occipital epilepsy* (EOCOE) and *benign childhood epilepsy with centrotemporal spikes* (BECTS) (sometimes called 'Rolandic epilepsy') have, in some ways, a good outlook. BECTS typically begins at around the age of 8 years, often with tonic–clonic seizures at night. In the daytime, motor seizures are often minor. Clinical changes frequently involve only facial changes such as motor aphasia and tingling of lips, face, or tongue. Consciousness is often preserved. Drugs for partial seizures (e.g. lamotrigine, carbamazepine) usually work.

BECTS usually resolves during adolescence, and it is appropriate to give reassurance that seizures in adult life are unlikely. Unfortunately, however, while the condition is 'benign' for seizure prognosis, it is far from benign for mental life. A prospective study by Massa et al. (2001) followed a group from the very first presentation and found that more than a quarter had problems in school progress and behaviour. ADHD is often present. Learning impairments are common and often improve greatly once the seizures remit—as they often do. Inter-ictal spikes are common, and may contribute to learning problems, but suppressing them does not seem to help much. Children with BECTS sometimes escape neurologists' surveillance because of the good prognosis. They still need their treatment and for progress to be monitored with cognitive and behavioural assessment. EEG should also be monitored, as the presence of a wider range of abnormalities than the defining centrotemporal spike activity is a predictor of problems in impulse control and attention. Antiepileptic therapy should not be withheld.

In EOCOE (Panayiotopoulos syndrome), otherwise normally developing children begin to have autonomic epileptic seizures (see chapter 2, Autonomic nervous system, Section2.10) often at ages 3 to 6 years. Nausea, retching, and vomiting dominate. Pallor or flushing, pupillary changes, altered body temperature, and incontinence can also occur. Sometimes, there is every appearance of a faint (ictal syncope). Sometimes, but not always, the seizure progresses to convulsive movements. Therefore, autonomic nervous system (ANS) epilepsy may masquerade in various ways and need differentiating from encephalitis, atypical migraine, cardiogenic syncope, or other unrelated medical conditions such as gastroenteritis (Baumgartner et al., 2019). Behavioural problems are seldom severe. The EEG usually helps by showing spike and wave activity during an episode. The prognosis of EOCOE is usually very good for eventual recovery (Panayiotopoulos, 2004).

Some syndromes seem to represent severe early-onset encephalopathies, which can occur alone or together.

Ohtahara syndrome presents in infancy, even in neonatal life. It is described as presenting with frequent and intractable minor generalized seizures, with severe and continuous epileptic EEG abnormality (Ohtahara & Yamatogi, 2006). It predicts to severe developmental problems and intellectual impairment, and can evolve to West and Lennox–Gastaut syndromes.

West syndrome arises early in development and is associated with tuberous sclerosis (see Section 6.2.1.2). It is characterized by infantile spasms (flexor or salaam spasms, extensor spasms or mixed spasms). The very severe EEG abnormality of hypsarrhythmia is typical. It describes a disorganized, high-amplitude EEG even between seizures. Random, irregular spikes and waves are continuously present. Intellectual impairment, Autism, and ADHD are all very common. Early treatment can make a big difference to developmental outcome later (O'Callaghan et al., 2011).

The *Lennox–Gastaut syndrome* presents with multiple severe seizure types. Tonic episodes and losses of awareness are both typical. The EEG is markedly abnormal, with slow spike-wave discharges. Behavioural and cognitive changes are those of a dementia (Kieffer–Renaux et al., 2001).

Rasmussen's syndrome is an encephalitis affecting only one of the cerebral hemispheres. Hemiparesis and hemianopia may accompany focal epilepsy. The damage is usually permanent. The affected hemisphere atrophies and cognitive deterioration is a feature. Anti-inflammatory therapy (steroids or immunoglobulins) is given. It can be a reason for hemispherectomy (Bien et al., 2005).

Juvenile myoclonic epilepsy (Janz syndrome) is characterized clinically by a combination of absence seizures, myoclonic jerks, and tonic–clonic seizures, particularly on awakening. Performance on tests of executive function is weaker than that of matched controls, but parents are of similar IQ to typically developing people (Lin et al., 2014). Correspondingly, the same study by Lin et al. found neuroimaging evidence of altered cortical volume of frontal and other structures in a fronto–thalamo–cortical network. This represents, on the face of it, a marked similarity with executive function disorders arising from other and unknown causes.

Acquired epileptic aphasia (Landau–Kleffner syndrome; LKS) is a rare condition, characterized by loss of language skills after apparently normal development, together with EEG evidence of epileptiform activity. The EEG changes occur especially at night, with continuous spike-waves in slow-wave sleep or even electrical status epilepticus in sleep. It typically begins in young people, up to the age of 18 years. An earlier onset implies a higher risk of long-term impairment. Hyperactivity and a decreased attention span are usually present—in about 80%. Rages, aggression, and anxiety are also common, probably secondary to the frustration and communication difficulties caused by language impairment. The communication problems can disrupt social relationships. While these seldom amount to a full picture of autism, LKS may account for some cases of apparent autistic regression (Besag, 2015). Treatment with steroids and/or antiepileptics is advised even if there are no daytime seizures (as is the case for about 30% of those with LKS). Multiple subpial transection is used by some neurosurgeons to isolate discharging centres, and there have been reports of excellent results in a few patients (Irwin et al., 2001).

Continuous spike-waves in slow-wave sleep (CSWS) is also present in some people who show other cognitive and behavioural problems rather than language impairment. Sleep EEG is therefore indicated for children with any kind of loss of cognitive ability.

6.2.7 Treatment of mental disorders in epilepsy

The commonest intervention is the control of seizures. This may achieve a better level of social and academic integration and be helpful. For many disorders, however, the lack of relationship between seizure frequency and psychological impact suggests that control of frequency is necessary for quality of life, but not a very promising treatment for psychological problems.

When inflammation of the brain is involved, therapies such as steroids and immunoglobulins may be added to anti-seizure therapies. Adverse mental effects can follow. (See 'Adrenal glands and steroids', Section 6.7.3.) Other treatments will follow the usual lines for those in whom mental disorders are not accompanied by seizures (see Chapters 8 and 9). The different pathways through which psychiatric conditions have arisen need to be included in individual formulation and case planning.

6.3 CEREBRAL PALSY

Cerebral palsy (CP) is a heterogeneous group of disorders affecting motor function. They arise early in development and the brain lesions are not progressive. About 1 child in 500 is affected, with males somewhat outnumbering females in a ratio of about 1.3 to 1.

The clinical picture varies from time to time: complications in muscle systems can increase impairment even if the underlying brain deficit is static. Pain is frequent. The traditional classification is based on the limbs that are paralysed or weak: diplegia, hemiplegia, quadriplegia (or -paresis to indicate weakness rather than paralysis). Congenital hemiplegia is a form of cerebral palsy in which only the right or left side of the body is affected.

This anatomical classification, however, does not do justice to the variability over time, the frequent coexistence of problems, or to impairments other than those of limb movements—such as in speech, swallowing, and articulation. Accordingly, the type of abnormal movement is also differentiated: spastic, dyskinetic ('athetoid'), or ataxic.

These indicate the brain structures most likely to be affected, and to some extent the types of disability likely to arise.

> *Spastic*: stemming from an upper motor neuron lesion in the brain and corticospinal tract. This damage impairs the ability of some nerve receptors in the spinal cord to receive gamma-aminobutyric acid properly, leading to excessive tone in the muscles controlled by those damaged nerves. Muscles and tendons can become shorter than they should be, or fibrotic or atrophied. A result of the stiffening and shortening is permanent contracture and consequent deformity of the bones to which they are attached.
>
> *Ataxic*: associated with damage to cerebellar structures. Ataxia refers to an uncoordinated and disorderly style of movement. In the legs, this means unstable and unbalanced walking, often staggering and entailing falls. In the arms, movements are shaky and finger movements clumsy. Speech is dysrhythmic and clumsy, and eye movements, too, can miss their target and be overcorrected.
>
> *Dyskinetic* (choreo-athetoid or dystonic): primarily associated with damage to the basal ganglia in the form of lesions that occur during brain development due to bilirubin encephalopathy or hypoxic-ischaemic brain injury. It is characterized by unwanted movements, either jerky (choreiform) or writhing (athetoid), and by an inability to control muscle tone.

Severity of all the types of cerebral palsy is usually graded by the need for support (i.e. the impact on the young person's functioning). Standard scales have been developed to assess the severity of gross movement problems (Palisano et al., 1997) and fine motor problems (Eliasson et al., 2006). These will give a better guide than diagnosis to the child's needs for assistance.

The course varies over time, even when the lesions are static. In the first few months of life, there may be no evident problem at all. The first recognition may be because one side does not move as much as the other or the legs seem stiff or the child cannot sit at the usual time (about 6 months). The full picture may not emerge even until 4 years, so premature assessments of needs can be mistaken.

Most of the risks for CP arise before birth, often well before. Sometimes, a specific cause can be found; often, not. Causes include:

- congenital malformations
- vascular events (e.g. middle cerebral artery occlusion)
- maternal infections during the first and second trimesters of pregnancy (rubella, cytomegalovirus, toxoplasmosis)
- infections of the fetal membranes (chorioamnionitis)
- maternal ingestion of toxins (e.g. mercury)
- maternal deficiencies (e.g. iodine)
- Rh blood type incompatibility (in which the mother's immune system attacks the baby's red blood cells)

- rare genetic
- death of a co-twin sharing a chorion.

Prevention is sometimes possible; for instance, maternal vaccination for dyskinetic CP due to kernicterus (Rh isoimmunization). Correction of maternal iodine deficiency, and removal of toxins such as lead from the environment are important everywhere, and especially in tropical countries. More often, any of many possible adversities have compromised fetal development in the womb. Placental dysfunction, slow fetal growth, and maternal illness or malnutrition can all contribute. The exact mechanisms are not clear, and many are associations rather than known causes. They are all associated with preterm birth, and rates of CP are high in small and premature babies: about 11% of those born before a gestational age of 28 weeks; about 6% in those weighing between 1 kg and 1.5 kg.

A short length of gestation, a low birthweight, and a low Apgar score are powerful predictors of CP. This strong association may reflect the results of prenatal adversity as much as or more than the risks of birth itself (such as intraventricular bleeds). Periventricular malacia is strongly associated with spastic CP, and points to a problem arising around 28 weeks of gestation. However, it is also found in babies born at term with CP, so the automatic attribution of birth injury in such cases is probably mistaken. Birth injury or hypoxia used to be considered as the major cause of CP. In fact, it is probably responsible only for a small minority of cases. Described perinatal factors are indicated in Box 6.1.

There has been a major change of understanding over the last two decades. The birth-damage theory energized big improvements in obstetric care, and the prevalence of CP was taken as the major indicator of care quality. The improvement in care resulted in a marked decline of still births and neonatal deaths, but CP rates did not improve (Braun et al., 2016). Other causes therefore play a larger part in current formulations. Public perceptions have been slower to change, and many compensation cases are still mounted based on a presumption that any obstetric negligence in a case must be responsible. Law courts deciding on compensation now usually require more evidence

---

Box 6.1 Perinatal factors associated with cerebral palsy

- Prolapsed cord
- Massive intrapartum haemorrhage
- Prolonged or traumatic delivery
- Prolonged second stage of labour
- Emergency Caesarean section
- Premature separation of the placenta
- Abnormal fetal position
- Neonatal encephalopathy

Many of these may reflect prenatal adversity rather than direct causality.

Box 6.2 Postnatal causes of motor impairment

- Physical brain injury (e.g. after motor vehicle accident)
- Abusive head trauma
- Severe hypoxia (e.g. after near drowning)
- Stroke; sickle cell
- Encephalitis or meningitis
- Toxins (e.g. lead poisoning)

---

than in the past that obstetric accidents were in fact responsible for an individual's plight and justify compensation payments.

After birth, other causes are indicated in Box 6.2.

6.3.1 Initial assessment

By the age of 8 months, inability to sit independently is a clinical sign requiring further monitoring. A full diagnosis should often be postponed until the age of 36 months, by which time motor function can be assessed more reliably. Intellectual impairment and fragile-X syndrome should be tested for routinely. Neuroimaging with magnetic resonance imaging (MRI) or computerized tomography (CT) should be undertaken when the cause is not known. MRI is preferred over CT, for its diagnostic yield. When abnormal, neuroimaging can also suggest the timing of the initial damage and reveal treatable conditions such as hydrocephalus, porencephaly, arteriovenous malformation, subdural haematomas and hygromas, and tumours.

6.3.2 Consequences

Sensory and perceptual problems are common. They often stem from the same occasions of brain injury that have caused the motor impairment. Around 5% of those with CP are impaired in hearing; around 10% in vision. Optic neuropathy and cerebral visual impairment can contribute. Coordinating the two eyes ('binocular fusion') is often difficult. Depth perception is frequently problematic and contributes further to difficulties in independent activity.

6.3.3 Complications of cerebral palsy

Some complications are particularly frequent for those with CP. They are indicated in Box 6.3. The stresses may be compounded by the effort required to cope with them.

Box 6.3 Complications of cerebral palsy

- Epilepsy
- Intellectual deficit
- Learning difficulties
- Language and communication
- Pain
- Fatigue
- Sleep
- Eating problems and poor nutrition
- School failure
- Problems with peers
- Deprivation of experience
- Dependence
- Family burden
- Psychiatric syndromes

6.3.3.1 *Epilepsy in cerebral palsy*

Seizures develop in about a third—especially those with spastic types of CP. When the CP can be attributed to white-matter injury, the commonest forms of seizures are the same as the commonest forms in the general population of young people (Cooper et al., 2017). In particular, the frequent syndromes of EOCOE and BECTS have a good outlook, and parents can be reassured that their children are unlikely to have seizures in adult life. If, however, the CP results from diffuse cortical malformations and injuries, then epilepsy can be expected to persist in as many as half. The effects of seizures on mental function are not different from those of epilepsy arising from other causes.

6.3.3.2 *Intellectual and learning disabilities*

Intellectual disability is more common than in typically developing populations and is present, to a significant degree, in about 20% of those with CP, and even more in those with severe and multiple motor problems. Nevertheless, many—even of those with severe CP—are as intellectually able as anyone else. Sometimes, intellectual ability is severely underestimated because of communication problems. A judgement of intellectual potential should be reserved until after school entry.

Specific learning difficulties are also quite common. They often come to light as school progresses, and emerge with written language and calculation. The reasons include a short attention span, motor planning difficulties (organization and sequencing of movement), perceptual difficulties, and language disability.

Both global and specific disabilities have comparable effects on behaviour and emotions to those occurring in people without CP. The effects are cumulative rather than dependent on aetiology.

6.3.3.3 *Language and communication*

The articulation of speech can be severely compromised. It calls for continuing therapy. Language in young people with hemiplegia has been extensively studied as evidence for hemisphere specialization and is considered under localized structural lesions (see Section 6.2.1.1).

6.3.3.4 *Pain*

Pain, especially for those with spastic motor tone, can dominate life. It can make sleep hard to achieve and maintain. At school, or in sedentary occupations, it can make the usual requirement for sitting still to be agonizing. It is sometimes underestimated, and does not always figure in training material, but should always be enquired about in assessment.

6.3.3.5 *Fatigue and sleep*

Feelings of being exhausted, tired, and lacking in energy are a frequent part of the experience of CP. These sensations are sometimes attributed to demoralization or a form of chronic fatigue syndrome. Much more commonly, however, they result simply from the much greater effort that is required to perform muscular actions and from greater muscle tone even at rest. Disturbed sleep, from pain and postural problems, can also play a part. Other factors include inadequate and unhealthy eating, and dehydration resulting from oropharyngeal difficulties. Some of the drug treatments given for spasticity or dystonia will have a sedative effect and therefore lead to feelings of fatigue or drowsiness.

6.3.3.6 *School failure*

The motor impairments can lead children to experience all kinds of difficulties in school, quite apart from any learning problems. Difficulties with handwriting, in carrying out school activities, in communicating verbally, and with interacting socially may all have to be explained to the school. Students with CP need to put more effort into concentrating on their movements and sequences of movements than others, so they may tire more easily. Teachers who have not been trained in the special educational needs that the children may present may well need support themselves.

6.3.3.7 *Deprivation of experience and dependency*

Physical restrictions on movement are also restrictions on the opportunities to learn. Active exploration of the environment is possible to all except the most severely impaired. Learning about space, effort, the social consequences of moving around other people, and the results of getting into mischief is very much available to those in wheelchairs as to those on foot. Nevertheless, and in spite of careful and sensitive efforts to promote independence, many barriers to participation remain. The sense of autonomy and self-efficacy can suffer. The amount of time that must be spent in the various therapies likely to be required comes at the expense of pleasurable activity and socializing. The adults running leisure activities have not always been taught the skills necessary to involve the young people who are less mobile.

Obvious inabilities evoke many kinds of reactions from other people. Some of them, including the struggles of some resourceful and solvent parents to find physical or medical fixes, can accentuate a feeling in the young people of being under external control. Other reactions include admiration for achievement over impairment, and self-esteem may be correspondingly spared (see 'Quality of life', Section 6.3.3.13).

6.3.3.8 Problems with peers

Many children with CP make very good relationships in an accepting peer group. The other children are still able to run faster and answer schoolwork questions faster, so there is still a risk of feeling left behind. In adolescence, self-esteem can slump, particularly in the context of developing romantic interests. Children with movement impairments are often the target of bullies, especially those who exploit people who are unlikely to defend themselves effectively.

6.3.3.10 Family burden

The burden of care is at least as great as in other developmental disorders (see Chapter 10, Section 10.6). Depending on the severity of physical problems, much of the day can be taken up with the everyday tasks of dressing, mealtimes, getting to school and clinics, and engaging in physiotherapy. Financial costs limit opportunities for other family members. The outcome of litigation is often uncertain and long-drawn-out. Parental distress is very often exacerbated by feelings of guilt and anger, as well as mourning.

6.3.3.11 Mental consequences

There are many possible consequences for emotions, learning, and behaviour, both as a result of brain dysfunction and consequent upon restriction of activities and the reactions of other people. Many of these adverse changes are common to many kinds of neurodevelopmental disorder. Experiences of bullying, stigma, and social exclusion are unfortunately so frequent as to be almost the rule. Chapter 10 considers them and other barriers to participation.

6.3.3.12 Psychiatric syndromes

Emotional and behaviour problems are common; more so than in the general population. A questionnaire survey of parents' reports was conducted in nine regions of Western Europe (Parkes et al., 2008). Over 40% of affected children aged 8 to 12 years had elevated scores based on problem counts (by comparison with approximately 18% of British general population samples). More than a quarter of the children with CP were rated by their parents at levels of behavioural and emotional problems that are considered to be a high risk for the presence of a diagnosable disorder. High levels of problems were predicted by the presence of low intellectual levels, chronic pain, having a brother or sister with a disability, and where they lived. In this survey, severe motor disability itself was not a strong predictor of psychological problems. Indeed, the worse their gross motor function, the less their behavioural and emotional problems were reported to impact their lives. Perhaps those with the most impaired motor function were the least likely to be able to show behaviours difficult for others to tolerate; perhaps the least impaired became more frustrated and distressed by comparisons with more mobile children.

The forms of psychiatric disorders in CP reflect a wide range of common mental health problems. Behavioural problems are usually oppositional (i.e. characterized by irritability and headstrongness). Conduct disorders, which involve deliberately anti-social behaviours such as stealing or bullying, are less common. Emotional disorders usually involve anxieties and fears; less frequently, depression.

Children with hemiplegia are usually less impaired in motor function and communication, but more prone to psychiatric problems—especially ADHD (Graham, 1996). A survey by Goodman & Yude (1996) found attention and executive function difficulties to be the usual ADHD presentation, but both pervasive and situational impulsiveness were also frequent difficulties. ADHD in hemiplegia was also highly predictive of other mental problems appearing (Goodman & Graham, 1996). The strongest single predictor of psychiatric problems was intelligence quotient (IQ), which was highly correlated with an index of neurological severity. Neurological severity was indexed by the degree of hemiparesis, presence and type of seizure disorder, presence of any signs of bilateral involvement, head circumference, and time of onset. Neither low IQ nor neurological severity could be regarded as total explanations of psychological problems. Even affected children with IQs in the normal range had a high rate of problems. Age, sex, and laterality of lesion had little or no predictive power. Family structure and size did not seem to contribute much.

Around 70% of the children with hemiplegia who had a psychiatric diagnosis initially were still psychiatric cases 4 years later (Goodman, 1998). In addition, around 30% of children who were not psychiatric cases initially had become so 4 years later. Those who persisted in having a psychiatric diagnosis were distinguished from those who developed out of it by the initial diagnosis and its severity, rather than by any specific neurological, demographic, or cognitive features. There were, however, other predictors in a population-based sample, such as chronic pain, family adversity, and maternal mental illness (Goodman & Graham, 1996).

6.3.3.13   *Quality of life*

Quality of life looks different to those who have the condition and those who observe it. A survey of quality of life in children aged 8 to 12 years in several European countries (Dickinson et al., 2007), and one of adolescents (Colver et al., 2015), asked the children and young people themselves about their perceptions of physical and psychological well-being. The children—or rather, those who were able to communicate their quality of life—were rather similar to their contemporaries in the general population. This is a tribute to the resilience of the human spirit. The children did not, for the most part, see themselves as pitiable, but as experiencing the challenges and pleasures of growing up in ways similar to anyone else. There were, to be sure, some particular aspects of life in that study that were reduced in quality—especially for those who experienced much pain. Intellectual impairment, too, was associated in that study with self-perception of lower mood, more anxiety, and less autonomy. The general finding should nevertheless encourage caregivers, educators, and clinicians to be positive about affected children's futures.

Parents' accounts of their children's quality of life tell a less encouraging story. They indicate that gross motor function and IQ are strong drivers of quality of life. They are also strong influences on the quality of life of the parents who are looking after them (which may be part of the reason for the disparity between what young people and their parents say).

6.3.4 Management

The goals of physical therapy are not only to fix individual physical impairments (such as spasticity in a limb) or even functional problems such as walking. Approaches to managing CP increasingly emphasize the wider goals of helping the individual to be as independent as possible and engaged with their community. Correspondingly, psychological help should also have broad goals of helping them to get along in a non-disabled world. Resolution of difficulties such as phobic fears of failure or ADHD can use the same approaches as in children without difficulties in movement (see Chapters 8 and 9).

6.3.5 Other disorders of movement control

The development of motor coordination and its pathology are described in Chapter 2. Developmental coordination disorder has been described, together with other learning impairments, in Chapter 5, Section 5.2. Catatonia is described in Chapter 4, Section 4.2.10 as a pathology of volition rather than motor control; cataplexy as a disorder of sleep. Tics and Tourette are described as psychiatric syndromes (Chapter 5, Section 5.1).

6.4 HYDROCEPHALUS

Hydrocephalus is a common disorder (about 1 in 800 babies) in which excessive pressure of cerebral spinal fluid (CSF) results in abnormally large ventricles of the brain. Infants develop large heads (macrocephaly). After about the age of 2 years, the skull has much less ability to expand, so by this age the usual sign is increasing pressure on the brain.

There are many causes, summarized by Kahle et al. (2016). Malformations of the brain, such as aqueduct stenosis, account for most cases arising prenatally. Neural tube defects (of which the most serious form is meningomyelocoele) are particularly important because they are linked to maternal folate deficiency, and folate supplementation in pregnancy has a major role in prevention. Perinatal onsets are often associated with bleeds; onsets later in childhood are often due to infections. Malignant tumours can also play a part. Some cases may develop because the brain has reduced compliance with pulsations as the heart beats.

The key part of management is surgical, and shunts are often inserted to help the cerebrospinal fluid to drain. Over time, the shunts can become blocked or infected, so continuing surveillance is essential.

A good quality of life is attainable, but many affected people will have long-term complications. Headaches are very common. Around a half of people with infantile hydrocephalus will develop mobility problems, often amounting to cerebral palsy; around a third will develop epilepsy. Learning difficulties will be apparent in as many as half—but somewhat fewer in those whose hydrocephalus was not apparent at birth (Persson et al., 2006).

Persistent cognitive changes have been described in case-control studies (Fletcher et al., 2000). No single pattern is to be expected—but non-verbal skills seem particularly likely to be affected. Visual motor, spatial, memory, attention, and executive dysfunctions are all described. Verbal fluency is often unimpaired, but comprehension of speech may be somewhat delayed.

In adolescence, sexual development is often accelerated. Precocious puberty brings particular stresses for girls. In adult life, some 45% of those who had infantile hydro cephalus were found to have needed treatment for depression, 43% were dependent on care, and 43% were unemployed (Gupta et al., 2007).

6.5 ACQUIRED TRAUMATIC INJURY TO THE BRAIN

Acute trauma affects many children all over the world, for many reasons. Motor vehicle accidents, abusive injury, falls, sports injuries, gunshot wounds, and other assaults all carry different implications for the young people most at risk and the social contexts in which they occur. Accordingly, understanding and managing abnormal mental states after head injury will need to consider the risk factors before the accidents, the nature and severity of the injury, and the direct and indirect consequences.

6.5.1 Epidemiology

Head injuries are the commonest cause of death in children and adolescents in affluent countries and are important causes of disability. Prevalence and incidence studies from

6.5.4.1.1 *Mild and moderate injury*

A single mild injury is likely to predict a good cognitive outcome. In one careful study of children hospitalized after head injury, 'mildly' affected children were defined as those with a post-traumatic amnesia of less than a week but more than an hour. They functioned at a somewhat lower level than children without injury or children with only orthopaedic injuries. Nevertheless, a detailed retrospective enquiry suggested that they would have functioned at a similarly low level before the injury. Furthermore, there was little evidence of improvement in the months after the injury. Both types of evidence suggested that a single mild injury is not usually very harmful to cognitive function but often reflects adversity that was present before the injury (Chadwick et al., 1981a).

Repeated mild injuries could still have longer-term effects. The issue has arisen particularly for brief concussions occurring frequently—for instance, in contact sports. Diagnosis is not very easy. The most prominent symptoms of concussions are amnesia and confusion, rather than loss of consciousness. They can be defined as the rapid onset of short-lived impairment of neurological function that resolves spontaneously.

Even when functional disturbance after an impact injury has recovered completely, and there is no decrement on test scores, a subsequent injury is more likely to produce cognitive impairment. Presumably, the first injury does indeed have consequences and limits the resilience of the brain. One possible mediator is a glutamate receptor, N-methyl-D-aspartate receptor (NMDAR). NMDA is released in the brain following concussion.

The extent to which repeated mild injury can cause long-term impairment is still disputed, but emerging consensus among sports psychologists recognizes the possible cumulative impact. Automated neurocognitive tests of memory, attention, and executive functions can be used to follow the development of athletes in sports, such as boxing, which involve violent impacts on the head. Young athletes are probably more susceptible than older ones to losing cognitive function. Young athletes are also prone to under-reporting injuries because of their wish to advance in the sport and not be restricted by the official preventive measures.

6.5.4.1.2 *Severe injury*

Children with severe brain injury show a different course over time. In a longitudinal study, they were seriously impaired shortly after the injury, to a degree dependent upon the severity of injury, and there was marked recovery in succeeding months (Chadwick et al., 1981a). Indeed, there was still some recovery proceeding in the second year after injury. The dose–response relationship was close, and non-neurological factors seemed to have little influence on IQ and reading later. Nor was there anything very specific in the profile of changes on IQ testing or on a set of neuropsychological tests. Indeed, there was a suggestion that tests of speed of visuomotor or visuospatial functioning could be more sensitive than other tests. Nevertheless, the changes were not specific enough to allow deductions backwards; for example, to say from the results of psychological testing alone that a child without a known history of severe trauma must nevertheless have suffered injury to the brain (Chadwick et al., 1981b).

The consequences for academic learning are substantial. Severely injured children and young people will be slow to learn reading and numeracy and social skills. The need for special intervention is often forgotten as they move into successive classes. If they do not have visible signs of motor disability, their special needs and disabilities may disappear from their records and be considered, it at all, only as moral failings.

6.5.4.2 *Behaviour and emotions after head injuries*

Psychiatric problems typically follow a more complicated course than the cognitive changes. In broad outline, they show a similar relationship to severity of brain damage but are also subject to other influences. Families and educators often identify emotional and behavioural changes as the most disabling alterations for the children. They involve various combinations of disinhibition, inattentiveness, impulsiveness, emotional lability, anger/aggression, anxiety, depression, apathy, and social withdrawal (Trenchard et al., 2013).

In a longitudinal prospective study, mild injuries did not usually affect psychosocial functioning in the short term and any impairments were static. After severe injury, by contrast, they were markedly impaired shortly afterwards but showed substantial and continuing recovery in succeeding months. The worse the injury, the more likely were behavioural and emotional changes. By contrast with cognitive changes, the trajectory of recovery was also influenced, for the worse, by socio-familial adversity and by behaviour problems before the injury (Brown et al., 1981).

Emotional and behavioural problems can result indirectly or directly from cognitive deficits. The children and young people may be vulnerable to the stresses of failure at school and altered family dynamics. If they cannot engage in the activities they wish, frustration can lead either to anger or sorrow. Stigma and discrimination can create a sense of unfairness or of low self-worth. The usual over-representation of boys in some behaviour problems, and of girls in some emotional problems, applies much less in the presence of neurological compromise.

New psychiatric diagnoses emerging after severe injury are quite common. Max et al. (1997) found a rate of 36% at the 2-year mark after injury. The range of mental health problems attributable to severe injury is wide. It includes ADHD, marijuana misuse, mood disorders, and various anxiety disorders including separation anxiety and obsessive-compulsive disorder. Social disinhibition and emotional dysregulation are often the key psychiatric problems. These, in combination with changes in executive function and impulse control, will often lead to meeting the full criteria for ADHD. This 'secondary ADHD' has similarities with frontal lobe syndromes but does not imply that the rest of the brain is intact. Secondary ADHD is also associated with oppositional and conduct problems in the same way as early-onset ADHD without a history of injury. Max et al. (1997) noted that 30–50% of school-age children developed symptoms of ADHD for the first time soon after injury. Depression is also a frequent consequence of injury. A systematic review by Li and Liu (2013) found that new depressive disorders occurred in some 10–25% of school-age children after traumatic brain injury, emerging up to 2 years later.

Social impairments have been reported to be very frequent in children with traumatic brain injury (Anderson et al., 2013). Both social outcome, and direct tests of the children's cognitive abilities important for social competence, are problematic in a large minority. Disinhibition, lack of awareness of social rules, lack of empathy, and subtle cognitive difficulties all play a part. Younger age at injury, severity of injury, current behaviour problems, low intelligence, and family dysfunction are all related to social impairment. Careful analysis of the difficulties is necessary for appropriate treatment.

Dollman et al. (2017) drew attention to the extent of unmet needs for managing behaviour problems and special educational needs after severe head injury in an under-resourced country (South Africa).

6.5.5 Processes of recovery

Recovery involves several processes. Immediate consequences, such as swelling and infection, can subside. There can be some regeneration of brain structures (e.g. with more sprouting of neurites), but this can also be counterproductive in leading to interference with other processes or to less controlled function. Sometimes, mildly damaged parts of the brain can recover some efficiency over time and aid recovery. Sometimes, other structures will take over the functions of the damaged ones—for instance, right hemispheres take over the language function of damaged left-sided structures. New strategies can be developed to solve problems in different ways. Parents and educators may vary in the extent to which they are able to support new learning.

Recovery is also influenced by the extent and localization of the injury, the age of the person, and brain plasticity.

6.5.6 Influences on recovery

The extent and severity of the initial injury continue to be a powerful influence, as described previously. In addition, the long-term outcomes vary greatly, depending on the age at injury, localization in the brain, level of psychological function before and after the injury, degree of social adversity, neuropsychological deficits, and neurological complications such as the advent of epilepsy. The ability of the family to remain supportive is important. Gender and ethnicity do not seem to be as significant in the genesis of psychological problems as they are in people who have not been injured.

6.5.6.1 *Age at injury and at assessment*
Early damage is more likely than late to leave a consequence of widespread brain dysfunction, but possibly less likely to result in localized psychological deficits.

A longitudinal study investigated the recovery, over a period of up to 30 months, of intellectual abilities of children sustaining traumatic brain injury (Anderson et al., 2005a). The injuries had occurred at various times between birth and 12 years of age. At 3 months after the injury, all children with severe damage had similar levels of impairment, whatever the age at damage. By 30 months, however, those with early injuries (before the age of 7 years) were performing significantly worse than those who had been injured at an older age. The clear implication is that services need to maintain a long-term follow-up of children injured in infancy and early childhood.

Several processes may contribute to early lesions being particularly damaging to later development of diffusely organized mental activity. There may be knock-on effects in which early disruption of control functions compromises the later development of abilities, such as those necessary for reading, that would have been more likely to recover if they were already established. The orderly development of brain function may be disrupted by the very processes of regeneration and substitution that are making for greater plasticity. The brain processes that are ongoing at the time of the injury might be particularly susceptible to disruption.

The age of assessment will also have an impact on what is found. If young people are assessed years after injury in childhood, there may be apparently new problems of psychological function. This can be simply because older children are now capable of carrying out more demanding tests and, therefore, of showing subtler dysfunctions than was the case when they were younger. It may also be because localization of function has shifted in the normal course of development, as when late-maturing frontal lobe structures have taken over the functions previously associated with other parts of the brain.

An influential series of experiments by Goldman–Rakic et al. (1983) demonstrated how findings can change as the brain changes. They described research on rhesus monkeys in which bilateral damage to dorsolateral parts of the frontal cortex in infancy seemed to produce little or no effect on delayed response learning, yet the same animals in adult life developed a deficit in frontal lobe-mediated delayed response learning that was very similar to that which appears in animals given the same lesions in adult life. Some specific effects of early localized damage were apparent in later development, not early.

6.5.6.2 *Brain plasticity*

'Plasticity' refers to the reshaping of brain architecture. It is exemplified by the effects of left- versus right-sided lesions on language development (see 'Effects of hemi-syndromes, Section 6.6.1). The evidence here is that young brains can develop language competence in right-sided structures in a way that is not open in adult life. In addition, local repair of left-sided structures allows distinctively left-sided abilities to be used (see Section 6.6). Experimental damage in animals has also indicated the potential for motor functions to be taken over by other brain structures.

6.5.6.3 *Localization*

The extent to which injury is localized will have a marked influence on its effects. The diffuse and widespread damage associated with closed injuries tends to have different effects on mental development from the effects of focal damage (e.g. in open injuries). The latter allow examination of the extent to which later sequelae can be specific to the area of the brain that has been affected.

A closely studied series was reported by Shaffer et al. (1975). They examined 98 children with circumscribed lesions that had caused neurosurgically verified dural tears. Most problems did not follow a pattern of association with site of damage. The clinical research did not find anatomical correlates of impairments in information processing, attention, language, or perceptual abilities. The investigation did, however, reveal some correlations between anatomical site and psychiatric syndrome. The most striking finding was an excess of affective symptoms in association with right frontal and left parieto-temporal sites of injury. The 33 depressed frontal fractures were associated with high rates of psychiatric disorder (80% for right-sided lesions, 65% for left-sided).

6.5.6.4 *Social and family influences*

The course of mental development after brain damage is subject to the reactions of others (Anderson et al., 2005b). Some influences bear forcefully upon those whose dysfunction has an immediate and obvious cause. Parents may themselves be traumatized from the agonies of fear and uncertainty that come from watching their child undergo a threat to life. They may react with bitter anger towards those held responsible for their child's predicament. Attitudes of parents and other caregivers can have strong effects. Parents may be deeply affected by grief or remorse, however unjustified. One typical result is overprotectiveness, limiting both the range of experience from which their children can learn and the confidence that comes from overcoming obstacles. Other possible results are overly indulgent or harshly demanding attitudes towards disciplinary problems or underachievement. Expectations should still be high, but realistic.

6.5.7 Management of acute brain injury

Treatment in the acute stage of a severe injury aims to reduce further damage. Adequate oxygen, support of blood flow to the brain, and control of raised intracranial pressure will all be goals. At a later stage, the goals may well shift to rehabilitation and support. An effective team will be able to call on occupational therapy, physiotherapy, or speech and language therapy as required. If there is persisting disability, special educational help may well be needed. Epilepsy will need to be watched out for. Psychiatric complications are as described previously. Sleeping problems are frequently reported, and it will be necessary to assess whether they are related to anxiety, depression, or post-traumatic disorder so that appropriate action can be taken.

Developing influences over time call for continuing evaluation and re-evaluation of mental functions. Clinicians should allow time before giving a prognosis. Continued monitoring and support for families are needed.

6.6 LOCALIZED STRUCTURAL LESIONS

The most frequent form of localized damage in childhood is hemiplegia due to a stroke. It occurs in young people, with a prevalence of about 1 in 1,000. Middle cerebral artery infarction or periventricular malacia (softening) is usually the pathology responsible for congenital cases, and the resulting circumscribed lesions can be visualized with neuroimaging techniques. Periventricular Sturge–Weber syndromes also result from readily visualized lesions. Other localized lesions, apart from CP and head injury, can give rise to cognitive, behavioural, and emotional dysfunctions. Tumours, bleeds, abscesses, and congenital malformations can all interfere with localized brain structures (Box 6.4).

Box 6.4 Causes of chronic hemiplegia in children

- Cerebrovascular accident (CVA; stroke): embolism, thrombosis, or haemorrhage
- Intraventricular haemorrhage (especially in premature babies)
- Head injury, including perinatal
- Brain tumour (primary or metastatic)
- Infections: encephalitis, meningitis, brain abscess
- Genetic disorders (e.g. leukodystrophies, leukoencephalopathies)
- Vascular diseases (e.g. Kawasaki)
- Inflammatory demyelinating diseases
- Congenital malformations: many rare conditions, including:
  - Sturge–Weber Syndrome (birthmark and brain angioma)
  - Arteriovenous malformations
  - Unilateral polymicrogyria
  - Hemi-megalencephaly
  - Unilateral hydrocephalus

6.6.1 Effects of hemi-syndromes

Localization of traumatic injury in adults was studied classically by Lishman (1973). He described intellectual impairments as resulting from left-sided damage, while right-sided injuries were more likely to result in emotional and behavioural changes. In children, there is much less evidence for laterality effects on mental changes. For instance, the behavioural effects of lateralized brain disease in childhood are not very specific to the side of injury or disease. Duval et al. (2002) compared children with left and right hemi-syndromes using a standardized rating scale (the Child Behaviour Checklist). The side of lesion did not predict the balance of internalizing and externalizing behaviour problems. Rather, the high rates of psychiatric difficulties could be partly attributed to social and familial influences. Chronic pain, family adversity, and maternal mental illness are key factors; so too is the severity of neurological damage.

In cognitive function, children take a somewhat different course from adults. Children with an early-onset hemiplegia have, as a group, a lower IQ than unaffected children (see Section 6.5.6.3). However, it is not true that low non-verbal IQ reflects right-sided brain damage, and low verbal, left-sided. Rather, both left- and right-sided lesions are characterized by lowered non-verbal IQ. This is usually attributed to the priority in natural development being given to language. The normally left-sided functions are partly taken over by right-sided structures, so that the spatial functions whose development is usually served by the right side are crowded out.

The greater recovery with early lesions seems to be a function of more plasticity, not less specialization. Indeed, studies of normal development are in keeping with specialization of hemisphere development from an early stage. Lateralizing features in responding to sounds, such as a right-ear advantage in dichotic stimulation, can be shown at ages right down to the first 3 months of life using experiments such as the power of speech sounds to change the non-nutritive sucking rate (Entus, 1977).

A complex conclusion came from studies of children who had received the extreme but effective treatment of surgical hemisphere destruction in a small number of cases of Sturge–Weber syndrome (Dennis & Kohn, 1975). There was no overall difference in IQ according to side, but the right hemisphere had not acquired quite the same syntactic abilities as the left. A residual right hemisphere was less well able than a left one to carry out tasks based on the internal phonological structure of heard language. Language and IQ were investigated in a population-based sample of 149 children with hemiplegia (Goodman & Yude, 1996). The major influence on IQ was an overall index of neurological severity. Performance IQ was an average of 13 points lower than verbal IQ—but this discrepancy was not related to the side of lesion. Neurological factors and social adversity had additive effects on IQ. Investigation of children's learning problems should include the full range of factors influencing cognitive impairments in the whole population, as well as the specific neurological lesions.

More recently, the advent of functional neuroimaging has enabled more direct study of localization. This has not exactly contradicted the notion of transfer of language functions from a damaged left hemisphere to an intact right one, but has suggested a more nuanced understanding. As an example, Raja Beharelle et al. (2010) were able to image lateralized activation in young people who had suffered right-sided congenital hemiplegia, due to a left-sided stroke, up to 29 years previously. The investigators used a verbal test requiring people to produce examples of a given category (e.g. types of animal)—which in typically developing people is particularly strongly associated with left-sided activation. They confirmed earlier findings of greater right-sided or bilateral activation than in typically developing people. This gave some support to the notion of transfer of language from left to right. They also found, however, that those with the best-preserved language were also those with the greatest left anterior (or bilateral posterior) activation. It seems that recovery of at least some linguistic functions is linked to preserved or recovered left-hemisphere structures.

In summary, there is evidence of early specialization of the hemispheres. Early damage to the left hemisphere is followed by greater development of language function than is the case in the adult brain. Some of the recovery is due to the right hemisphere taking over language function. It manages well, but may be limited in some syntactic abilities.

6.6.2 Right hemispheres

The consequences in childhood of damage to 'right-sided' functions such as spatial perception, face and music recognition, attention, and emotional control after right hemisphere damage is less well established than in adults. Unilateral right-sided cerebral damage is classically associated with deficits in visuospatial skills, directed attention, and modulation of affect. Classic symptoms in adults include:

- Disorientation in time and place
- Left-sided neglect (in which there is reduced responsiveness to stimuli presented on the person's left side)
- Anosognosia (lack of awareness of the impairment of function)
- Visuospatial deficits such as failure to recognize faces or to integrate details into a whole
- High-level communication compromise: when unilateral right-hemisphere damage affects communication, it does not lead to gross deficits in syntax or word finding; rather, high-level aspects of discourse (e.g. understanding humour, metaphors, sarcasm, facial expression, and prosody) are compromised
- Related cognitive deficits, such as inference, working memory, and theory of mind

Localized problems in adolescents and young adults are broadly similar, but persistence and the process of recovery are not yet clear. Spatial neglect in younger children can be assessed by the search habits of children (e.g. the Teddy Bear Cancellation Test, in which pictures of teddy bears must be crossed out on a sheet containing many other images).

The localization of omissions on that test was skewed significantly to the left in children with right-sided lesions compared to children with left-sided lesions (Laurent–Vannier et al., 2006). The distinction, however, was not strong enough to be useful in diagnosis.

Weintraub and Mesulam (1983) claimed a syndrome of 'introversion, poor social perception, chronic emotional difficulties, inability to display affect, and impairments in visuospatial representation' that was associated with motor and/or neuropsychological evidence of right-sided brain dysfunction. Their 14 adult cases had been selected from clinical referrals for social difficulties and visuospatial deficits: 'The prosodic quality of speech, maintenance of eye contact, and the use of gestures received special notice'. All of the described features read today very like features of ASDin adult life; yet autism research bears little trace of a unique role for the right hemisphere. Selection of cases could well have generated the apparent neurological specificity. Assessment of any right-hemisphere dysfunction in autistic presentations would have to be based initially on neurological examination, and definitively on neuroimaging, usually with MRI.

6.6.3 Frontal lesions

Localized frontal disorders typically have multiple effects at high levels of coordination. The structure and function of the prefrontal cortex follow an unusually protracted course in ordinary development. Synaptic density in layer III of the middle frontal gyrus proceeds more slowly than in most of the rest of the brain and is not at its maximum until after the age of 15 months (Huttenlocher & Dabholkar, 1997). Connections in the corpus callosum between frontal structures are still developing through childhood, and peak growth rates proceed from rostral to caudal (Thompson et al., 2000). Myelination in the prefrontal cortex continues into adult life. The elimination of synapses is still continuing in the prefrontal cortex until middle adolescence (Huttenlocher & Dabholkar,1997). Diseases of the frontal lobes are dependent on these complex dynamics of brain development. The immature brain may use quite different strategies from the mature one in achieving the same goal (see 'Age at injury and at assessment', Section 6.5.6.1).

Animal experiments have suggested that certain periods in brain development (e.g. in postnatal synaptic proliferation) are particularly sensitive to brain damage (e.g. Kolb et al., 2000). This has been influential in leading researchers to consider possible developmental changes in susceptibility to lesions of the brain. Some human research (not all) has come to a similar conclusion. As an example, a study examined the development of executive function deficits in children with circumscribed frontal lobe conditions (Jacobs et al., 2007). The lesions were of several kinds—strokes, trauma, tumours, abscesses, and bleeds. Results, like the animal research on experimental damage, suggested a complex relationship between age of onset and eventual outcome. They described some 'critical periods' during development in which insults to the frontal lobes were particularly likely to give rise to behavioural or cognitive impairment. Children with lesions sustained between the ages of 2 and 10 years showed less impairment in executive functions than those with onsets earlier or later. Older children were starting to show some of the clear and specific brain–behaviour correlations described in adults.

6.6.4 Multiple and frontal strokes

6.6.4.1 *Sickle cell disease*

Sickle cell disease (SCD) is the most common group of genetic haemoglobin disorders. Results include chronic haemolytic anaemia; recurrent, painful episodes; increased risk of infections and absences from school; and vaso-occlusive complications including multiple strokes. Arterial blockage in the anterior and middle cerebral arteries can result both in neurological syndromes and in infarcts that are only apparent on neuroimaging. The neurological effects of these strokes can be subtle and need continuing psychological surveillance. Furthermore, and even apart from evident strokes, there is an elevated risk of cognitive impairment, shown in lower IQ, poor attention and executive function, and lower levels of academic achievement than in matched controls.

Frontal lobe abnormalities are associated (Berkelhammer et al., 2007). Psychiatric interview with affected individuals has suggested not only a very high rate of ADHD (40%) but also moderate levels of diagnosable anxiety and depression, as expected for young people with chronic physical illnesses (Benton et al., 2011). Psychiatric supervision and consultation are therefore advised.

6.6.5 Corpus callosum

Some children are born with a totally or partially undeveloped corpus callosum. The anomaly is one of the most frequent brain malformations (about 1 in 3,000 live births). It is usually detected in pregnancy by routine scanning, and therefore gives rise to anxiety about future development and decisions about termination.

Any abnormalities in learning, cognition, or behaviour are related to the extent of other brain abnormalities. When agenesis is the only abnormality, the outlook is good. Most affected young people are in the normal range of IQ and do not have marked emotional or behavioural problems. Some researchers have found subtle abnormalities of function: Moutard and colleagues (2012) describe a possibly increased rate of educational problems. Even then, however, it is not clear that reduced function of the callosum is responsible, rather than associated abnormalities even in these 'isolated' cases. The existence of any specifically localized impairment of performance has been hard to demonstrate. Ettlinger et al. (1972, 1974) found no difference between cases and controls in visual and tactile tests that are presumed to involve interhemispheric transfer of information and do show alterations in adults after surgical interruption of the commissures.

It is counterintuitive that the great bridge between hemispheres can be dispensed with at so little cost. Presumably, the developing brain finds other routes for transferring information, or possibly efficient ways of processing information in a single hemisphere. Even when the corpus callosum is divided surgically, to reduce intractable seizures in young people with epilepsy, disconnection syndromes are mild and transient—less prominent than in adults (Graham et al., 2016).

6.7 ENDOCRINE AND METABOLIC DISORDERS WITH NEUROPSYCHIATRIC EFFECTS

6.7.1 Thyroid disease

Several diseases of the thyroid gland result in either too much or too little of the hormones produced (thyroxine, T^4 and tri-iodothyronine, T^3). These hormones contain iodine and have very widespread effects on the cells of the body, regulating growth and metabolic activity.

6.7.1.1 *Hypothyroidism*

Hypothyroidism (underfunctioning thyroid) may be due to disease of the thyroid or secondary to disease elsewhere, especially of the pituitary gland, which produces a thyroid-stimulating hormone (TSH). A lack of iodine in the diet can also be responsible (see Chapter 7, Section 7.8.2.1). The effects on the brain can result in disturbances of activity level, attention, intellectual development, anxiety, and mood. If these disturbances present to child and adolescent mental health services, the disease is occasionally missed by clinicians unfamiliar with its signs. There is nothing very specific about the mental changes, so clinicians need to be alert to the possibility that they are secondary to the physical illness. The possibility will be raised by the occurrence of characteristic physical changes, mentioned here and well described in a review by Hanley et al. (2016).

6.7.1.1.1 *Congenital hypothyroidism*

Clinical presentations in the neonate include feeding difficulties, sleepiness, constipation, and jaundice. At this age, however, most cases should be detected by routine screening before any symptoms are apparent. All babies born in the UK are screened for congenital hypothyroidism at about 5 days old, using a blood spot test, and the same should be true in other countries with developed health systems. The commonest causes are dysgenesis of the gland (incomplete development) or a failure of the normal process of development in the womb, in which the thyroid gland moves from the back of the tongue to its postnatal position in the neck. The chance of parents having another baby who is affected in the same way is very low.

Another rare type of congenital hypothyroidism is inherited. In this form, the child's thyroid gland is anatomically correct, but it cannot produce thyroxine. In another rare inherited condition, the thyroid gland itself is normal but the tissues of the body do not respond to the hormones it produces. Thyroid dysfunction and hearing problems can both be part of another rare inherited condition (Pendred syndrome), in which there is also a malformation of the inner ear and sensorineural impairment of hearing.

Whatever the cause, the effects on body and brain development can be severe. During development in the womb, the fetus does not make its own thyroxine at sufficient levels but relies, in part, on that from its mother. During the first trimester, the fetus is entirely reliant on mother's hormones crossing the placenta. After that time, the fetus is making some of its own but is still dependent on thyroid hormones crossing the placenta. After birth, however, infants make enough hormone themselves. Hypothyroidism in pregnant mothers can therefore influence the prenatal brain development of their children. Subclinical maternal hypothyroidism and isolated hypothyroxinaemia are associated with fetal loss, prematurity, and impaired cognitive function in offspring. There is also evidence that maternal thyroid autoimmunity could be a potential risk factor for fetal loss. The incidence of overt hypothyroidism in pregnancy ranges from approximately 0.2% to 0.6%, whereas subclinical hypothyroidism, with elevated TSH and normal free thyroxine (FT^4) concentrations, occurs in 2% to 3% of pregnancies. Isolated hypothyroxinaemia, defined as a normal TSH and low FT^4, occurs in about 2% of pregnancies.

6.7.1.1.2 Acquired hypothyroidism

Hashimoto's thyroiditis is the most common type of acquired thyroid underactivity in young people. It is an autoimmune condition in which the body makes antibodies to pieces of the thyroid peroxidase and thyroglobulin proteins. Young people may experience slower growth and development. The mental changes can develop so insidiously that they are not noticed by people in everyday contact with them. The physical changes include:

- Short stature or slow growth
- Rough, dry skin
- Constipation
- Cold intolerance
- Fatigue and decreased energy
- Sleeping more
- Bruising easily
- Bone fractures or delayed bone age on X-ray
- Swelling of the gland in the neck (goitre)
- Early or delayed puberty

6.7.1.1.3 Diagnosis

Diagnosis is made by testing for hormone levels in the blood. Thyroxine (T^4) is reduced (except that in cases of decreased responsiveness of the body tissues to thyroxine, T^4 may be increased). In primary thyroid disease, TSH is increased as a result of feedback at the pituitary. If the primary cause is pituitary deficiency, then the TSH is normal or low.

6.7.1.1.4 *Treatment*

Treatment of hypothyroidism is with levothyroxine. In congenital hypothyroidism, this is usually successful in preventing cognitive dysfunction—provided that the replacement hormone is given promptly, regularly, and in sufficient dosage (Bongers–Schokking & de Muinck Keizer–Schrama, 2005; Simoneau–Roy et al., 2004). Before the advent of routine neonatal screening in the 1970s, there was typically intellectual disability, often with specific defects in verbal and visuomotor development and in behaviour, especially in attention and aggression.

6.7.1.2 *Hyperthyroidism (thyrotoxicosis)*

An excess of thyroid hormones can also be a risk for mental problems. It should be borne in mind as a possible cause of anxiety and ADHD presentations (see Box 6.5). As with other endocrine conditions, recognition is based on physical symptoms and signs on examination and on hormone tests.

Mental changes of emotional lability, crying easily, irritability, and excitability are common and can mimic the similar problems of very anxious children and children with ADHD. A recent case-register study among military families in the USA noted high rates of all these mental problems, and a fivefold increase in suicidality (Zader et al., 2019). These mental changes often, but not always, resolve after thyroid function is restored to normal, and they are often present before the condition is recognized. The pathogenesis is not established.

Box 6.5 Thyrotoxicosis: signs and symptoms

- Tremors
- Increased appetite
- Weight loss
- Growth acceleration
- Enlarged thyroid gland (goitre) and protruding eyes (exophthalmos) in Graves' disease
- Flushed skin
- Excessive sweating
- Muscle weakness
- Tachycardia (rapid heartbeat) and palpitation (an unpleasant sense of feeling the heart beating)
- High blood pressure
- Thyroid hormones (T^3 and T^4) ordinarily both raised—often T^3 first in early cases, so it should be tested for specifically. TSH is suppressed by the antibodies of Graves' disease, so blood levels can be low in that condition. The antibodies to the thyroid can also be measured in the blood.

Treatment in young people usually begins with anti-thyroid drugs such as carbimazole or methimazole. A few will have permanent remission, but many will eventually wish to progress to definitive treatment with surgery to the gland or (after the age of 10 years) with radioiodine. Both the definitive treatments will aim to produce hypothyroidism that might need replacement hormones.

Some aspects of therapy can produce psychiatric problems. Steroids, if used, may produce mood change. Beta blockers given to reduce tachycardia or anxiety can produce depression and sedation.

6.7.2 Diabetes mellitus

Most children and young people with diabetes have Type 1 of the condition (Type 1A of the American Diabetes Association). This form is caused by autoimmune attack on the islet cells of the pancreas which secrete insulin and thus regulate blood sugar levels and utilization. Treatment with insulin is required, and there is a complex regimen of multiple doses, diet control, exercise, and monitoring. Specialist clinics aim at close control to reduce complications in blood vessels, eyes, kidneys, and nerves.

There is also an association with small reductions in IQ and cognitive performance on testing, by comparison with their non-diabetic siblings. This is usually attributed to loss of schooling and other social disadvantage, although there are also direct effects on the brain. Early onset, by comparison with later-onset cases of Type 1, carries a stronger association with cerebral atrophy (Ferguson et al., 2005). Hippocampal volumes were larger in an imaging study by Hershey et al. (2010). Early onset, frequent hypoglycaemic episodes, and chronic severe hyperglycaemia are all risk factors for cognitive impairment in later life.

The main psychiatric problems in childhood and adolescence arise from the interactions between the emotional life of the young person and the stresses of living with diabetes. The fears of coma and medical complications, the need for careful calculation of personal and social life, and the restrictions imposed on social life by the constraints of diet and regular hours—all pose real challenges to the resilience of the young person and coping by their families. Overt emotional and behavioural disorders can supervene.

A sinister development is the combination of an eating disorder with diabetes. All too many young people, especially female adolescents, are tempted to restrict insulin in order to lose weight (so-called 'diabulimia'). Unexplained high blood sugar readings are an early sign. Feelings about diabetes, food, body appearance, autonomy, and weight become bound up together. This challenges the skills of the therapists and the liaison between services. The ethos of the diabetes clinics, which is usually to foster the autonomy and decision making of the young person, can clash with that of mental health professionals trying to encourage parents to take control.

Type 2 diabetes can also occur, especially in young people with ASD for whom atypical antipsychotics have been prescribed. There is also an association with

ADHD. A report from the national health register in Taiwan has identified more than 35,000 young people with ADHD and found a disproportionately high number with Type 2 diabetes: incidence was 0.83 per 1,000 person years, versus 0.21 in typically developing people (Chen et al., 2018). Those who had received atypical antipsychotics were at the highest risk, but this did not account for the whole risk. Other potential reasons for Type 2 developing in ADHD include obesity and, possibly, immune dysregulation. Stimulant drugs, however, do not seem to be involved.

6.7.3 Adrenal glands and steroids

6.7.3.1 *Cushing syndrome*

Cushing syndrome describes the bodily effects of an excess of glucocorticoids. Affected children become obese and hairy; there may be striae in their skin; their growth is delayed; and they are prone to high blood pressure. Their mental state can also be affected, especially through mood disorder and increased aggression. It is much rarer than in adults, but can result from a growth in the pituitary gland that makes an excess of adrenocorticotrophic hormone (ACTH)—the hormone that stimulates the adrenal cortex (Cushing disease). There are also some very rare genetic conditions with similar physical results (Lodish, 2015).

In young people, however, excess states are not usually the result of disease, but due to exogenous substances—anabolic androgenous steroids (AASs), taken either to treat disease or, more commonly, without prescription and in large doses to enhance athletic performance and competitiveness and increase body mass, appearance, and self-esteem (Cunningham et al., 2013). This recreational use is a dangerous practice, especially around the time of puberty when the adolescent remodelling of the brain is strongly influenced by adrenal hormones. Neurotransmitter function and dendritic spine density in limbic structures are altered. Furthermore, long-term use (e.g. by weightlifters and bodybuilders) can lead to severe acne, sexual problems, gynaeco-mastia, altered sperm motility, infertility, and liver and kidney problems. The AAS does not directly give users a 'high', and dopamine metabolism is not much affected—but depression and fatigue on lowering the dose are commonplace and sometimes contribute to dependent use.

The most typical mental change from steroid misuse is aggression. Even in rodents (in which it has been most studied), the aggression is not indiscriminate but modified by context and the victim. It can be described as a heightened response to challenge. Manic excitement and paranoid jealousy can also appear in humans. Medical use of steroids can have complex neuropsychiatric effects. In acute treatment, irritability and euphoria appear and can reach psychotic proportions. Reduction of dosage classically results in depression of mood. Changes, however, are complex and hard to predict. Prolonged treatment carries a risk of mood depression.

6.7.3.2 *Adrenal insufficiency (Addison's disease)*

Adrenal insufficiency seldom presents to child psychiatric clinics, but fatigue and generalized weakness are typical and can lead to a diagnosis of chronic fatigue syndrome if there is a failure to recognize the underlying cause. (Slow weight gain, low blood pressure, reduced blood sodium, and cravings for salt are also characteristic; additionally, the skin may become darker, especially at the skin creases.) Diagnosis is by blood tests of cortisol level and its response to ACTH injection.

The usual causes are diseases affecting the adrenal gland, especially congenital adrenal hyperplasia due to enzyme deficiency or autoimmune attack, or diseases affecting the pituitary gland in the brain and causing deficiency of ACTH (a hormone regulating cortisol secretion). It is a part of a rare inherited condition that also causes dementia: X-linked adrenoleukodystrophy (see Chapter 7, Section 7.3).

Treatment is with replacement of hydrocortisone (and sometimes aldosterone). There is a continuing responsibility for families, not only to ensure regular dosing, but to be prepared for sudden crises when an infection or episode of vomiting precipitates life-threatening collapse and the need for intravenous treatment.

6.8 Functional neurological disorders

Medically unexplained presentations, such as seizures, paralyses, and anaesthesias, are confusingly described in classifications under various headings such as 'conversion disorders', 'hysteria', 'somatizing disorders', 'dissociative illnesses', and 'psychogenic disorders'. They have in common that a set of symptoms, usually attributed to a brain disorder, proves on examination not to have an organic cause and, sometimes, to make one very unlikely. Examples include dissociative convulsions, chronic fatigue syndromes, and disturbances of voluntary motor and sensory function that do not correspond with neuroanatomy.

They can be very worrying to families, and often present as emergencies. Minor stresses immediately beforehand are usual. Proving a negative about causality can be very difficult. Many physical illnesses do go unrecognized in early stages. Total exclusion of all possibilities can be impossible, and doubt often remains about the nature of the illness. Uncertainty, itself, can limit a child's opportunities to engage in ordinary activities.

Functional disorders often clear up rapidly after reassurance and, in some cultures, will do so after suggestion. However, a good deal of education can be missed until the true nature of the symptoms is appreciated. In the long term, the conditions are not altogether benign. A long-term follow-up of children with medically unexplained neurological symptoms found 'only' 21% to have continued with the problems originally mentioned on their medical charts (Raper et al., 2019).

Exhaustive investigations can cement parents' belief that there is an obscure or wilfully unrecognized physical illness. Wise management involves both physical and mental health professionals from an early stage. A positive diagnosis of functional disorder should be communicated empathetically, and with agreement between those involved professionally with physical and mental aspects. It is then possible for families to plan constructively.

Total certainty that there is no physical illness is often impossible. Functional and physical problems often coexist (see Section 6.2). Families usually recognize this more readily than clinicians think, and appreciate honesty in communications and a clear plan of psychological treatments (Heyman, 2019). The opposite is a reluctance by some paediatric specialists to entertain a psychogenic contribution until everything else has been 'ruled out'. Psychiatric or psychological referral is then delayed and seen as a kind of defeat. Families become not only confused but skeptical of the competence of the professionals advising them, and reluctant to engage in psychologically informed rehabilitation (Hulgaard et al., 2020).

References

Epilepsy

Asadi-Pooya, A. A., Bahrami, Z., & Homayoun, M. (2019). Natural history of patients with psychogenic nonepileptic seizures. *Seizure, 66*, 22–25.

Austin, J. K., Harezlak, J., Dunn, D. W., Huster, G. A., Rose, D. F., & Ambrosius, W. T. (2001). Behavior problems in children before first recognized seizures. *Pediatrics, 107*(1), 115–122.

Baumgartner, C., Koren, J., Britto–Arias, M., Schmidt, S., & Pirker, S. (2019). Epidemiology and pathophysiology of autonomic seizures: a systematic review. *Clinical Autonomic Research, 29*(2), 137–150.

Besag, F. M. (2015). Current controversies in the relationships between autism and epilepsy. *Epilepsy & Behavior, 47*, 143–146.

Bien, C. G., Granata, T., Antozzi, C., Cross, J. H., Dulac, O., Kurthen, M., Lassmann, H., Mantegazza, R., Villemure, J.–G., Spreafico, R., & Elger, C. E. (2005). Pathogenesis, diagnosis and treatment of Rasmussen encephalitis: a European consensus statement. *Brain, 128*(3), 454–471.

Bolton, P. F., Carcani–Rathwell, I., Hutton, J., Goode, S., Howlin, P., & Rutter, M. (2011). Epilepsy in autism: features and correlates. *British Journal of Psychiatry, 198*(4), 289–294.

Budman, C. L., Rockmore, L., Stokes, J., & Sossin, M. (2003). Clinical phenomenology of episodic rage in children with Tourette syndrome. *Journal of Psychosomatic Research, 55*(1), 59–65.

Burns, T. G., Ludwig, N. N., Tajiri, T. N., & DeFilippis, N. (2018). Cognitive and behavioral outcomes among seizure-controlled children with partial epilepsy on antiepileptic drug monotherapy. *Applied Neuropsychology: Child, 7*(1), 52–60.

Chong, L., Jamieson, N. J., Gill, D., Singh–Grewal, D., Craig, J. C., Ju, A., Hanson, C. S., & Tong, A. (2016). Children's experiences of epilepsy: a systematic review of qualitative studies. *Pediatrics, 138*(3), e20160658.

Clancy, M. J., Clarke, M. C., Connor, D. J., Cannon, M., & Cotter, D. R. (2014). The prevalence of psychosis in epilepsy: a systematic review and meta-analysis. *BMC Psychiatry, 14*(1), 75.

Dunn, D. W., Austin, J. K., & Perkins, S. M. (2009). Prevalence of psychopathology in childhood epilepsy: categorical and dimensional measures. *Developmental Medicine & Child Neurology*, *51*(5), 364–372.

Fiest, K. M., Sauro, K. M., Wiebe, S., Patten, S. B., Kwon, C. S., Dykeman, J., Pringsheim, T., Lorenzetti, D. L., & Jetté, N. (2017). Prevalence and incidence of epilepsy: a systematic review and meta-analysis of international studies. *Neurology*, *88*(3), 296–303.

Fisher, R. S., Cross, J. H., French, J. A., Higurashi, N., Hirsch, E., Jansen, F. E., Lagae, L., Moshé, S. L., Peltola, J., Roulet Perez, E., Scheffer, I. E., & Zuberi, S. M. (2017). Operational classification of seizure types by the International League Against Epilepsy: Position Paper of the ILAE Commission for Classification and Terminology. *Epilepsia*, *58*(4), 522–530.

Hesdorffer, D. C., Ludvigsson, P., Olafsson, E., Gudmundsson, G., Kjartansson, O., & Hauser, W. A. (2004). ADHD as a risk factor for incident unprovoked seizures and epilepsy in children. *Archives of General Psychiatry*, *61*(7), 731–736.

Irwin, K., Birch, V., Lees, J., Polkey, C., Alarcon, G., Binnie, C., Smedley, N., Baird, G., & Robinson, R. O. (2001). Multiple subpial transection in Landau–Kleffner syndrome. *Developmental Medicine and Child Neurology*, *43*(4), 248–252.

Kieffer–Renaux, V., Kaminska, A., & Dulac, O. (2001). Cognitive deterioration in Lennox–Gastaut syndrome and Doose epilepsy. In I. Jambaqué, M. Lassonde, O. Dulac (Eds.), *Neuropsychology of childhood epilepsy* (pp. 185–190). Springer.

Krishnamoorthy, E. S., Trimble, M. R., & Blumer, D. (2007). The classification of neuropsychiatric disorders in epilepsy: a proposal by the ILAE Commission on Psychobiology of Epilepsy. *Epilepsy & Behavior*, *10*(3), 349–353.

Lewis, D. V., Shinnar, S., Hesdorffer, D. C., Bagiella, E., Bello, J. A., Chan, S., Xu, Y., MacFall, J., Gomes, W. A., Moshé, S. L., Mathern, G. W., Pellock, J. M., Nordli, D. R., Jr., Frank, L. M., Provenzale, J., Shinnar, R. C., Epstein, L. G., Masur, D., Litherland, C., ...& FEBSTAT Study Team. (2014). Hippocampal sclerosis after febrile status epilepticus: the FEBSTAT study. *Annals of Neurology*, *75*(2), 178–185.

Lin, J. J., Dabbs, K., Riley, J. D., Jones, J. E., Jackson, D. C., Hsu, D. A., Stafstrom, C. E., Seidenberg, M., & Hermann, B. P. (2014). Neurodevelopment in new-onset juvenile myoclonic epilepsy over the first 2 years. *Annals of Neurology*, *76*(5), 660–668.

Massa, R., de Saint–Martin, A., Carcangiu, R., Rudolf, G., Seegmuller, C., Kleitz, C., Metz-Lutz., M. N., Hirsch, E., & Marescaux, C. (2001). EEG criteria predictive of complicated evolution in idiopathic rolandic epilepsy. *Neurology*, *57*(6), 1071–1079.

O'Callaghan, F. J., Lux, A. L., Darke, K., Edwards, S. W., Hancock, E., Johnson, A. L., Kennedy, C. R., Newton, R. W., Verity, C. M., & Osborne, J. P. (2011). The effect of lead time to treatment and of age of onset on developmental outcome at 4 years in infantile spasms: evidence from the United Kingdom Infantile Spasms Study. *Epilepsia*, *52*(7), 1359–1364.

Ohtahara, S., & Yamatogi, Y. (2006). Ohtahara syndrome: with special reference to its developmental aspects for differentiating from early myoclonic encephalopathy. *Epilepsy Research*, *70*, 58–67.

Ott, D., Siddarth, P., Gurbani, S., Koh, S., Tournay, A., Shields, W. D., & Caplan, R. (2003). Behavioral disorders in pediatric epilepsy: unmet psychiatric need. *Epilepsia*, *44*(4), 591–597.

Panayiotopoulos, C. P. (2004). Autonomic seizures and autonomic status epilepticus peculiar to childhood: diagnosis and management. *Epilepsy & Behavior*, *5*(3), 286–295.

Pericall, M. L., & Taylor, E. (2010). Psychosis and epilepsy in young people. *Epilepsy & Behavior*, *18*(4), 450–454.

Pericall, M. T. L., & Taylor, E. (2017). Factors associated with psychiatric disorder in children with epilepsy (CWE): a systematic review. *Journal of the American Academy of Child & Adolescent Psychiatry*, *56*(10), S287.

Plioplys, S., Dunn, D. W., & Caplan, R. (2007). 10-year research update review: psychiatric problems in children with epilepsy. *Journal of the American Academy of Child & Adolescent Psychiatry*, 46(11), 1389–1402.

Raper, J., Currigan, V., Fothergill, S., Stone, J., & Forsyth, R. J. (2019). Long-term outcomes of functional neurological disorder in children. *Archives of Disease in Childhood*, 104(2), 1155–1160.

Reilly, c., Atkinson, P., Das, K., Chin, R., Aylett, S., Burch, V., Gillberg, C., Scott, R. & Neville, B. (2014). Neurobehavioral comorbidities in children with active epilepsy: a population-based study. *Pediatrics*, 133, e1586–1593.

Rutter, M., Graham, P., & Yule, W. (1970). *A neuropsychiatric study in childhood*. Heinemann Medical.

Shorvon, S. D. (2011). The etiologic classification of epilepsy. *Epilepsia*, 52(6), 1052–1057.

Thomas, S., Hovinga, M. E, Rai, D., & Lee B. K. (2017). Brief report: prevalence of co-occurring epilepsy and autism spectrum disorder: the U.S. national survey of children's health 2011–2012. *Journal of Autism and Developmental Disorders*, 47, 224–229.

Strasser, L., Downes, M., Kung, J., Cross, J. H., & De Haan, M. (2018). Prevalence and risk factors for autism spectrum disorder in epilepsy: a systematic review and meta-analysis. *Developmental Medicine & Child Neurology*, 60(1), 19–29.

Sundelin, H. E., Larsson, H., Lichtenstein, P., Almqvist, C., Hultman, C. M., Tomson, T., & Ludvigsson, J. F. (2016). Autism and epilepsy: a population-based nationwide cohort study. *Neurology*, 87(2), 192–197.

Suurmeijer, T. P., Reuvekamp, M. F., & Aldenkamp, B. P. (2001). Social functioning, psychological functioning, and quality of life in epilepsy. *Epilepsia*, 42(9), 1160–1168.

Trinka, E., Cock, H., Hesdorffer, D., Rossetti, A. O., Scheffer, I. E., Shinnar, S., Shorvon, S., & Lowenstein, D. H. (2015). A definition and classification of status epilepticus—report of the ILAE Task Force on Classification of Status Epilepticus. *Epilepsia*, 56(10), 1515–1523.

Cerebral palsy, hydrocephalus, strokes, head injury, endocrine and functional disorders

Anderson, V., Beauchamp, M. H., Yeates, K. O., Crossley, L., Hearps, S. J., & Catroppa, C. (2013). Social competence at 6 months following childhood traumatic brain injury. *Journal of the International Neuropsychological Society*, 19(5), 539–550.

Anderson, V., Catroppa, C., Morse, S., Haritou, F., & Rosenfeld, J.(2005a). Functional plasticity or vulnerability following early brain injury? *Pediatrics*, 116, 374–82.

Anderson, V., Catroppa, C., Morse, S., Haritou, F., & Rosenfeld, J. (2005b). Identifying factors contributing to child and family outcome 30 months after traumatic brain injury in children. *Journal of Neurology, Neurosurgery & Psychiatry*, 76, 404–408.

Anderson, V., Spencer–Smith, M., & Wood, A. (2011). Do children really recover better? Neurobehavioral plasticity after early brain insult. *Brain*, 13, 2197–2221.

Benton, T. D., Boyd, R., Ifeagwu, J., Feldtmose, E., & Smith–Whitley, K. (2011). Psychiatric diagnosis in adolescents with sickle cell disease: a preliminary report. *Current Psychiatry Reports*, 13(2), 111–115.

Berkelhammer, L. D., Williamson, A. L., Sanford, S. D., Dirksen, C. L., Sharp, W. G., Margulies, A. S., & Prengler, R. A. (2007). Neurocognitive sequelae of pediatric sickle cell disease: a review of the literature. *Child Neuropsychology*, 13(2), 120–131.

Bongers–Schokking, J. J., & de Muinck Keizer–Schrama, S. M. (2005). Influence of timing and dose of thyroid hormone replacement on mental, psychomotor, and behavioral development in children with congenital hypothyroidism. *Journal of Pediatrics*, 147(6), 768–774.

Braun, K. V. N., Doernberg, N., Schieve, L., Christensen, D., Goodman, A., & Yeargin–Allsopp, M. (2016). Birth prevalence of cerebral palsy: a population-based study. *Pediatrics*, *137*(1), 1–9.

Brown, G., Chadwick, O., Shaffer, D., Rutter, M., & Traub, M. (1981). A prospective study of children with head injuries: III. Psychiatric sequelae. *Psychological Medicine*, *11*(1), 63–78.

Chadwick, O., Rutter, M., Brown, G., Shaffer, D., & Traub, M. (1981a). A prospective study of children with head injuries: II. Cognitive sequelae. *Psychological Medicine, 11*(1), 49–61.

Chadwick, O., Rutter, M., Shaffer, D., & Shrout, P. E. (1981b). A prospective study of children with head injuries: IV. Specific cognitive deficits. *Journal of Clinical Neuropsychology*, 3, 101–120.

Chen, M. H., Pan, T. L., Hsu, J. W., Huang, K. L., Su, T. P., Li, C. T., Lin, W. C., Tsai, S. J., Chang, W. H., Chen, T. J., & Bai, Y. M. (2018). Risk of Type 2 diabetes in adolescents and young adults with attention-deficit/hyperactivity disorder: a nationwide longitudinal study. *Journal of Clinical Psychiatry, 79*(3).https://doi.org/10.4088/jcp.17m11607

Colver, A., Rapp, M., Eisemann, N., Ehlinger, V., Thyen, U., Dickinson, H. O., Parkes, J., Parkinson, K., Nystrand, M., Fauconnier, J., Marcelli, M., Michelson, S. I., & Arnaud, C. (2015). Self-reported quality of life of adolescents with cerebral palsy: a cross-sectional and longitudinal analysis. *Lancet, 385*(9969), 705–716.

Cooper, M. S., Mackay, M. T., Fahey, M., Reddihough, D., Reid, S. M., Williams, K., & Harvey, A. S. (2017). Seizures in children with cerebral palsy and white matter injury. *Pediatrics*, *139*(3), e20162975. https://doi.org/10.1542/peds.2016-2975

Cunningham, R. L., Lumia, A. R., & McGinnis, M. Y. (2013). Androgenic anabolic steroid exposure during adolescence: ramifications for brain development and behavior. *Hormones and Behavior, 64*(2), 350–356.

Dennis, M., & Kohn, B. (1975). Comprehension of syntax in infantile hemiplegia after cerebral hemidecortication: left hemisphere superiority. *Brain and Language*, 2, 472–482.

Dennis, M., Lovett, M., & Wiegel-Crump, C. A. (1981). Written language acquisition after left or right hemidecortication in infancy. *Brain and Language, 12*(1), 54–91.

Dickinson, H. O., Parkinson, K. N., Ravens-Sieberer, U., Schirripa, G., Thyen, U., Arnaud, C., Beckung, E., Fauconnier, J., McManus, V., Michelsen, S. I., Parkes, J., & Colver, A. F. (2007). Self-reported quality of life of 8–12-year-old children with cerebral palsy: a cross-sectional European study. *Lancet, 369*(9580), 2171–2178.

Dollman, A. K., Figaji, A. A., & Schrieff–Elson, L. E. (2017). Academic and behavioral outcomes in school-age South African children following severe traumatic brain injury. *Frontiers in Neuroanatomy, 11*, 121.

Duval, J., Braun, C. J., Daigneault, S., & Montour–Proulx, I. (2002). Does the child behavior checklist reveal psychopathological profiles of children with focal unilateral cortical lesions? *Applied Neuropsychology, 9*(2), 74–83.

Eliasson, A. C., Krumlinde–Sundholm, L., Rösblad, B., Beckung, E., Arner, M., Öhrvall, A. M., & Rosenbaum, P. (2006). The Manual Ability Classification System (MACS) for children with cerebral palsy: scale development and evidence of validity and reliability. *Developmental Medicine and Child Neurology, 48*(7), 549–554.

Engberg, A., & Teasdale, T. W. (1998) Traumatic brain injury in children in Denmark: a national 15-year study. *European Journal of Epidemiology*, 14, 165–173.

Entus, A. K. (1977). Hemispheric asymmetry in processing of dichotically presented speech and nonspeech stimuli by infants. In S. Segalowitz & F. Gruber (Eds.), *Language development and neurological theory* (pp. 63–73). Academic Press.

Ettlinger, G., Blakemore, C. B., Milner, A. D., & Wilson, J. (1972). Agenesis of the corpus callosum: a behavioural investigation. *Brain*, 95, 327–346.

Ferguson, S. C., Blane, A., Wardlaw, J., Frier, B. M., Perros, P., McCrimmon, R. J., & Deary, I. J. (2005). Influence of an early-onset age of type 1 diabetes on cerebral structure and cognitive function. *Diabetes Care*, 28,1431–1437.

Fletcher, J. M., Dennis, M., & Northrup, H. (2000). Hydrocephalus. In K. O. Yeates, M. D. Ris, & H. G. Taylor (Eds.), *The science and practice of neuropsychology. Pediatric neuropsychology: research, theory, and practice* (pp. 25–46). Guilford Press.

Goldman–Rakic, P. S., Isseroff, A., Schwartz, M. L., & Bugbee, N. M. (1983). The neurobiology of cognitive development. In P. Mussen (Ed.), *Handbook of child psychology, biology and infancy development* (pp. 281–344). John Wiley.

Goodman, R., & Graham, P. (1996). Psychiatric problems in children with hemiplegia: cross sectional epidemiological survey. *British Medical Journal*, 312(7038), 1065–1069.

Goodman, R., & Yude, C. (1996). IQ and its predictors in childhood hemiplegia. *Developmental Medicine & Child Neurology*, 38(10), 881–890.

Goodman, R. (1998). The longitudinal stability of psychiatric problems in children with hemiplegia. *Journal of Child Psychology and Psychiatry and Allied Disciplines*, 39(3), 347–354.

Graham, D., Tisdall, M. M., & Gill, D. (2016). Corpus callosotomy outcomes in pediatric patients: a systematic review. *Epilepsia*, 57(7), 1053–1068.

Gupta, N., Park, J., Solomon, C., Kranz, D. A., Wrensch, M., & Wu, Y. W. (2007). Long-term outcomes in patients with treated childhood hydrocephalus. *Journal of Neurosurgery: Pediatrics*, 106(5), 334–339.

Haarbauer–Krupa, J., Lee, A. H., Bitsko, R. H., Zhang, X., & Kresnow–Sedacca, M. J. (2018). Prevalence of parent-reported traumatic brain injury in children and associated health conditions. *Journal of the American Medical Association: Pediatrics*, 172(11), 1078–1086.

Hanley, P., Lord, K., & Bauer, A. J. (2016). Thyroid disorders in children and adolescents: a review. *Journal of the American Medical Association: Pediatrics*, 170(10), 1008–1019. https:/doi.org/10.1001/jamapediatrics.2016.0486

Hershey, T., Perantie, D. C., Wu, J., Weaver, P. M., Black, K. J., & White, N. H. (2010). Hippocampal volumes in youth with type 1 diabetes. *Diabetes*, 59, 236–241.

Heyman, I. (2019). Mind the gap: integrating physical and mental healthcare for children with functional symptoms. *Archives of Disease in Childhood*, 104 (12),1127–1128.

Hulgaard, D. R., Rask, C. U., Risør, M. B., & Dehlholm, G. (2020). 'I can hardly breathe': exploring the parental experience of having a child with a functional disorder. *Journal of Child Health Care*, 24(2), 165–179.

Huttenlocher, P. R., & Dabholkar, A. S. (1997). Regional differences in synaptogenesis in human cerebral cortex. *Journal of Comparative Neurology*, 387(2), 167–178.

Jacobs, R., Harvey, A. S., & Anderson, V. (2007). Executive function following focal frontal lobe lesions: impact of timing of lesion on outcome. *Cortex*, 43(6), 792–805.

Kahle, K. T., Kulkarni, A. V., Limbrick Jr, D. D., & Warf, B. C. (2016). Hydrocephalus in children. *Lancet*, 387(10020), 788–799.

Kolb, B., Coie, J., & Wishaw, I. (2000). Is there an optimal age for recovery from motor cortex lesions. I. Behavioral and anatomical sequelae of anatomical bilateral motor cortex lesions in rats on postnatal days 1, 10, and in adulthood. *Brain Research*, 882, 62–74.

Laurent–Vannier, A., Chevignard, M., Pradat–Diehl, P., Abada, G., & De Agostini, M. (2006). Assessment of unilateral spatial neglect in children using the Teddy Bear Cancellation Test. *Developmental Medicine and Child Neurology*, 48(2), 120–125.

Li, L., & Liu, J. (2013). The effect of pediatric traumatic brain injury on behavioral outcomes: a systematic review. *Developmental Medicine & Child Neurology*, 55(1), 37–45.

Lishman, W. A. (1973). The psychiatric sequelae of head injury: a review. *Psychological Medicine*, 3, 304–318. https://doi.org/10.1017/S003329170004959X

Lodish, M. (2015). Cushing's syndrome in childhood: update on genetics, treatment, and outcomes. *Current Opinion in Endocrinology, Diabetes, and Obesity*, 22(1), 48.

Max, J. E., Robin, D. A., Lindgren, S. D., Smith, W. L., Sato, Y., Mattheis, P. J., Stierwalt, J. A. G., & Castillo, C. S. (1997). Traumatic brain injury in children and adolescents: psychiatric disorders at two years. *Journal of the American Academy of Child & Adolescent Psychiatry*, 36, 1278–1285.

Moutard, M. L., Kieffer, V., Feingold, J., Lewin, F., Baron, J. M., Adamsbaum, C., Gélot, A., Isapof, A., Kieffer, F., & de Villemeur, T. B. (2012). Isolated corpus callosum agenesis: a ten-year follow-up after prenatal diagnosis. (How are the children without corpus callosum at 10 years of age?) *Prenatal Diagnosis*, 32(3), 277–283.

Palisano, R., Rosenbaum, P., Walter, S., Russell, D., Wood, E., & Galuppi, B. (1997). Development and reliability of a system to classify gross motor function in children with cerebral palsy. *Developmental Medicine & Child Neurology*, 39(4), 214–223.

Parkes, J., White–Koning, M., Dickinson, H. O., Thyen, U., Arnaud, C., Beckung, E., Fauconner, J., Marcelli, M., McManus, V., Michelsen, S. I., Parkinson, K., & Colver, A. (2008). Psychological problems in children with cerebral palsy: a cross-sectional European study. *Journal of Child Psychology and Psychiatry*, 49(4), 405–413.

Persson, E. K., Hagberg, G., & Uvebrant, P. (2006). Disabilities in children with hydrocephalus—a population-based study of children aged between four and twelve years. *Neuropediatrics*, 37(06), 330–336.

Raja Beharelle, A., Dick, A. S., Josse, G., Solodkin, A., Huttenlocher, P. R., Levine, S. C., & Small, S. L. (2010). Left hemisphere regions are critical for language in the face of early left focal brain injury. *Brain*, 133(6), 1707–1716.

Raper, J., Currigan, V., Fothergill, S., Stone, J., & Forsyth, R. J. (2019). Long-term outcomes of functional neurological disorder in children. *Archives of Disease in Childhood*, 104(12), 1155–1160.

Shaffer, D., Chadwick, O., & Rutter, M. (1975). Psychiatric outcome of localized head injury in children. In R. Porter & D. FitzSimons (Eds.), *Outcome of severe damage to the central nervous system* (Vol. 34, pp. 191–213). Excerpta Medica Amsterdam.

Simoneau–Roy, J., Marti, S., Deal, C., Huot, C., Robaey, P., & Van Vliet, G. (2004). Cognition and behavior at school entry in children with congenital hypothyroidism treated early with high-dose levothyroxine. *Journal of Pediatrics*, 144(6), 747–752.

Teasdale, G., Maas, A., Lecky, F., Manley, G., Stocchetti, N., & Murray, G. (2014). The Glasgow Coma Scale at 40 years: standing the test of time. *Lancet Neurology*, 13(8), 844–854.

Thompson, P. M., Giedd, J. N., Woods, R. P., MacDonald, D., Evans, A. C., & Toga, A. W. (2000). Growth patterns in the developing brain detected by using continuum mechanical tensor maps. *Nature*, 404(6774), 190–193.

Thurman, D. J. (2016). The epidemiology of traumatic brain injury in children and youths: a review of research since 1990. *Journal of Child Neurology*, *31*(1), 20–27.

Trenchard, S. O., Rust, S., & Bunton, P. (2013). A systematic review of psychosocial outcomes within 2 years of paediatric traumatic brain injury in a school-aged population. *Brain Injury*, *27*(11), 1217–1237.

Weintraub, S., & Mesulam, M. M. (1983). Developmental learning disabilities of the right hemisphere: emotional, interpersonal, and cognitive components. *Archives of Neurology*, *40*(8), 463–468.

Zader, S. J., Williams, E., & Buryk, M. A. (2019). Mental health conditions and hyperthyroidism. *Pediatrics*, 144 (5), e20182874. https://doi.org/10.1542/peds.2018-2874

CHAPTER 7

GENETIC AND ENVIRONMENTAL INFLUENCES ON EARLY DEVELOPMENT

7.1 BEHAVIOURAL GENETICS

CLASSIC studies have indicated that genetic influences on neurodevelopmental disorders are strong. Until recent years, these mostly focused on the individual psychiatric syndromes of autistic spectrum disorder (ASD), attention deficit hyperactivity disorder (ADHD), and chronic tic disorders. The behavioural similarities between individuals were considered in the light of their degree of biological relatedness. Several designs were applied. Identical twins were compared with non-identical, full siblings with half-siblings, siblings with unrelated stepsiblings growing up in the same family, and so on. In several cases, the methods were used to study the reasons for the associations between different disorders. The results are described in the sections on 'Risks' for the individual syndromes in the respective chapters.

7.1.1 Heritability

One result of such methods was an appreciation of the high levels of heritability associated with these neurodevelopmental disorders. The balance between genetic (G) and environmental (E) influences has been argued intensively (e.g. on the development of 'intelligence'). It is important to realize both that G and E interact, and also that heritability (h^2) is not a fixed property of individuals. Rather, h^2 is an attribute of a population. It is, technically, the proportion of variance in the phenotype that is explained by genetic factors. In other words, it is about the *differences* between people, and depends on the population. In a population of identical twins, nearly all the difference between people would be due to their environments, and therefore heritability would be close to zero. By contrast, in a depriving institution where the environment is homogeneous, most of the differences (say, in IQ) would be due to G, and h^2 would be very high.

Heritability is high for most neurodevelopmental conditions. Exact figures vary with methodology. The figure for ADHD, for example, is particularly high when based on clinical diagnosis that integrates several sources of information: 88% in a large Swedish twin register of both children and adults (Larsson et al., 2014a). Shared environmental effects were negligible. The figures for ASD are also high: from 64% to 91% in a meta-analysis of twin studies (Tick et al., 2016), in which shared environmental influences only reached statistical significance when the most restrictive diagnosis was applied. A current estimate for schizophrenia is comparably high, at 79%, when based on a similar methodology of comparing monozygotic with dizygotic twins identified from a nation-wide (Danish) twin register (Hilker et al., 2018).

7.2 MOLECULAR GENETICS

In recent years, it has become possible to study directly the individual genes involved in psychopathology. Results have been rapid.

Individual people have millions of variations in their DNA by comparison with a reference genome. Of the variants, 95% are shared with 5% or more of the population and are therefore called 'common variants'. By contrast, about 1% of variants are 'rare' or even unique to one person (and possibly their immediate family).

Modern molecular genetics seeks to relate these variants to the risk for disorder. Altered structure at the level of the whole chromosome (such as the extra chromosome 21 in Down syndrome) was easier to detect than the much smaller changes at the level of an individual gene, and correspondingly was identified earlier. Candidate gene approaches followed; they were based on a small number of variants in genes that were already known to be involved in relevant processes. For instance, the genes coding for the dopamine transporter (DAT) and dopamine-4 receptor (DRD4) were of interest for ADHD because those protein molecules are a significant part of the process of dopaminergic transmission of nerve impulses, and therefore of stimulant drug effects on behaviour. It turned out, however, that even when the selection of genes to study was intelligent, the associations with behaviour were very small and correspondingly hard to interpret.

Replicable associations with schizophrenia, autism, and ADHD are now being achieved by high throughput microarray and whole-genome sequencing platforms, and by the recruitment of very large numbers of subjects. Candidate gene studies have given way to studies in which the whole genome, or the whole exome, is scanned. These are not hypothesis-driven but systematically examine the whole of the DNA to look for satellite markers that are associated with the condition. Several hundred thousand such comparisons are often made. The chances of false positive associations are therefore very high. Very stringent levels of statistical significance have to be applied, and therefore very large sample sizes are required. The satellite markers are single nucleotides, and indicate where on the chromosome the association is to be found. The existence of detailed chromosome maps then facilitates the search for the altered gene—but there is still much research to do before the molecular basis is clear.

This chapter will start by illustrating the power of genetic influences to alter mental function with descriptions of the effects of large-scale alterations in chromosomes, and the syndromes arising from single genetic changes. These are for the most part rare disorders, but the total of rare conditions makes up a substantial part of the aetiology of intellectual disorders. The chapter will proceed to illustrate the complexity of influences by considering the common neurodevelopmental disorders that are linked to common genetic variants, and genetic influences that do not depend on altered DNA structure.

Knowledge is advancing rapidly, and clinicians should be aware of the possibility of consulting up-to-date information at the Genetic and Rare Diseases Information Center (GARD). A striking example is that of a rare neurological condition: spinal muscular atrophy. This has been shown to be due to mutation of the gene *SMN1* at chromosome 5q13. It can now be treated, for example with an antisense nucleotide called nusinersen.

Genes typically work in combination with environmental influences. This chapter will go on to describe some environmental influences on early development that can be considered as parts of the cause of disorders. Environmental risks in later childhood can also be very influential on the course of a disorder. The pathways from impairment of function to restrictions on life are considered in Chapter 10.

7.3 CONSEQUENCES OF LOCALIZED CHROMOSOMAL AND SINGLE-GENE ABNORMALITIES

Several chromosomal conditions give rise to complex and characteristic changes in mental and physical development; a listing and guide is provided by Winter and Baraitser (2013). The changes include well-known alterations on chromosomes X, 7, 15, 21, and 22. Most cases are not inherited but represent accidents in very early development.

7.3.1 21 trisomy (Down syndrome)

Extra material of chromosome 21 gives rise to a syndrome of multiple but characteristic physical changes and cognitive difficulties. It is a genetic, but not usually an inherited disorder. The great majority of cases have an extra chromosome 21, for which the causes are not completely known. There is also a proportion of cases in which material from chromosome 21 has been incorporated into another chromosome, so that the total number of chromosomes remains at the usual 46. A fraction of these 'translocation' cases prove to be inherited from a parent who themselves carry the translocation, so genetic counselling is still important. There are also cases in whom only some of the cells of the body carry the extra material—'mosaics'—and the clinical features are then sometimes milder.

Prevalence rates vary with parental decisions about termination of pregnancy, with maternal age, and with quality of medical care. After allowance for these factors, prevalence at birth has been similar across countries (Carothers et al., 1999). About 1 in 700 live births are affected in the USA; the survival rate is rising. In England and Wales, as in many European countries, the figure is around 1 in 1,000.

The diagnosis is usually made prenatally or in early postnatal life, often by paediatricians. Physical findings include hypotonia; small brachycephalic head; epicanthal folds; flat nasal bridge; upward-slanting palpebral fissures; small white spots on the edge of the iris ('Brushfield spots'); small mouth; small ears; excessive skin at the nape of the neck; single transverse palmar crease; a short, inward-curving fifth finger, with clinodactyly and wide spacing; and, often, a deep plantar groove between the first and second toes.

Subsequent supervision of progress and prevention of complications involves several disciplines, including mental health professionals or learning disability specialists. Both primary care professionals and several types of specialists therefore need to understand the basics of medical supervision and how it needs to change over development (Bull & the Committee on Genetics, 2011). Box 7.1 provides an (incomplete) list of disorders in other systems of the body.

Clinicians should be aware not only of the possible medical complications, but also of the real possibilities for healthy, productive lives of people with Down syndrome. They should convey a balanced approach to families, and not allow their personal attitudes towards the condition to colour the advice they give. Current printed materials and websites (e.g. Down Syndrome International Education: www.downsed.org) should be made available. It is very helpful for families to meet other families where the children have Down syndrome. There are usually local support organizations. The same influences that affect the mental health and intelligence of neurotypical children also apply to those with a chromosomal condition such as Down.

7.3.2 Williams–Beuren syndrome (WBS)

WBS is a multisystem disorder, caused by a deletion of some 26 to 28 genes in the 'Williams–Beuren syndrome chromosome region' on chromosome 7. It is estimated to occur in approximately 1 in 10,000 persons (Pober, 2010).

The effects include morphological changes ('elfin facies'), slow growth, developmental delay, and cardiovascular anomalies (aortic and pulmonary stenosis, attributable to the missing elastin gene). Young children are often described as cute or pixie-like, with a

---

Box 7.1 Conditions associated with 21-trisomy that require surveillance

Cognitive impairment of greater or lesser degree: mild (IQ 50–70), moderate (IQ 35–50), or (but only occasionally) severe (IQ 20–35)

Hearing loss

Obstructive sleep apnoea

Otitis media

Eye disease, including cataracts and severe refractive errors

Congenital heart defects

Neurological dysfunction, including seizures but seldom involving autism

Intestinal obstruction from areas of underdevelopment

Coeliac disease

Hip dislocation

Thyroid disease

Blood diseases, including transient myeloproliferative disorders and later leukaemia

Atlantoaxial instability (dislocation of the neck)

Alzheimer's disease in later life

---

flat nasal bridge, short upturned nose, periorbital puffiness, long philtrum, and delicate chin; older patients tend to have full lips and a wide smile.

Psychological and motor changes are usually described as:

- Mild intellectual disability, with strengths in language
- Endearing, friendly personality that can amount to overfriendliness to strangers, and confer vulnerability to inappropriate advances
- Impulsivity and short attention span (ADHD)
- Anxiety and phobias
- Obsessive–compulsive traits
- Hyperacusis
- Poor pencil control

Anxiety and obsessional traits develop over time and are present in a majority of adolescents and adults. Mild intellectual disability is the most frequent cognitive change; it typically combines strengths in language skills and auditory rote memory (e.g. digit recall) with marked weaknesses in visuospatial and visuomotor skills (the ability to spatially relate objects, such as in assembling a jigsaw puzzle) (Udwin et al., 1987).

Other researchers have reported similar results in smaller series. Expert assessments find that 50–90% of adolescents and adults meet the diagnostic criteria of DSM-IV for anxiety disorder, phobic disorder, ADHD, or a combination thereof. Almost all have prominent anticipatory anxiety about upcoming events but little social anxiety (e.g.

about meeting strangers). Many are socially isolated in spite of their seeming friendliness. People with WBS also show diminished amygdala activation when viewing threatening or angry faces, but increased activation in response to threatening stimuli of a non-social nature, suggesting that impaired limbic circuitry may underlie their distinctive anxiety profile (Meyer–Lindenberg et al., 2005).

There seems to be a phenotype here, but it is a pattern describing a group rather than every individual. Any one child may show a different pattern: some have performance abilities superior to verbal. Even if there is a specific impairment at a deep level of neuropsychological function, then many other factors will determine how it appears in an individual.

Idiopathic infantile hypercalcaemia (IIH) was initially important in the recognition and description of WBS, and found to be very similar in its manifestations (Martin et al., 1984); so that IIH and WBS became near synonyms. Increasing knowledge and experience, however, have separated the conditions, and they are now regarded by many as genetically and clinically distinct.

Hypercalcaemia is a feature only in a minority of those with WBS, and it is not usually very severe. The diagnosis of WBS is now made pathologically, not on the basis of blood calcium; usually of fluorescent in situ hybridization (FISH) involving elastin-specific probes. Very high levels of calcium in the blood are dangerous and uncommon. They are often a feature of vitamin D intoxication, but most children exposed to large doses of vitamin D do not develop the syndrome. Those who do develop IIH carry missense mutations of *CYP24A1*, which is the gene coding for 25-hydroxyvitamin D3-24-hydroxylase, a key cytochrome enzyme for converting 25-hydroxyvitamin D_3 to 1,25-dihydroxyvitamin D_3. The effect of the mutations is to render those who possess them hypersensitive to vitamin D.

Udwin et al. (1987) applied Wechsler scales and behavioural ratings to 44 children and teenagers with 'IIH'. Their account, however, makes it clear that the subjects did also meet the morphological criteria of WBS. The children all showed some degree of learning disability; verbal skills were superior to visuospatial and motor abilities. Coding and arithmetic subtests were particularly impaired. Behavioural rating scales showed a somewhat different pattern of deviance from that in mixed groups of intellectually handicapped children. Irritability, solitariness, fussiness, tearfulness at school, complaints of aches and pains, destructiveness, tantrums, worries, and eating, sleeping, and wetting problems were all common.

7.3.3   22q11.2 deletion syndrome (velocardiofacial syndrome; DiGeorge syndrome)

A missing portion of a chromosome 22 gives rise to multiple and variable problems in physical and mental development. The individual genes involved are not completely identified and can also be variable: they probably include COMT and TBX1. Only about

10% of cases are inherited from a parent; the rest are of unknown origin. They can usually be identified by chromosomal microarray but are not part of universal screening. Recognition often arises from prenatal ultrasound scanning that has detected the cardiac problems.

The clinical problems can include (but are not confined to) some of the following:

- Facial changes, including cleft palate
- Heart defects, including abnormalities of the aortic arch, pulmonary valve, and/or atrial septum
- Abnormal development of the larynx, trachea, and/or oesophagus
- Immune deficiency and recurrent infections
- Hearing impairment
- Kidney abnormalities
- Low calcium levels
- Hearing loss
- Developmental delays and learning disabilities

Current estimates of prevalence vary between approximately 1 in 4,000 and 1 in 6,000; the true rate may be greater as it is likely that some cases are not detected. The neuropsychiatric problems can be extensive and may present late in development (i.e. in adolescence or early adult life). The deletion is second only to Down syndrome as a chromosomal cause of intellectual disability (which is usually borderline or mild). ASD and schizophreniform disorders are noteworthy. About 25% of affected individuals will develop schizophrenia-type problems; about 60% will develop that or another mental disorder. These neurodevelopmental problems figure largely in the information on websites, and correspondingly in parental concerns, but are often not part of the initial professional giving of information to families.

The risks for autism spectrum and schizophrenia spectrum disorders are accompanied by disproportionately high rates for anxiety and attention deficit. Current knowledge does not allow for prediction about which people with the chromosome disorder will develop them. There is, accordingly, a need for continuing surveillance to allow for prompt treatment. Management is no different from that of the same conditions arising in the general population.

7.3.4 Chromosome 15 deletions (Prader–Willi and Angelman syndromes)

A region of chromosome 15 (15q11-13) is involved in neuropsychiatric syndromes that are also characterized by distinctive physical changes. The result is determined by sex specificity and imprinting. If there is a deletion of paternal copies of genes in this region (e.g. *SNRPN* and *NDN*), then the result is the condition of Prader–Willi syndrome

(PWS). It is also possible for an individual to have two copies of the chromosome from the mother and none from the father, and again the result can be PWS. A few cases are reported with an inherited abnormality of imprinting.

PWS is a rare condition, affecting about 1 in 20,000. The striking and troublesome feature is extreme and insatiable appetite, with consequent risks for extreme obesity and diabetes mellitus. Management has to involve restriction of access to food (e.g. with locks on anywhere food is stored). There is also a high level of risk for inflexibility, stubbornness, emotional dysregulation (especially, temper tantrums), controlling behaviour, rigid routine, and compulsions. These problems (though not the overeating) tend to become worse in adult life. Cognitive changes involve some degree of intellectual disability (typically of verbal ability), with preservation of visual and motor skills. All the changes, including the overeating, present as a continuum of severity (Manzardo et al., 2018).

Deletion of the same region of the chromosome coming from the mother brings about the very different pattern of Angelman syndrome. Intellectual disability is often severe and accompanied by problems in motor development. Typically, there are hand flapping movements, and walking is accompanied by arms being raised and flexed. Emotionally, affected young people are easily excitable, but have a cheerful demeanour and often appear very sociable. The same pattern can arise if the individual has both of their 15 chromosomes stemming from the father (as the normal process of sex-specific epigenetic imprinting blocks the expression of some paternal genes such as UBE3A).

7.3.5   Chromosome 17p11.2 deletion (Smith–Magenis syndrome)

The major features of this condition include mild to moderate intellectual disability, sleep disturbances, and behavioural problems. There may be distinctive facial features, with a broad and rather flattened appearance. The changes in the face can also be subtle and not apparent at all in early years.

The region of the chromosome that is deleted would ordinarily contain multiple genes. One of them—*RAI1*—which is usually considered responsible and, indeed, the cause of the syndrome, is occasionally not a full deletion but a mutation in that particular gene. As with the other chromosomal abnormalities, it is not usually inherited from a parent.

Emotional and behavioural problems are mostly not very specific. Frequent tempers, high anxiety, impulsive and inattentive behaviour, and self-injury can all add to the clinical picture and the burden of care. Rituals of repetitively hugging oneself, licking fingers, and flipping pages of books can be distinctive. Most affected children have a sleep disorder, even more than in other types of developmental delay. Sleepiness in the day and sleeplessness at night are typical, and some children have a corresponding abnormality of melatonin secretion during the day. Difficulty in falling asleep, however, is not typical, by comparison with nocturnal waking which is. The logical intervention of giving melatonin is not always effective. Sometimes, aggressive outbursts in the daytime can be linked to the sleep problem—as they can be in other types of sleep disorder.

7.3.6 Sex chromosome anomalies

Two or more copies of the X chromosome in males (Klinefelter syndrome; prevalence about 1 in 1,000 males) can result in low testosterone and mild cognitive difficulties, especially in executive function. There are occasionally delays in motor or language development. Most affected young people, however, have unremarkable lives. Gynaecomastia can lead to bullying and shame. Cognitive and behavioural changes are inconstant, but more common with increasing numbers of X chromosomes. Mental health problems are not necessarily attributable to the syndrome in itself; stigma and self-stigma can be key influences.

Complete or partial absence of the X chromosome in females (Turner syndrome; prevalence about 1 in 2,000 females) is not usually associated with altered cognition or behaviour, but some people have problems in mathematics and spatial awareness.

7.3.7. Other chromosomal anomalies

Chromosomal microarray methodology is identifying an increasing number of deletions and duplications that are also considered to contribute to risks for mental disorders. They include deletions at 1q21.1, 15q13.3, and 17q12; and duplications at 1q21.1, 2q13, 15q11-q13, 16p13.11, and 22q11.2—which have all been associated with the development of schizophrenia (Wapner et al., 2012). It seems likely that increased use of this and polygenic DNA profiling will equip clinicians with more precise knowledge of the risks for the individual. The principal value of making a chromosomal or genetic diagnosis is to guide additional medical and developmental evaluations. An established cause helps to exclude other possible explanations for the features and allows more accurate recurrence risk estimates. When some of the known risks in a disorder can be discounted for the individual, then the benefits for families could include a reduction in onerous multiple visits to clinics with different specialisms.

7.4 SYNDROMES FROM SINGLE (OR FEW) GENETIC CHANGES

Many individually rare conditions can follow from both heritable and non-heritable alterations in single genes that have rare but large effects on neuropsychiatric function. Descriptions and illustrations can be found in texts such as *Fenichel's Clinical Pediatric Neurology* (Piña–Garza, 2013). They are worth study for the generalist, even when they are very rare, because of the light they shed on the processes through which they lead to neurodevelopmental deficits and disorders and how those processes can, in principle, be corrected. They emphasize the power and the complexity of genetic changes and the high level of assessment that is required.

7.4.1 Inborn errors of metabolism correctable at birth

Hundreds of heritable errors—mostly inherited as single-gene autosomal recessives—are known. Many of them are screened for at birth. The numbers detected are increasing, especially for those conditions where effective treatment by diet is available. Details of screening vary between nations (Loeber et al., 2012; Villoria et al., 2016), but many Western European countries screen for at least some of those indicated in Box 7.2.

Box 7.2 Amino acid and organic acid disorders often screened in neonates

Amino acid disorders

Phenylketonuria

Homocystinuria

Maple syrup urine disease

Citrullinaemia type I

Argininosuccinic aciduria

Tyrosinaemia type I

Organic acid disorders

Propionic acidaemia

Methylmalonic acidaemia

Methylmalonic acidaemia with homocystinuria

Glutaric acidaemia type I

3-Methylcrotonyl-glycinuria

3-Hydroxy-3-methyl glutaric aciduria

Holocarboxylase synthetase deficiency

Beta-ketothiolase deficiency

Isovaleric acidaemia

In addition to amino acid and organic acid disorders, some regions test more widely and include testing also for mitochondrial fatty acid β-oxidation disorders and galactosaemia in newborns.

Source: data from *J Inherit Metab Dis.*, 35(4), Loeber JG, Burgard P, Cornel MC, et al., Newborn screening programmes in Europe; arguments and efforts regarding harmonization. Part 1–From blood spot to screening result, pp. 603–611, Copyright (2012), John Wiley and Sons; *Semin Pediatr Neurol.*, 23(4), Villoria JG, Pajares S, López RM, et al., Neonatal screening for inherited metabolic diseases in 2016, pp. 257–272, Copyright (2016), Elsevier Inc.

7.4.1.1 *Phenylketonuria (PKU) (phenylalanine hydroxylase deficiency)*

PKU has been the paradigm for inherited metabolic disorders. It is due to mutations in the *PAH* gene, which results in low levels of the enzyme phenylalanine hydroxylase. The normal conversion of phenylalanine into tyrosine is therefore compromised. Toxic levels of phenylalanine (and, probably, deficiency of tyrosine and other amino acids) can then cause major neuropsychological effects, including widespread white-matter degeneration, seizures, and intellectual disability.

Treatment is with a diet low in foods that contain phenylalanine. It needs to start in early infancy and be strictly maintained. It is effective, and allows normal mental development for some, but is disagreeable for most. Phenylalanine levels are regularly monitored by collecting blood from a finger prick. Supplementation with other amino acids, including tyrosine, is usually included. Possible enhancements to treatment include pegvaliase, an enzyme which metabolizes phenylalanine. It is not yet available in the UK, pending results of a trial on whether it justifies the high cost. Tetrahydrobiopterin is a cofactor in the conversion of amino acids such as phenylalanine, tyrosine, and tryptophan to the precursors of dopamine and serotonin. It is sometimes prescribed, at great expense, to overcome the deficiencies in PKU, but unfortunately is not effective for most people.

7.4.1.2 *Other metabolic disorders*

Other metabolic disorders exert their influences through several mechanisms. Chronic energy deficit in the brain can cause growth delay and neurological symptoms, such as seizures and strokes. Accumulation of toxic compounds and lack of precursors of essential compounds can be responsible for inefficient processing of information. Hypoglycaemia and metabolic acidosis can be responsible for many problems, including autonomic changes and seizures.

7.4.2 Fragile-X (Martin–Bell syndrome)

Alterations of the *FMR1* gene (in chromosome band Xq27.3) give rise to conditions inherited in an X-linked dominant fashion. The most frequent alteration in the gene is a variation in the number of times a particular sequence of base pairs (CGG) is repeated. The usual number of repetitions in the general population is between 5 and 40. Fragile-X syndrome (fraX) occurs when there are more than 200. An intermediate number of repeats is called a 'premutation' and acts as a carrier status. The length of the CGG repeat frequently increases over generations, arising during meiosis in female premutation carriers.

FraX is the commonest single-gene cause of intellectual impairment, and the commonest inherited cause. Prevalence is approximately 1 in 2,000. It should be sought in the investigation of neurodevelopmental disorders—not only autism. Physical changes may include a long and narrow face, large ears, flexible fingers, and large testicles. Seizures occur in about 10%. Males are usually more affected than females.

The neuropsychiatric features are very variable in type and severity. Autism was the first to be described, but the full range of changes is wider (Budimirovic & Kaufmann, 2011). Typically, there are problems of social anxiety or avoidance, and often an aversion to looking into other people's eyes. Poor face recognition can be associated. Probably more than half of those with fraX will show some level of social impairment, but full ASD is decidedly less common. Stereotypic behaviours such as hand flapping are also common, and some affected people will talk repetitively on a narrow range of topics. Sensory hypersensitivity can contribute to their irritability. Nevertheless, most affected children do not have the extremes of rigidity that characterize severe ASD, and many are affectionate and sociable.

The commonest psychiatric diagnosis is ADHD, and some level of that spectrum is usually present. Cognitive changes include a diminished IQ by contrast with unaffected peers, but the intellectual level can be anything from normal to severe impairment; mild impairment is the commonest level in males. Attention and executive function are sometimes very weak.

Knowledge of the pathogenesis is increasing rapidly. The lack of the gene product (FMR protein) is associated with altered binding of RNA. Abnormal dendritic spines are considered to be a structural consequence, with effects on synaptic function. This could lead to impaired neuroplasticity, increased local connectivity, and decreased long-range connectivity (Bassell & Warren, 2008). The condition may also be involved in signalling pathways. Telias (2019) reviews the likely metabolic pathways, which include:

- the group 1 metabotropic glutamate receptor (mGluR) pathway, involved in learning;
- dopamine pathways in the prefrontal cortex involved in impulse control;
- GABA pathways involved in the maintenance of anxiety.

7.4.3 Single-gene disorders with progressive course

The term 'dementia' is seldom used about conditions with an early onset; 'developmental regression' is preferred. Nevertheless, some inherited presentations appear after only the first years of life and run a progressive course including loss of cognitive and motor skills and increasing incapacity.

7.4.3.1 Rett syndrome

Rett syndrome is a rare brain disorder, caused by mutations in the gene coding for methyl cytosine binding protein 2 (MECP2, pronounced 'mec-pea-too'). The gene is on the X chromosome and usually modifies the expression of many other genes. The great majority of Rett syndrome patients are female, raising the probability that the condition is usually lethal in males. The disorder is not inherited but arises through random mutation.

Development in the first year of life is usually like that of other children. Sometimes, there are subtle signs reminiscent of autism or motor dysfunctions. Around the second year, however, speech and motor function start to deteriorate. Walking is unsteady. Functional use of the hands is lost, followed by repetitive and stereotyped hand movements such as wringing and washing. There is retardation of growth, dystonia, and cognitive problems. Respiratory problems include overbreathing and breath-holding, and supplementary oxygen is sometimes necessary. In later childhood, the signs and symptoms often stabilize and the course is one of intellectual deficit, with social skills frequently improving.

7.4.4 Storage diseases

Many of the rare progressive conditions are caused by storage diseases, in which metabolic abnormalities lead to a gradual build-up of toxic substances. They are mostly classified by the substances involved.

7.4.4.1 *Neuronal lipofuscinoses*

Neuronal lipofuscinoses are a class of diseases differing in age of onset and pattern of inheritance. Each is due to changes in one of several single genes. Collectively, they are the most frequent neurodegenerative disorders to affect children.

Batten disease (juvenile ceroid neuronal lipofuscinosis) (CLN3) is one such, caused by mutations in the gene CLN3 on chromosome 16. For historical reasons, it is often termed simply 'childhood dementia'. It is inherited as an autosomal recessive. The gene product is battenin. Loss of vision develops between the ages of 4 and 7 years, with macular degeneration and optic atrophy. Children go on to develop learning and behaviour problems, and there is a slow cognitive decline. In later childhood and adolescence, there is a progression to seizures, motor retardation, and loss of language, balance, and independence. EEG and electroretinography have been important in diagnosis, but nowadays the diagnosis is mostly made by DNA analysis.

7.4.4.2 *Lipid storage diseases*

Lipid storage diseases (LSDs) are diseases in which toxic fatty materials slowly accumulate. LSDs are generally classified by the nature of the primary stored material involved.

Sphingolipidoses: for example, Gaucher disease. Caused by a recessively inherited mutation in the *GBA* gene located on chromosome 1. Deficiency of glucocerebrosidase causes build-up of glucocerebroside. Neurological and psychiatric symptoms occur only in some types of Gaucher's and include intellectual deficit, seizures, and myoclonus.

Gangliosidoses: for example, Tay–Sachs disease. Caused by a recessively inherited mutation of the HEXA gene on chromosome 15. Neurones become distended with GM2 ganglioside. There is—in the most severe forms starting in infancy— progressive motor delay and loss of hearing and vision.

Mucopolysaccharidoses: for example, Hunter disease (autosomal recessive with severe multisystem changes and distinctive physical appearance), Hurler disease (with less marked physical changes and X-linked recessive inheritance). SanFilippo (MPS Type III) is a group of single-gene disorders noteworthy for marked cognitive and behavioural problems, often starting before or shortly after school entry and running a progressive course. The other physical abnormalities of the mucopolysaccharidoses may be absent. The toxic substances are different in different forms and include heparan sulphates.

Some forms of glycoprotein storage disorders and mucolipidoses can also cause developmental delays.

7.4.5 Leukodystrophies

Leukodystrophies involve degeneration of myelin, which provides insulation for conducting nerve fibres. The effects typically include decreased motor function, muscle rigidity, and degeneration of sight and hearing.

7.4.5.1 *Adrenoleukodystrophy*

Adrenoleukodystrophy (ALD) is a degenerative disorder that can be caused by mutations in the ATP-binding cassette transporter D1 gene (**ABCD1**) on the X chromosome. Very long-chain fatty acids accumulate in tissues throughout the body. White matter in the brain containing myelin deteriorates. ALDs occur as random mutations and are not inherited. The conditions are rare—about 1 in 20,000. Affected boys present with emotional instability, hyperactivity, and disruptive behaviour at school. It proceeds to dementia. Affected girls have a less severe and later-onset course. 'Lorenzo's oil' can correct some of the chemical changes but does not seem to alter the neurological course. Stem-cell therapy is sometimes applied.

7.4.5.2 *Metachromatic leukodystrophy*

Metachromatic leukodystrophy (MLD) deserves particular mention for its capacity to cause severe psychiatric disorder and dementia in previously undiagnosed adolescents and young adults. It is caused by a deficiency of the enzyme arylsulfatase A. The enzyme activity in leukocytes can be less than 10% of that in normal controls.

MLD can occur in the second year of life with difficulty walking, muscle wasting, weakness, and rigidity. There is progressive loss of vision leading to blindness, convulsions, impaired swallowing, paralysis, dementia, and early death. Later childhood-onset forms can present initially with decline in school performance. Age of death is variable, but normally within 10 to 15 years of symptom onset, although some patients can live for several decades after onset. Adolescent and adult presentations run a more protracted course and should be considered in the differential diagnosis of psychotic disorders and early-onset dementias.

Bone marrow transplantation (including stem-cell transplantation) can be considered. It may slow down progression of the disease in the central nervous system.

7.4.6 Wilson disease

Wilson disease is inherited as a rare autosomal recessive disorder. The gene responsible is *ATP7B*, on chromosome 13, coding for copper-transporting ATPase 2. The protein plays a major role in copper transportation and metabolism. As a result, there is a risk for problems in the liver, eyes, kidneys, and brain. Presentation to neurology or psychiatry is usually in late childhood, adolescence, or early adult life. Disorders such as parkinsonism, ataxia, or dystonia are typical. Psychiatric problems such as personality disorder and schizophrenia can occur without other neurological signs.

The condition is treatable by removal of copper with chelating agents such as penicillamine. Copper studies in blood and urine, and examination for a ring of copper in the eye (Kayser–Fleischer ring), should therefore be undertaken routinely in the investigation of psychosis.

7.4.7 Lesch–Nyhan syndrome

Lesch and Nyhan described a very rare but severe X-linked recessive disorder (Nyhan, 1976). Mutations in the *HPRT* gene cause a deficiency of the enzyme hypoxanthine-guanine phosphoribosyl transferase (HGPRT). Uric acid therefore builds up. Neurological problems include intellectual disability and dystonias reminiscent of athetoid cerebral palsy. Self-mutilation is very striking, and the distinctive pattern is biting one's own lips and fingers. There are also serious gout and kidney problems.

Treatment includes reduction of uric acid (through dietary restriction and allopurinol). Baclofen is used for spasticity, and gabapentin to reduce self-injury. Self-mutilation often requires restraints, which individuals may actively seek. It can be accompanied by other forms of self-harm such as rejecting pleasurable experiences and deliberate failures to achieve.

7.4.8 Huntington disease

Mutations in a gene called *huntingtin* on chromosome 4 are inherited as an autosomal dominant or (in about 10%) arise as a random mutation. There is an increased number of repeats in a CAG (cytosine–adenine–guanine) triplet sequence. The onset is usually in adult life but can also affect children and young people. In the juvenile form, it usually starts insidiously with a drop in school performance and loss of cognitive skills, together with a stiff gait, and progresses to muscle twitches, rigidity, and, eventually, to dementia and paralysis.

7.4.9 Tuberous sclerosis (TS)

Two genes—TSC1 on chromosome 9q34 and TSC2 on chromosome 16p13.3—each give rise to a severe condition involving non-malignant growths (hamartomas) in the brain, skin, kidneys, and other organs. Prevalence is estimated at about 1 in 6,000 live births. A third of cases are inherited as autosomal dominants; most of the others arise as a new mutation. Diagnosis requires a combination of the genetic change with two or more clinical features from a long list of possible structural abnormalities.

Epilepsy arises early in 70–90% of affected children. Infantile spasms (West syndrome) are classic. The psychiatric changes are very variable, and inconsistent even between siblings and in individuals over time. Alterations in social competence, executive function, attention, and intellect are frequent. In motor systems, both repetitive behaviour and overactivity are typical. Challenging behaviours and emotional dysregulation are especially likely to make them hard to care for.

More than half of those with intellectual delay will receive a diagnosis of ASD. Even in those with a normal IQ, ASD is ten times more likely to be present than in those without TS. ADHD, similarly, is more often diagnosed in TS than in those without it, and especially so in those with intellectual disabilities. The development of a low IQ and psychiatric conditions is closely linked to the severity of the TS itself and of epilepsy. Other potentially mediating influences—such as male gender and family adversity—do not seem to have much further effect.

7.4.10 Cornelia de Lange syndrome

This rare condition is caused by any one of several known genetic changes, mostly arising from random mutation rather than being inherited from parents. The gene most likely to be involved (in 60% of cases) is *NIPBL*, but there are at least four others, and sometimes none is identified. *NIPBL* codes for the protein Delangin, which is involved in cell division and DNA repair.

The genetic change affects many bodily systems including the brain. The syndrome is recognizable from unusual bodily features including short stature, microcephaly, hirsutism, synophris (heavy eyebrows growing together), malformed arms, and small, widely spaced teeth. However, no one feature is constant. The neuropsychological changes include intellectual disability, seizures, ASD, and self-injury.

7.4.11 Variable expression of single-gene and defined chromosomal disorders: phenotypes and stereotypes

It will be clear from the preceding text that simple genetic changes can have complex and variable results. One unusual instance is of a boy with skeletally and cytogenetically typical Prader–Willi syndrome who nevertheless showed, not obesity, but extreme emaciation (Miike et al., 1988).

Where there is a clear behavioural phenotype, it can clarify case description and aid early diagnosis and identifying patterns of transmission. It is none the less important to avoid its being corrupted, in the mind, to a stereotype. Some children with Klinefelter syndrome, for example, may conform to the 'classical' picture of nervousness, shyness, and immaturity with intermittent aggression (Caldwell & Smith, 1972), but many have quite different psychiatric presentations. It is important that professionals do not allow their knowledge of what characterizes the group to change their attitude to the individual. This would be part of the process of stigma, and it can distort the lives of individuals who are judged for their disorder and not for themselves.

An occasional family carrying a genetic change may show a uniform presentation. One such, with 16 members showing severe verbal dyspraxia, was described by Hurst et al. (1990). It is, however, much more usual for a multiply-affected family to show many variations on a common theme. Perhaps their altered gene has variable effects on the structure of the brain. Perhaps the result of the structural change produced by the gene is a disposition to any of a wide range of impairments. Perhaps environmental influences or other genetic changes complicate the presentation.

7.5 SYNDROMES FROM COMMON GENETIC VARIANTS

By contrast with the chromosomal and rare gene alterations of large effect, which have been considered earlier, most neuropsychiatric conditions with substantial heritability are associated with DNA variants that are frequent in the general population. The vast majority of these variants do not show one-to-one correspondence with specific changes in behaviour, cognition, and emotion. Rather, they each appear to have very small but multiple effects, and many of those effects are similar to those of other variants. Effects on brain function are dependent on complex interactions with each other and with environmental influences. Correspondingly, the results are probabilistic.

Knowledge is increasing rapidly. Genome-wide association studies (G-WAS) have involved correlations of genetic structure with the clinical syndromes described in Chapters 3 to 5, and the growing number of reliably associated genes are therefore described in the sections on those syndromes. For ASD, and to a lesser extent for ADHD and chronic tic disorders, the yield from testing individuals is high enough for many clinics to recommend routine genome-wide chromosomal microarray. The practical results include improved genetic counselling, identification of related medical risks, a deeper understanding of how conditions have arisen, and access to specialized support groups. Clinicians therefore need to keep informed about current knowledge.

7.5.1 Polygenic risk profiling

The results of scanning the whole genome in G-WAS have included identifying substantial numbers of genetic variants that are individually associated with conditions such as ASD, ADHD, and schizophrenia, even after allowing for the very large number of comparisons that are made. It is possible to combine these potential genetic influences into a polygenic risk score (Sugrue & Desikan, 2019). The resulting mathematical aggregates (there is no single accepted way of weighting them and calculating the score) offer a potentially strong prediction of an outcome such as a diagnosis. The prediction is probabilistic. It raises the likelihood of an outcome but should not be taken to describe a destiny.

Previous sections have illustrated the potential of the method for answering research questions such as the relationship between ASD and ADHD. A recently published study has, for instance, used the genetic liability to ADHD to predict the likelihood of exposure to psychosocial adversity (Zwicker et al., 2020). It falls well short of providing a complete explanation for the association: 4% of the variance in adversity was uniquely explained by genetic risk for ADHD. Nevertheless, the prediction was statistically very significant. It supports the complex approach to psychosocial challenges as both the cause and effect of psychiatric disorder (see 'Adverse outcomes', Chapter 10, Section 10.1).

7.5.2 Inherited influences not based on DNA variants

'Epigenetics' refers to the mechanisms through which gene expression is altered without changes in the DNA sequence. As examples, the DNA can be methylated, or the shape of the histone proteins modified. The result can be to activate or silence the effect of the gene on the cell. These modifications can themselves be passed down the generations. Most of the direct evidence that this happens comes from research on animals, but the phenomenon could still become highly relevant to human problems. Babies who were in the womb when their mothers starved during the Dutch Hunger Winter of 1944–1945 have a high rate of illness in adult life—including schizophrenia (Lumey et al., 2011). This has been attributed to silencing of genes by epigenetic processes (Tobi et al., 2014).

In *genomic imprinting*, a specific allele from one parent or the other is preferentially expressed in somatic cells of the offspring because of DNA methylation or histone modifications. It can lead to notably different phenotypes, according to which parent it derives from. The clearest known influences are on Prader–Willi and Angelman syndromes, described earlier.

7.5.3 Gene–environment correlations

The effects of genetic influences work in transaction with the environment. Many environmental influences on neuropsychiatric function are described in the next section.

They include toxins, infections, trauma, physical ill health, abuse, and chronic psycho-social adversity. They do not arise in complete independence from the individual's nature. Life events themselves can be inherited. They may be brought about by qualities of the child open to genetic influence, and qualities of the caregivers who may share some of the genetic influences.

Chapter 10 will describe some of the ways in which genetically influenced neurodevelopmental disorders can expose young people to environmental risks that further impair psychological function. A straightforward example is that impulsive behaviour in children with ADHD can bring their fingers, and hence their mouths, into close contact with old paint containing lead—and so contribute to lead-induced problems of cognition. In so far as genes influence impulsiveness, this is often termed *active* (or *evocative*) *gene–environment correlation*. The full picture is not simple. In this instance of impulsiveness and exposure to toxins, the trait in the child can both bring about and reflect qualities of parenting. Parents can model calm and reflective behaviour, practice delayed gratification, teach self-control skills, and encourage coping with potential dangers. The extent to which they do so will in part be genetically influenced, like other aspects of parenting (Oliver et al., 2014). Both the genes and the family culture will be transmitted to children. The correlation between parental genotype and the environment is called *passive gene–environment correlation*.

It is often necessary to include genetic thinking to understand environmental effects. As an example, advanced age of the father is a risk for his child developing ASD. This can be a direct physical influence brought about by changes in ageing sperm. It can also be subject to the different, and potentially heritable, reasons for conception later in the father's life.

7.5.4 Gene–environment interactions

Sometimes, individuals' reactions to their environment are altered by their genes. This would be the case if, for instance, the methylation patterns of DNA were to magnify the damaging effects of alcohol exposure in the womb. (This is put as a hypothetical example because, even though there is evidence from Lussier et al. (2018) that that is the case, it is still to be replicated.) Another possible example from psychopathology is the effect of cannabis use in adolescence to create a risk for schizophrenia later. The risk may be moderated by a functional polymorphism in the catechol-O-methyl transferase gene (COMT) (Caspi et al., 2005).

One kind of potential G–E interaction is differential susceptibility (Belsky & Pluess, 2009). The idea, as applied to psychopathology, is that the constitution of some individuals makes them vulnerable not only to the influence of harmful environments but also to that of beneficial ones. These 'plastic' individuals would be, for instance, more prone than their peers in similar circumstances to develop behaviour problems in response to harsh and insensitive parenting, but also *less* likely to develop antisocial behaviour if their parents have been stable, warm, sober, and competent.

7.5.5 Clinical significance of genetic understanding

Our understanding of genetic influences has grown remarkably but has not simplified. The advice given to families should still be that genetic influences are strong—but they are multiple. The scientific difficulty in specifying the precise influences responsible makes genetic counselling inexact for most affected families. For the moment, investigation of chromosomes and DNA for individual patients is recommended only when there are specific reasons—such as a phenotype suggesting a large gene effect (e.g. Williams syndrome), or the presence of many affected family members, or the existence of other neurodevelopmental problems (e.g. intellectual disability) that are enough in themselves to indicate genetic evaluation.

Besides the practical utility for counselling on risks of recurrence, genetic evidence is increasing our understanding of development and informing attitudes towards affected individuals. Life events can be inherited, so the environmental hazards to be considered in the next sections have to be judged in the context of the personal development of the individual.

7.6 Early environmental hazards

7.6.1 Prenatal programming

Chapters 3 and 4, on ADHD and ASD, have identified several types of environmental influences on pregnant mothers that predict persisting neurodevelopmental problems in their children's postnatal life (see Box 7.3 and Chapter 6, Section 6.3).

7.7 Infections

7.7.1 Prenatal infections

Infections of children before they are born have profound effects on the public health. They remain major causes of developmental delays for children in low- and middle- income countries.

Many infections are very common, especially in tropical countries, and have only trivial or no effects on most healthy adults. The same infections of pregnant women can have devastating effects for the fetus, which has little immune defence. They should therefore be considered for all cases of developmental disability, whether or not there is a history of maternal infection. Serological testing of the mother does not help much: in

Box 7.3 Environmental influences in pregnancy

Toxins

Maternal smoking

Maternal alcohol consumption

Maternal drug use (therapeutic or illicit)

Lead, mercury, insecticides

Deficiencies

Maternal hypothyroidism

Malnutrition

Micronutrient deficiencies (folate, iron, iodine)

Antibodies to fetal antigens

Kernicterus

Placental insufficiency

Underprovision of oxygen and nutrients to fetus

Diabetes mellitus, hypertension, anaemia, clotting disorders

Placentopathies (e.g. poor attachment to uterine wall)

Infection and inflammation

Toxoplasmosis, rubella, cytomegalovirus, herpes, syphilis

Other viral infections (e.g. influenza, HIV, Zika virus, varicella, and parvovirus)

Psychological problems in mothers

Acute or chronic stress

Depression and anxiety

Socioeconomic problems affecting families

many communities the infections are ubiquitous. Rather, screening of all with intellectual disability (ID) should include TORCHES and some other conditions. TORCHES is a mnemonic to remind clinicians of the importance of detecting and, where possible, preventing congenital infections: TO(toxoplasma); R(rubella); C(cytomegalovirus); HE(herpes); S(syphilis). The list should be expanded to include human immunodeficiency virus (HIV), varicella, and parvovirus.

7.7.1.1 *Congenital toxoplasmosis*

Toxoplasma gondii is a parasite very commonly present in many animals, including cats, humans, and many others. Transmission is by ingestion of excreted cysts in faeces via food that has been contaminated and not thoroughly cooked. In healthy mothers, the illness produced, if any, is minor and often overlooked. It is a very different story for the offspring who have been infected through the placenta because the mother does not have immunity herself. Mothers who do not have immune protection should be advised to guard against infection, and to be careful when preparing food. They should avoid contact with animal excrement—especially from cats, which are the definitive host and the only animals in which the parasite can reproduce sexually. (It is possible that toxoplasma parasites can manipulate the behaviour of their hosts. Infected rodents tend to lose their fear of novel situations. In particular, rats with toxoplasmosis lose their typical aversion to the odour of cat urine and develop a perverse attraction to it. This could be seen as an advantage to the parasite's ability to spread.)

An embryo does not have much immune defence and is likely to be infected and have brain involvement. A classic triad of chorioretinitis, intracranial calcifications, and hydrocephalus is accompanied by a range of other problems (McAuley, 2014). Later results include ID, epilepsy, encephalopathy, and visual problems. Such problems can appear even after a period of normal development, if the cysts in the brain are activated by a later immune failure. Treatment is urgent—before birth, usually with spiramycin; afterwards, with a prolonged course of pyrimethamine/sulfadiazine.

People with schizophrenia are at increased risk of having antibodies to toxoplasma (Torrey et al., 2006). The odds ratio is about 2.7. However, the causal role of toxoplasma is not established.

7.7.1.2 *Congenital rubella*

Maternal infection with the rubella virus in the first 12 weeks of gestation carries around an 80% risk of involving the fetus. Sensorineural deafness, structural abnormalities of the heart, and various eye problems, including cataracts and retinopathies, are typical. Intellectual deficit and microcephaly are frequent. Later, schizophrenia spectrum disorders are more frequent than in other children (Brown, 2006).

Prevention by vaccination should be universal. In the UK, the NHS provides it in combination with vaccines against mumps and measles (MMR), as a single injection to babies within a month of their first birthday. A second injection follows shortly before starting school, usually at 3 years and 4 months.

7.7.1.3 *Congenital cytomegalovirus*

Cytomegalovirus (CMV) is ubiquitous. The majority of humans are infected. Primary infection in individuals with normal immune function usually produces no symptoms at the time, but the virus enters long latency in various host cells unless and until immune function is suppressed and no longer keeps it under control. If, however, a pregnant mother, who is not protected by previous infection and immunity, develops the infection, then the fetus is infected too in about 50% of cases. About 30% of infected babies will show problems as a result. The problems are usually in multiple systems. Hearing impairments and ID are frequently the key outcomes. CMV may well be a cause of many cases of developmental delays that are not yet recognized as such (Griffiths & Walter, 2005).

Vaccines are pressingly awaited (Bernstein, 2017). The fetus can be protected with hyperimmune globulin. Molecular testing can detect the DNA in blood from the neonate. Hearing loss can be significantly decreased by ganciclovir given in the first week.

7.7.1.4 Herpes simplex

The herpes simplex virus can also be transmitted from mother to child, usually towards the end of pregnancy when the baby is passing through the birth canal. Correspondingly, it behaves in a similar way to postnatally acquired herpes—with a skin rash and the possibility of encephalitis or disseminated illness involving the whole body. Signs usually appear in the first month of life. When the brain or whole body is affected, the outlook is grave. All infected babies should receive an antiviral such as intravenous acyclovir.

Herpes simplex infection in postnatal life can cause a devastating encephalopathy. In the absence of effective antiviral treatment, about 70% of patients die. This very high rate should be reduced by acyclovir to less than 20%—but this is still very high, and a large minority of those who recover will have persisting neurological disability.

The virus typically infects through damaged mucosae and migrates up nerve axons (e.g. olfactory nerve) to cause localized brain damage (e.g. in temporal lobes). Localized lesions may be seen on magnetic resonance imaging. Long-term neuropsychiatric sequelae of encephalopathy involve language, memory, and personality changes, but with no pathognomonic profile. Case histories suggest that autistic syndromes can result. There is, however, no good evidence for the widely circulated suspicion that herpes infection is a frequent cause of ASD or a cause in those without signs of infection.

Diagnosis, which used to be based on brain biopsy, is now made from molecular tests (e.g. via a polymerase chain reaction) for the presence of herpes DNA in the cerebrospinal fluid.

7.7.5 Congenital varicella

Varicella is a herpes-type virus responsible for the frequent childhood illness of chickenpox. Most pregnant mothers will be immune because of previous illness or vaccination. If one is in contact with a case of chickenpox, her immune status should be tested. If she has not been vaccinated and is seronegative, then treatment should be given (with varicella zoster immunoglobulin and/or antiviral drugs) to reduce the risk to the fetus.

Most transplacental infections are asymptomatic, but they can cause the rare congenital varicella syndrome with multisystem abnormalities including skin lesions, neurological defects, eye diseases, limb hypoplasia, and/or skeletal anomalies (Ahn et al., 2016). Neonatal chickenpox can itself be a serious illness.

7.7.1.6 *Congenital syphilis*

The spirochaete bacterium, Treponema pallidum, remains sensitive to penicillin. The fetus can be infected from the mother at any stage. Serological testing is effective for diagnosis. Pregnant women with syphilis should be treated promptly, which is an effective intervention for the fetus, especially if given before the sixteenth week of gestation.

The postnatal manifestations are manifold, and many of them only appear in later childhood. Early signs include seizures, rhinitis, and generalized skin rash. If not detected and treated early, syphilis can enter a latent stage, emerging later with damage to brain, bones, teeth, eyes, and ears. Neurosyphilis can be detected by analysis of cerebrospinal fluid. Penicillin cannot be expected to reverse damage done but should prevent it.

7.7.1.7. *Influenza virus*

Much research has investigated the possibility that schizophrenia can also be a result of congenital infection with the influenza virus. Some but not all epidemiological studies have found a relationship between season of birth and rates of non-affective psychosis in adult life. This has been interpreted as evidence for an aetiological role. An excess of psychosis in people born in the summer does not, however, automatically imply that a greater likelihood of influenza in early stages of pregnancy is responsible. It often represents a non-specific risk of being among the youngest children in the class (see also 'Cerebral palsy', Chapter 6, Section 6.3).

The evidence most often cited is serological. The evidence from antibodies, however, is flawed and inconclusive (Selten & Termorshuizen, 2017).

7.7.1.8 *Congenital human immunodeficiency virus (HIV)*

The child of an infected mother has a 25–40% chance of acquiring the infection if there is no medical intervention. Transmission can be transplacental, in the course of delivery, or via breastfeeding. It can be drastically reduced by effective antiretroviral therapy (ART) given in pregnancy. Delivery by Caesarean section can reduce infant transmission from the birth canal. Infected mothers are advised not to breastfeed unless no other feeding option is available. Infection of children is therefore usually a consequence of ineffective antenatal care. It is still common in regions where antenatal health services are weak.

Brain involvement can result from an encephalopathy. The virus crosses the blood–brain barrier and invades brain cells—especially the microglia, rather than the neurones themselves. Progressive white-matter degeneration and brain atrophy can follow and eventually result in neurological motor symptoms, microcephaly, and developmental delays. Neuroimaging changes include cranial ultrasound altered signals from lenticulostriate vessels, computerized tomography evidence of calcifying microangiopathy, and/or magnetic resonance evidence of white-matter lesions and central atrophy.

7.7.2 Postnatal infections

Chronic infections cause failures of growth and mental blunting. Some multisystem diseases—notably acquired immune deficiency syndrome (AIDS), malaria and measles—carry strong implications for neurodevelopment. AIDS and malaria are examples of the many chronic and infective diseases that still devastate poor tropical countries.

7.7.2.1 *Acquired immune deficiency syndromes*

HIV causes many syndromes of acquired immune deficiency. The consequences of the infection are not only for developmental regression, and more broadly for mental disorders; and not only for other bodily systems; but for the whole ecology. Impoverishment, bereavement, illness in caregivers, stigma, associated traumas such as rape, and a lack of access to education and healthcare—all combine to produce complex pathogen–pathogen interactions. Even children who have been exposed but not infected are at risk for adverse cognitive and psychiatric outcomes. Infection in childhood and adolescence can result from blood transfusion, drug injection, and sexual transmission. The commercial sex worker industry in countries such as Thailand and the Caribbean Islands is responsible for high levels of HIV transmission to young women and girls.

The advent of antiretroviral drugs has had a profound effect and, for many, they have transformed the outlook to one of a normal life span, albeit one of chronic illness and a need for long-term medication. Nevertheless, many young people, and especially those living in sub-Saharan Africa, do not have access to the drugs. Many more still lack the educational, social, and mental health support that is called for.

7.7.2.2 *Malaria*

Like HIV, malaria causes both serious illness in children and impairment of care-giving through effects on adults. Transmission of the parasite species, most seriously Plasmodium falciparum, is through the bites of female Anopheles mosquitoes, or via blood transfusion. Many organs can be affected. In the brain, diffuse and potentially lethal pathology comes from infected blood cells sticking to each other and the walls of blood vessels and causing obstructions. Multiple strokes and inflammation result. Cytokines, and neurotoxins such as nitric oxide, are released. Prostration, coma, and convulsions characterize acute infection. Prolonged seizures can cause neurocognitive problems in their own right.

In the longer term, cerebral malaria causes many types of psychological deficit. Nearly all the functions described in Chapter 2 can be involved. Motor coordination, executive function, language, attention, and learning difficulties have all been described (Boivin et al., 2007). After recovery, a minority of patients can develop a 'post malaria neuro-logical syndrome' (Nguyen et al., 1996). Acute confusional states, psychoses, visual hallucinations, catatonia with waxy flexibility, and generalized convulsions are part of it. No parasites are necessarily found in the blood and the pathogenesis is unclear.

Antimalarial drugs bring their own risks of neuropsychiatric disorders, including psychotic disturbances.

7.7.2.3 Cysticercosis

Cysticercosis is a major cause worldwide of epilepsy, especially in countries where humans and pigs live close to each other. If the eggs of the pork tapeworm are ingested, the resulting larvae invade muscles, eyes, skin, and brain. The multiple small cysts in the brain can readily be seen on computerized tomography or magnetic resonance imaging.

Treatment with antiparasitic drugs can be effective but can also produce cerebral oedema and hydrocephalus. Antiepileptics are recommended for seizures. Surgical intervention can be indicated to remove expanding cysts or insert shunts to relieve hydrocephalus.

7.7.2.4 Tuberculous infection

Tuberculosis, once the 'Captain of all these men of death', remains a scourge. The World Health Organization (WHO) estimates that a quarter of the world is infected. Initially invading the lungs, it can spread to many parts of the body and often complicates AIDS. Meningitis and encephalitis are often lethal, and for those who recover, the neurological complications can be devastating (Chin & Mateen, 2013). The mycobacterium is developing resistance to antibiotics. Rifampicin is increasingly given in high doses and in combination with isoniazid, pyrazinamide, and ethambutol.

7.7.2.5 Measles virus

Subacute sclerosing panencephalitis (SSPE) is a rare but very serious complication of measles. Patients show cognitive losses, disruptive behavioural changes, visual disturbances, and pyramidal and extrapyramidal signs. The disease has a gradual progressive course, leading through dementia to death within 1–3 years. Brain biopsies or post-mortem histopathological examination show evidence of astrogliosis, neuronal loss, degeneration of dendrites, demyelination, neurofibrillary tangles, and infiltration of inflammatory cells.

Treatment is attempted with antiviral drugs and drugs that modulate the immune system. They are not cures, but sometimes prolong life.

7.7.2.6 Common infective illnesses in childhood

There have been many attempts over the years to understand the long-term effects on mental life of common physical illnesses in childhood. Infections have been implicated as causes of mental illness in postnatal as well as prenatal life.

In the specific instance of schizophrenia, cohort studies have received a competent meta-analysis (Khandaker et al., 2012). When the child has suffered an infection of the central nervous system, their subsequent risk for schizophrenia is almost doubled (relative risk 1.8). It appears that viral meningitis or encephalitis is a bigger risk than bacterial. CMV, mumps, and varicella zoster were the main culprits in the one study that defined the causative agents.

To move from the well-studied case of schizophrenia to the commoner mental disorders, there is an association between contracting severe infections and neurodevelopmental problems later. A recent population study, of more than a million people born in Denmark between 1995 and 2012, has used case registers to estimate the frequency of psychological sequelae of infections that were serious enough to require admission to hospital (Köhler–Forsberg et al., 2019). The risks of developing a mental disorder (diagnosed in hospital) were increased by 84% and those for use of psychotropic medication by 42%. Even less severe infections (defined as having been treated in the community with anti-infective agents) increased the risks somewhat: by 40% for diagnosed mental disorder and 22% for psychotropic drug use.

The increased risk applied to a wide range of neurodevelopmental and other disorders, including obsessive-compulsive disorders, tics, schizophrenia spectrum disorders, personality and behaviour disorders, ASD, and ADHD. Association does not by itself imply cause. There could be many confounders, including associations in common—such as poverty and help-seeking behaviour. Anti-infective agents might be risky by altering the blood–brain barrier or the microflora of the gut. There could be reverse causality if the risks for mental disorder should also increase susceptibility to infection. The same population study in Denmark, however, was able to control for possible confounders by recording also the risks for siblings who did not have infections. The increase of risk for later mental illness then fell—but not to zero. The increase, when compared to that for siblings, fell from 84% to 21%.

There is, therefore, a reasonable case that some of the results of everyday infection include direct neurocognitive effects. The mechanisms are receiving current research attention. Altered family relationships and inflammatory and allergic reactions are all strong candidates for the processes involved. The research findings, however, are not yet robust enough to indicate routine detailed enquiry about the history of common infections. Inflammation, in particular, is receiving much current research attention. Metabolic and immune consequences of infection may directly compromise brain function. Infective agents can cross the blood–brain barrier and produce meningitis (inflammation of the membranes that surround the brain) and encephalopathies (in which the substance of the brain itself is compromised). Anti-infective agents may lead to a disturbed microflora of the gut and alterations in the blood–brain barrier.

7.7.2.7 *Streptococcus pyogenes and autoantibodies*

Streptoccoccal throat infections can give rise to neurological problems. Abnormal movements after streptococcal infection (Sydenham's chorea) have long been recognized. More recently, it was realized that the condition was often accompanied by tics and by obsessional, anxiety, and ADHD-type symptoms. There was a clear analogy with a newly described syndrome of explosive onset of obsessional and other neuropsychiatric symptoms. This analogy created the terminology of 'paediatric autoimmune neuropsychiatric disorders associated with streptococcal infections' (PANDAS) (Swedo et al., 1998).

> ## Box 7.4 Suggested NIMH criteria for diagnosis of PANDAS
>
> - Presence of obsessive-compulsive disorder and/or a tic disorder
> - Paediatric onset of symptoms (age 3 years to puberty)
> - Episodic course of symptom severity
> - Association with group A beta-haemolytic streptococcal infection (a positive throat culture for streptococcus or a history of scarlet fever)
> - Association with neurological abnormalities (physical hyperactivity, or unusual, jerky movements that are not in the child's control)
> - Very abrupt onset or worsening of symptoms
>
>   Antibody tests were not a criterion, but 'If the symptoms have been present for more than a week, blood tests may be done to document a preceding streptococcal infection'.
>
> Source: data from *Am J Psychiatry*, 155(2), Swedo SE, Leonard HL, Garvey M, et al., Pediatric autoimmune neuropsychiatric disorders associated with streptococcal infections: clinical description of the first 50 cases, pp. 264–271, Copyright (1998), American Psychiatric Association

Antibodies raised to beta-haemolytic streptococci can cross-react with brain structures such as the basal ganglia. PANDAS was quite difficult to diagnose reliably (see Box 7.4). Autoantibodies were not consistently detected, and some cases developed without them. There was very often uncertainty about the link with the streptococcus in individual cases. The clinical evidence needed to come from throat cultures. If, as is often the case, these were uninformative, then clinicians relied on antistreptolysin tests (ASOTs), which have uncertain relationships in time to the putative symptoms. The diagnosis led to immune therapies (such as steroids and globulins), cytotoxic drugs, removal of antibodies with dialysis, and antibiotic cover to eliminate streptococci. The full package did not survive a lack of replicated trial evidence for its value.

The diagnostic criteria suggested in Box 7.4 (Swedo et al., 1998) did not get universal support. Difficulties arose particularly in linking the clinical course to an acute streptococcal infection (e.g. in relying on antibody tests such as the ASOT when throat culture was not informative). A more recent evolution of the concept has been to 'paediatric acute-onset neuropsychiatric syndrome' (PANS) (Swedo et al., 2012) (see Box 7.5).

A presentation defined as in Box 7.5 can indeed be distinctive and serious. Case series have been reported at the clinical level (Johnson et al., 2019). No unifying pathology or treatment, however, has yet been found. The recognition of a case should therefore lead clinicians to a search for specific conditions that may present in this way—including systemic lupus, NMDAR encephalitis, cerebral vasculitis, and streptococcal infection. Treatment is therefore symptomatic (psychotropic drugs and/or cognitive behavioural therapy (CBT)) or directed at an underlying pathology.

Box 7.5 Suggested criteria for PANS

PANS describes a condition whose hallmark is a very rapid, even explosive, onset of obsessive-compulsive symptoms (or sometimes of severely restrictive eating disorder); together with at least two out of seven other neuropsychiatric problems:

1. Anxiety

2. Emotional lability and/or depression

3. Irritability, aggression, and/or severely oppositional behaviours

4. Behavioural (developmental) regression

5. Deterioration in school performance

6. Sensory or motor abnormalities

7. Somatic signs and symptoms, including sleep disturbances, enuresis, or urinary frequency

Source: data from *Pediatr Therapeut.*, 2(2), Swedo SE, Leckman JF, Rose NR, From research subgroup to clinical syndrome: modifying the PANDAS criteria to describe PANS (pediatric acute-onset neuropsychiatric syndrome), pp. 1000113, 1–8, Copyright (2012), Swedo SE, et al. Reproduced under the terms of the Creative Commons Attribution License (CC BY). https://doi.org/10.4172/2161-0665.1000113

7.7.2.7.1 *Immune encephalopathies*

Encephalopathies can result from many external causes affecting the brain. Several are associated with immune changes. *Systemic lupus* (SLE) can attack most organs of the body, and the brain is no exception. Its manifestations include cognitive blunting ('lupus fog'), fatigue, headaches, seizures, depression, and acute psychotic disturbances.

Hashimoto's encephalopathy describes a diffuse set of brain problems, affecting most of the functions described in Chapter 2, that are associated with autoimmune inflammation of the thyroid gland (Hashimoto's thyroiditis, see Chapter 6, Section 6.7). It is a rare condition. The pathogenesis is thought likely to come from immune attack on the brain. The association with thyroid antibodies is suggestive, and autoantibodies to alpha-enolase have sometimes been found. (Enolase is the penultimate step in glycolysis, so widespread effects on cell function would be expected.) The course is very variable. Treatment with steroids is indicated, and often effective.

Some types of severe encephalopathy (*NMDAR encephalitis*)—often presenting with seizures, coma, psychotic features, and/or motor and/or cognitive changes—are thought to be autoimmune in origin because of association with circulating levels of antibodies; for example, to the N-methyl-D-aspartate (NMDA) receptor, or to the voltage-gated potassium channel, which is differentiated into LGI1 (leucine-rich glioma inactivated 1) and CASPR2 (contactin-associated protein 2). NMDAR encephalitis in adults is now widely known from a fine personal account by Susannah Cahalan (2018). Cases have been reported of affected adolescents who present with psychiatric problems including hallucinations, delusions, and catatonic motor changes. The pathogenesis is often uncertain, and it remains possible that the antibodies could be present because of neurological disease or of tumours elsewhere—rather than being the primary cause of the illness.

The diagnosis is mostly made by suspecting it in acute-onset organic psychosis and going on to laboratory investigation. EEG and magnetic resonance imaging (MRI) testing are often abnormal but non-specific. The antibodies sometimes appear in the blood or cerebrospinal fluid only weeks after the clinical onset—so suspicion should not be dispelled by early negative results. Anti-immune therapies (e.g. steroids) can help. They are severe neurological illnesses and can result in lasting impairments.

7.8   Environmental deficiencies

7.8.1 Malnutrition

Malnutrition in children is defined by height and weight compared to the WHO child growth standards, which take into account age and gender. Deficiencies of calories, protein, and micronutrients are all involved. Underweight (low weight for age) comprises both stunting and wasting.

Wasting is a result of acute nutritional deficiency or illness and can usually be corrected rapidly. It represents a body weight of two (or more) standard deviations less than the average. *Stunting* represents chronic poor nutrition from an early age and is difficult to correct. Height for age is below two standard deviations of the WHO references. Infections and inflammation are also involved, and damage to the intestinal mucosa from polluted environments also play a part. Cognitive loss is frequent, and infections add to the loss of human potential.

International joint estimates of the UNICEF/WHO/World Bank report continuing surveys of the prevalence of both wasting and stunting in children under 5 years (WHO & UNICEF, 2009). Figures are frequently updated at https://data.unicef.org/topic/nutrition/malnutrition/. Rates have been declining, but not disappearing. In March 2019, the countries studied (many of them low- and middle-income countries) had, for the under fives, rates of wasting at about 7.5% (49 million) and, for stunting, about 22% (149 million).

Fatigue, depression, anxiety, and selective vitamin deficiencies are widespread in all kinds of generalized malnutrition.

7.8.2 Selective malnutrition: micronutrient deficiencies

7.8.2.1 *Iodine*

The thyroid gland and the hormones it secretes are vulnerable not only to the diseases described earlier, but also to dietary deficiency of iodine. Such deficiency is very common, and in fact considered to be one of the biggest causes of intellectual slowing worldwide. International surveillance has suggested, on the basis of urinary iodine levels, that some 30% of countries have insufficient iodine intakes: 76 million people in South-East Asia and 58 million in Africa are exposed (Andersson et al., 2012). Much of the damage is likely to be done during fetal life.

Mild cases in other countries are unlikely to be a major public health issue. In Norway, possible minor problems were detected by Abel et al. (2017) investigating maternal intakes of iodine below the estimated average requirement during pregnancy. There were some signs of suboptimal language, noticeable behaviour problems, and backward fine motor skills when children were 3 years old. Supplementation, however, did not help.

The effects can be dramatic in iodine-deficient areas. Qian et al. (2005) have summarized all the studies of correction of parts of China with severely low iodine. There is persuasive evidence of population increases of IQ of up to 10 points. Feyrer et al. (2017) have used historical evidence to argue that the iodization of salt in the USA in the 1920s had a major impact on the great increase in IQ seen there between the wars. This was larger in areas known to be low in iodine because of a high prevalence of goitre. There was a cost though: a sizeable increase in death, presumably due to thyrotoxicosis triggered by the relief of iodine deficiency.

7.8.2.2 *Iron and zinc*

Iron deficiency is very frequent and can result from many causes. Chronic infections, inflammation, bleeding, malignancy, malnourished mothers, and social deprivation can all be responsible (Lozoff, 2007). It has many pathological results, including anaemia (Lozoff et al., 2008). It has correspondingly been difficult to go beyond the observation that many anaemic children have poor concentration and learning. Any brain reactions leading to altered mental function are therefore hard to specify. Zinc may contribute; hippocampal involvement is suspected.

Supplementation with iron and zinc in infancy has received some support. Mental and psychomotor development were somewhat improved in a group of Bangladeshi infants given iron and zinc by comparison with riboflavin (Black et al., 2004)

7.8.2.3 *Vitamins*

Selective malnutrition of essential vitamins can arise in impaired children as a result of extreme faddiness, dogmatically imposed diets, and coincident illness. Some of the vitamins are essential for mental welfare. Not all candidates will be mentioned in detail; the focus is on those capable of causing mental changes.

Vitamin B1 (thiamine) is needed throughout life. Low levels have been found in refugee populations, people with high carbohydrate intakes (e.g. of polished rice), and neglected babies. Low levels can give rise to fatigue and depression, poor memory and concentration, and neuropathy. Diets as poor as this have been found, in the past, in residential schools and young people's institutions.

Vitamin B6 (pyridoxine) has, in low levels, been responsible for outbreaks of fatigue, poor attention, and depression. Deficiency is found in people with renal impairment or autoimmune disorders. Some young children with seizures show pyridoxine dependency. PLP, a metabolite, is a cofactor in the metabolism of tryptophan, gamma aminobutyric acid, and niacin, and therefore in the synthesis of many neurotransmitters.

Vitamin B12 (cyanocobalamin) and *folate* deficiency can each cause fatigue, poor memory, neuropathy, depression, and blunting of mental faculties. Autoimmune disorders, poor diet, and Crohn's disease (an inflammatory disease of the bowel) are all possible causes. Folic acid fortification of flour and bread is known to reduce neural tube defects significantly in fetuses, by raising folate levels in women who could become pregnant.

7.8.2.4 *Deficiencies in a normal diet*

Vitamin deficiencies usually have to be severe before they have neurological effects. Some recent accounts, nevertheless, concern the possibility that mild and frequent deficiencies of micronutrients in an 'industrial' diet play a substantial role in learning and behaviour impairment. The possibility, if real, would increase the role of dietary advice and supplementation for cognitive problems in children. Overall, however, trials of adding extra vitamins and minerals to an otherwise normal diet have not given strong results. Crombie et al. (1990) carried out a randomized, double-blind, placebo-controlled trial extended over a school year, involving 86 schoolchildren aged 11–13. None of the tests of verbal or non-verbal ability showed a significant gain attributable to the supplement.

7.8.2.5 *Polyunsaturated long-chain fatty acids*

A controversy regarding the need for 'essential fatty acids' has generated many research trials and reviews, with strikingly different results. Improvements in methodology and meta-analyses have led to a widely accepted, though perhaps not an unchallenged consensus. There are probably real but small effects in reducing the ADHD behaviours that have been researchers' main target.

Long-chain fatty acids are considered 'unsaturated' if they contain a double bond between a pair of their carbon atoms, and are classified by the position of that bond in the chain (e.g. at n-6 or n-3). The modern Western diet has a high amount of n-6 and a low amount of n-3 polyunsaturated fatty acid. The many trials have focused on enriching diets of children with ADHD with extra n-3. Fish oils contain two n-3 (or 'omega-3') compounds: eicosapentaenoic acid (EPA) and docosahexaenoic acid (DHA). Flaxseed oil contains EPA. Both compounds can inhibit the release of chemicals that promote inflammation. There are several applications in physical medicine. Trials in conditions affecting mental health, however, have been based on proprietary formulations.

DHA is widely distributed in cell membranes in the brain; EHA less so. A systematic review by Sonuga–Barke et al. (2013) covered 11 competent trials of supplementation in ADHD. The overall analysis was positive, with an effect size of 0.17, for children whose treatment had not also included medication. This is a small effect only, and the cost of the proprietary preparations is not inconsiderable. The results were not enough to persuade health authorities to provide the treatment free on prescription. Nevertheless, the effect was large enough to maintain statistical significance even when the raters were probably blinded to the treatment given. The mechanism of effect is not yet clear. Other, non-pharmacological interventions (neurofeedback, cognitive training—see Chapter 8, Section 8.6) were less promising for the reduction of hyperactivity impulsiveness and inattention. Trials have not indicated a therapeutic effect of fatty acids in ASD, learning impairments, or chronic tics.

7.9 Toxins, allergens, and immune influences

7.9.1 Lead

Lead is a poison, found all over the world as a result of industrial pollution. It damages many organ systems. The neurological effects in young people include dullness, irritability, poor attention span, headache, muscular tremor, loss of memory, and hallucinations (Wani et al., 2015). Cellular actions include inactivation of glutathione and inhibition of many enzymes, including the antioxidants that are part of the body's defences against the oxidative stress of reactive oxygen species.

The main sources of lead are:

- industrial plants, such as smelters and battery recyclers, contaminating the dust and air in their neighbourhood,
- petrol fumes (e.g. from vehicles using organic lead compounds as anti-knock measures),
- water, especially where old lead piping has not been replaced and soft water allows lead to dissolve,
- old lead-based paint in domestic housing.

Understanding its role is complicated by confounding factors. Most of the sources of exposure are associated with deprived areas and poverty, which have their own effects on intellectual development and antisocial behaviour. Furthermore, reverse causality is a real possibility in the case of hyperactive behaviour. Inquisitive children with ADHD may well get their hands contaminated with dust and transfer it to their mouths and bodily systems. It has not yet been definitively shown that public health measures to reduce the burden of lead will also reduce neuropsychological damage. Nevertheless, and despite the doubts that can be raised, the clear dose–response relationship between higher blood levels, lower IQ, and more hyperactive behaviour supports both a causal role for lead exposure and the public health case for restricting exposure (Wani et al., 2015).

Level of current exposure is best assessed from blood levels. Whole blood is needed (not serum or plasma) and blood samples need to be drawn with the proper needles (stainless steel), syringes (polypropylene), and approved sample containers, to avoid contamination. Even low exposure levels (i.e. those causing blood levels of 5–9 µg/dL) are associated with cognitive deficits. Whether blood lead should be included in the routine assessment of neurodevelopmental disorders will depend on the likelihood of useful results, and therefore on the area. Clinicians should inform themselves about the level of pollution in their community in order to make the decision.

For most children with raised blood levels, the main action required is to limit exposure. A long scientific argument about its role in causing ADHD and lowering IQ was eventually resolved by cumulative evidence and enquiries that found the association probably to be causative. Remedial action has included public funding to remove lead compounds from petrol. The main sources of contamination now are old paint, the combination of old lead water pipes and soft water, lead toys or toys coated with leaded paint, and battery recycling. When renewal of house paint is not feasible, it can be sealed. A major immediate route is from curious children's fingers being contaminated and then sucked. Lead itself may add to the risks: one of its bodily consequences is to induce children to eat inedible objects (pica).

At high blood levels (>45 mcg/dL), chelation will be advised, to complex with lead and remove it from the body. Suitable chelating agents include racemic-2,3-dimercapto-1-propanesulfonic acid (DMPS) and penicillamine, which can be given orally. Acute lead poisoning may produce encephalopathy in children. Ataxia, altered states of consciousness, and seizures have been reported in children with blood lead concentrations over 80 mcg/dL. At this level of severity, children should be hospitalized and given intravenous calcium disodium edetate.

The blood lead level is the best guide to current exposure, but does not inform about historical exposure or the possibility that neurodevelopmental disorders may have been initiated by early exposure (e.g. in prenatal life or infancy). Lead remains in the blood for 35 days; 40 days in soft tissues; 3 to 4 years in trabecular bone; and 16 to 20 years in cortical bone. The greater the body lead burden, the slower the rate of disappearance from the tissues, including blood.

7.9.2 Mercury

Mercury is better absorbed, and therefore more dangerous, when in organic compounds such as methylmercury. A negligent release of industrial chemicals at Minamata, Japan was followed by an outbreak of neurological problems in children including, but not confined to, autistic symptomatology. The severity of neurological impairment was directly related to the level of mercury in children's blood (Harada et al., 1999). Within the range occurring commonly in the population, higher levels of mercury have been linked to higher levels of autistic symptoms (Kern et al., 2016). The evidence is, however, some-what inconsistent and in some studies, in some places, no relationship has been found.

One source of mercury in the general population is an ethyl mercury-based preservative called thimerosal, used to prevent infection of vaccines. It has been the subject of claims that it is involved in the causation of ASD (Bernard et al., 2001). The claim was discredited by extensive investigation, including epidemiological evidence from countries that first excluded it and then reintroduced it. It made no difference to the incidence of ASD (US Institute of Medicine, 2012). Massive media exposure, however, still discourages many families, in many countries, from the highly desirable procedure of routine vaccination.

7.9.3 Manganese and other metals

Manganese occurs naturally in the diet and is needed for human health and some industrial processes. High blood levels, however, have been associated in Bangladesh, Italy, and Canada with cognitive problems and poor school achievement; and at the extreme, with extrapyramidal neurological signs (Henn et al., 2010). Infant formula milks sometimes contain very high levels.

Body burdens of cadmium, arsenic, nickel, uranium, and tin have sometimes been found to be elevated in people with ASD (Rossignol et al., 2014). The studies do, however, contain many possibilities of bias and confounding. Routine estimates in blood or hair are not advised unless there is specific local public health concern.

7.9.4 Pesticides and other chemicals

Potentially harmful chemicals in agriculture or food wrappings are topics of intense debate. It raises broad issues about the generalizability of animal studies to humans, the quality of evidence needed for decisions about banning compounds, and the ethical responsibilities of large corporations.

7.9.4.1 PCBs and DDT

Polychlorinated biphenyls (PCBs) and the pesticide dichlorodiphenyl trichloroethane (DDT) are widespread in the environment, even after public health moves to reduce them. Other halogenated pesticides, such as lindane, have appeared with hopes to reduce hazards for mental health. They can all be neurotoxic after both acute intoxication (Hsu et al., 1985) and chronic exposure (Mariussen & Fonnum, 2006). Children exposed to PCBs prenatally and/or during the breastfeeding period are particularly at risk for motor abnormalities and defects in short-term memory. Animal studies have indicated effects on brain turnover of dopamine, noradrenaline, and serotonin.

The effects of other pesticides have been reviewed and meta-analysed (Liu & Schelar, 2012). Some studies have investigated risks for ASD specifically and reported an increased risk being associated with prenatal exposure to organochlorine pesticides such as dicofol and endosulfan. Overall, there are only inconsistent findings about an association with mental dysfunction in children. Nevertheless, cautious practice will educate parents and teachers about washing and changing clothes after using pesticides.

7.9.4.2 *Chemicals from the plastics industries*

Bisphenols, phthalates, and perfluoroalkyl chemicals are used to manufacture plastic containers and food and beverage packing. They have aroused concern, but not yet rigorous evidence, about effects on human development.

7.9.5 Prenatal fluoride

Fluoride is routinely added to water in many countries in the interests of dental health. A long-running controversy queries whether this is safe for other organ systems. For instance, an association has been reported between fluoride levels in pregnant women in Mexico and cognitive problems, including ADHD, in the offspring (Bashash et al., 2017). No scientific consensus has yet been achieved.

7.9.6 Air pollution

Air pollution related to traffic is reviewed by Rossignol et al. (2014). Many studies have used retrospective case-control studies of autism, in which the main evidence is estimates of local pollution in the area where the child was born or grew up. They are not conclusive, but add to the arguments for keeping air clean.

7.9.7 Food additives

Artificial food colours and preservatives are often added to products that appeal to children, such as juice drinks and sweets. They have acquired a reputation for worsening ADHD, but research so far has not been conclusive. Some additives are restricted in some countries. In Europe, packaging will often display a warning if the food contains any 'E numbers'. There is particular concern about:

- E102 (tartrazine)
- E104 (quinoline yellow)
- E110 (sunset yellow FCF)
- E122 (carmoisine)
- E124 (ponceau 4R)
- E129 (allura red)

There is some scientific evidence for an association with ADHD. Meta-analysis (e.g. by Sonuga–Barke et al. (2013)) has brought together a disparate set of randomized trials of elimination diets. The overall conclusion was for a small but statistically significant effect of reducing hyperactive behaviour in children with ADHD. It may well be that the children who become subjects for the trials are preselected by having an idiosyncratic response to the dyes.

When such a trial was done with a different type of preselection, then a different pattern appeared. From the general population, 277 3-year-olds were selected on the basis of whether or not they showed an atopy as a marker to altered immune response, and, separately, on whether or not they were hyperactive (Bateman et al., 2004). A disguised drink of colourings and sodium benzoate was given in crossover with placebo, and the children showed a tendency to be more hyperactive than when they had a drink without incriminated substances. Neither those who were hyperactive to start with, nor those with atopies, were disproportionately affected.

The same investigators later replicated the findings with 8–9-year-old children as subjects. There was an association between a good response to elimination of artificial colours/benzoate and polymorphisms in two genes involved in histamine degradation (HNMT Thr105Ile and HNMT T939C), and also in one dopamine polymorphism.

The National Institute for Health and Care Excellence (NICE) has recommended trials of exclusion of foods for people with ADHD only if there is clear evidence of an adverse reaction to a specific food or foods, and if a dietitian is advising. It seems likely that there will be more developments.

7.9.8 Tobacco

The offspring of women who smoke are more likely than other children to be of low birthweight and to show behavioural and cognitive abnormalities, including attentional deficits, impaired learning and memory, and lowered IQ (Han et al., 2015). The observation is accepted, and various studies have examined the possible reasons.

- Possibly there is a confounding effect of other kinds of pregnancy problems being related both to smoking and to risk for behaviour problems. A comparison between mothers who continued to smoke during pregnancy with those who did not was indeed taken to suggest a direct effect on brain development (Roza et al., 2009). This association, however, between maternal smoking during pregnancy and children's behaviour disappeared when national origin, parental socioeconomic status, and parental psychiatric symptoms were taken into account. Parental smoking during pregnancy could, therefore, be a vulnerability marker and not a direct causal factor.
- Direct effects of maternal smoking on fetal brains would predict that the association would be found not only in community studies but also within families. The odds ratio for mental problems in children who were exposed to smoking as fetuses was 2.86 by comparison to unexposed children in the general community, in a large population

sample of nearly a million reported by Lindblad and Hjern (2010). This odds ratio fell to 1.56 when the comparison was with unexposed siblings, so the risk is probably due not only to direct effects on the brain but includes a direct component.

- Genetic factors could lead both to mothers being likely to smoke in pregnancy and to their children having behaviour and emotion problems. Attempts to disentangle the genetic and environmental effects have been made, for instance by studies of artificial insemination and studying the offspring of non-smoking mothers who are the twins of mothers who smoke. In the case of ADHD, an offspring-of-twins design indicated that the monozygotic twins of mothers who used tobacco regularly were as likely as their smoking sisters to have a child with ADHD, even if they did not themselves smoke (Knopik et al., 2006).

Conclusions are not final: genetic influences are probably part of the story, but there may indeed be direct harmful effects of mothers smoking in pregnancy on the birthweight and later neurodevelopmental outcome of the child (Knopik, 2009). The evidence favours complex patterns of transmission. It is still wise to advise pregnant women to avoid smoking completely.

The way that smoking works is likely to include an effect of nicotine in disrupting the development of nicotinic cholinergic receptors, which are present very early in the developing brain of rodents (embryonic day 10) and humans (4–5 weeks of gestation). Nicotinic signalling is part of the normal development of the brain, and its disruption is likely to have extensive effects.

7.9.9 Alcohol

Fetal alcohol syndrome (FAS) includes poor growth, cranial and other bodily defects, and a range of neurodevelopmental consequences. There is an excess of psychopathology (including hyperkinetic disorders, emotional disorders, sleep disorders, and abnormal habits and stereotypies) with a strong persistence over time. Cognitive functioning is marked by a large proportion of intellectually impaired children, and also does not change considerably over time. There is a dose–response relationship in that the physical stigmata correlate with the psychological impairment.

The incidence of FAS is not securely known. The best assessed figures, and certainly the highest, come from the USA, where prospective surveillance suggests an incidence of 1.95 per 1,000 live births (Abel, 1998). This is very high by international standards, and particularly striking because the consumption of alcohol per head is not particularly high in the USA. Sweden and France have relatively high levels of alcohol use but report incidence rates a little lower than that of the USA. The UK, with quite high alcohol use, does not undertake systematic surveillance of FAS because of the uncertainties about accuracy.

Lesser levels of alcohol exposure for the fetus are much more frequent and can also be harmful. Meta-analysis of studies testing children who were exposed in the womb to the effects of mothers drinking alcohol has defined the association (Flak et al., 2014).

Heavy drinking in pregnancy and binge drinking on occasions (more than four drinks in a day) are both associated with a wide range of adverse behavioural and cognitive outcomes. Moderate levels of drinking (less than one drink daily) are not consistently associated with ID or diagnosed neurodevelopmental problems in the offspring, but there remains a possibility of subtle effects. Some exposed children demonstrate other behaviours of concern, including increased demand for attention, behaviour regulation problems, and poorer interactive play skills.

This wider problem of alcohol-related neurodevelopmental problems, if added to the rate of full FAS, yielded a combined prevalence of 9 per 1,000 in an earlier study in Seattle, USA (Sampson et al., 1997). We do not, unfortunately, know how far this high risk applies internationally.

Genetic influences could contribute to the widespread risk to the public health. The alcohol dehydrogenase 1B genotype is a rate-limiting step in the degradation of ethanol. Studies have been reported in which mothers with genotypes making for faster metabolism of ethanol are protected against their offspring showing FAS (Green & Stoler, 2007). However, the evidence is not unequivocal and there is no case for including such a test in the counselling of pregnant women. The safest advice for pregnant women remains to abstain from alcohol altogether.

In the case of ADHD, some of the association with early alcohol exposure may be due to genetic influences determining both mothers' drinking and children's ADHD. An offspring-of-twins design has indicated that the monozygotic twins of mothers who misuse alcohol are as likely as their drinking twins to have a child with ADHD, even if they do not use alcohol in pregnancy themselves (Knopik et al., 2006).

More research is needed. Some advocates argue that there is no point in alarming mothers with the possibility that their drinking has damaged their child, since there is, in any case, no curative treatment. Informing the mother does, however, give her the opportunity of avoiding another child being affected. There is reason to think that this information is sometimes not given.

7.9.10 Cocaine

Prenatal exposure to cocaine is associated with compromised mental development, even in adolescence (Richardson et al., 2015). However, it has been hard to show, with any consistency, that this reflects a direct causal effect after allowing for potentially confounding influences such as maternal mental disorder and exposure to other substances (Frank et al., 2001).

7.9.11 Cannabis

Δ9-tetrahydrocannabinol (THC), the main psychoactive component of *Cannabis sativa*, can have adverse effects on mental health, against which cannabinol protects

(Niesink & van Laar, 2013). Several studies have demonstrated that adolescent cannabis users are at heightened risk for a range of adverse psychological outcomes, including psychotic symptoms and neurocognitive impairments (review by Lubman et al., 2015).

7.10 Early psychosocial adversity

7.10.1 Maternal stress in pregnancy

There is epidemiological evidence from several countries that various kinds of stress on pregnant mothers are associated with neurodevelopmental diagnoses in the offspring. Class et al. (2014) reported a study from Swedish population registers in which the death of a first-degree relative in the course of pregnancy raised the risk of ASD and ADHD in the offspring. MacKinnon et al. (2018) used data from the Avon Longitudinal Study of Parents and Children (ALSPAC) cohort in England and reported that adverse life events during pregnancy increased the risks for hyperactivity and conduct disorders in the offspring. Grizenko et al. (2012) reported a case-control study in Canada, comparing the perinatal histories of referred children with ADHD with those of their unaffected siblings: those with ADHD were more likely to have come from pregnancies marked by high stress. Ramchandani et al. (2010) took data from a longitudinal study in a township in South Africa. They could therefore study mothers of children who would later develop behaviour problems at the age of 4 years, at a point before their children were born. The stressed mothers-to-be had secreted high levels of hypothalamic–pituitary–adrenal (HPA) axis hormones in their response to stress. These hormones can affect fetal brain development. The sources of stress in this group were marital stress, family stress, economic stress, societal stress, and violence. Family stress (e.g. fighting within the family; family member with a drug problem, a disability, or in conflict with others) was the most likely to be impacting on the children at age four.

It is much less clear what processes are involved in the associations between mothers' stress and offspring's disorders. 'Stress' is a complex idea and is used to describe many kinds of adverse experience, and both mental and physical reactions to them. Anxiety and depression are common in pregnancy, as are changes in the bodily reactions of the HPA axis and the immune system. Poor maternal glucocorticoid–immune coordination is increasingly guiding research on these early developmental influences on prenatal life. Many influences could therefore be responsible for the impact of maternal stress and/or emotional disorders on the children (reviewed by Newman et al., 2017). Perhaps the presence of stressful events is a marker to other kinds of disadvantage, including some that operate in the postnatal life of the children and are described in the next sections. Perhaps the association is attributable to anxiety/depression rather than stress itself. Perhaps there are direct physical influences crossing the placenta. The clinical implications would depend upon the processes that are responsible—from treating mothers' anxiety/depression while they are pregnant, to assisting parenting during infancy or later childhood, and to physical interventions for the newborn. The evidence endorses antenatal services providing emotional support for expectant mothers.

Some evidence supports the notion of direct effects of mothers' mental state on the fetus. O'Connor et al. (2003) were able to use data, from a longitudinally followed population cohort, to examine whether anxiety in pregnancy predicted behavioural/emotional problems when the offspring were 4 years old, and again at 81 months of age. It did. Furthermore, the association was still present after controlling for obstetric risks, psychosocial disadvantage, and postnatal anxiety and depression (odds ratios after adjustment about 2). This made it unlikely that the effects on children were entirely due to postnatal disruptions of parenting, such as those caused by mothers' anxiety persisting after pregnancy, or to the coexistence of other types of disadvantage. It gave some support to the conclusions from research on animals that prenatal programming can have enduring influences on the trajectories of brain development. There may well be transplacental transmission of exaggerated glucocorticoid and cytokine levels that disrupt fetal brain development (Hantsoo et al., 2018).

There could also be influences from medication effects. Indeed, a meta-analysis of studies, examining the effects of maternal exposure to antidepressants while pregnant, has estimated an increased risk in the offspring for ASD (relative risk about 1.5) and for ADHD (around 1.4) (Morales et al., 2018).

7.10.2 Psychosocial adversity in early postnatal life

After the period of infancy, many psychosocial stressors are potentially harmful to the developing brain. There are known associations, especially for ADHD, with several types of psychosocial disadvantage. Children in families of low socioeconomic status are at an approximately doubled risk of developing ADHD (Russell et al., 2016). No single risk such as low income dominates the association.

Children who were growing up for their first 5 years in Swedish families with the lowest income levels were at an approximately doubled risk of being diagnosed with ADHD later (Larsson et al., 2014b). Cash poverty, however, could be a marker to early causal influences (already described) rather than an active cause itself. The more types of disadvantage that are present, the greater the links between them and ADHD. Other and later behavioural and emotional disorders are also more likely in the children of disadvantaged families (Reiss, 2013). (For the effects of economic disadvantage in later childhood and adolescence, see also Chapter 10, Section 10.5.)

Adversity in early childhood can cast a long shadow. The sequelae of maltreatment include both injury to the brain and enduring neuropsychological and physiological changes (Danese & McCrory, 2015). At an extreme, the children who have spent years of their early childhood in depriving orphanages are at risk for ASD-like disturbances of social contact and ADHD-like changes in attention and impulse control in later childhood. The changes persist even after they have been rescued into benign family environments, and are still present in early adult life (Kennedy et al., 2016). The changes in the multiply-deprived children are linked to structural brain alterations that can be visualized by MRI (McLaughlin et al., 2014). Widespread cortical thinning—affecting the lateral orbitofrontal cortex, insula, inferior parietal cortex, precuneus, superior temporal cortex, and lingual gyrus—is associated both with institutional rearing and with inattention/impulsivity.

More commonly encountered aspects of maltreatment include maternal rejection, harsh discipline, disruptive caregiver changes, physical abuse, neglect, and sexual abuse. They predict lower IQ, poorer declarative memory, and less effective executive function than is seen in individuals with no such background (Pechtel & Pizzagalli, 2011). The mechanisms are not certainly established. The 'biological embedding' of harmful experiences is reviewed by Danese et al. (2011). At a psychological level, the experience of living in a frightening world might well condition a young child's beliefs about safety and increase the risk of developing phobias and aversions.

At a brain level, smaller hippocampal volume is associated with a history of deprivation and changes in declarative memory. Post-traumatic deficits in executive function seem to be related to functional and structural prefrontal cortex abnormalities (Danese & McEwen, 2012). A causal relationship is supported by studies of similar changes in animals experimentally exposed to early-life stress (Brunson et al., 2005). Blunted subjective responses to reward-predicting cues after maltreatment have been associated with blunted activation in the basal ganglia during reward anticipation (Dillon et al., 2009). Oversensitivity to threat is linked with selective heightened amygdala activation (van Harmelen et al., 2013).

At a physiological level, inflammatory changes are becoming increasingly recognized as mediators of early stress on brain development. In a longitudinally studied cohort, cumulative exposure to childhood maltreatment predicted significant elevation in inflammation levels at the age of 32 (Danese et al., 2007). The alterations are apparently similar to those involved after childhood infections (see Section 7.7.2). They include:

- neuroendocrine changes in the system of HPA axis hormones,
- immune and inflammatory changes, reflected for instance in cytokine levels,
- autonomic nervous system changes, with release of catecholamines from sympathetic nerves and the adrenal medulla.

All these physiological alterations interact with each other. Chronically elevated cortisol is associated with insulin resistance, hyperlipidaemia, and altered effects of interleukin and other immune components.

Allostatic load refers to chronic overactivation of these regulatory systems and their cost to the functioning of organs, including the brain. In studies on adult volunteers, effects on the brain can be seen experimentally. Administration of lipopolysaccharide triggers a release of cytokines that cross the blood–brain barrier and promote an inflammatory response. The results in brain function include reduction in verbal and non-verbal memory, reduction in ventral striatal responses to reward, and enhanced amygdala activation in response to fearful faces (Schedlowski et al., 2014). (See also Chapter 10 for long-term implications of stress and disadvantage in people with altered brain function.)

7.11 RISK OF MALE SEX AND GENDER IN EARLY DEVELOPMENT

Male sex is associated with higher rates of neurodevelopmental disorders. The reasons arise early in development and are largely physical.

7.11.1 Brain injury and masculinity

There is probably a constitutional vulnerability of males to the damaging effects of pre-term birth (Johnston & Hagberg, 2007). Male brains are somewhat more vulnerable than female to early brain disease and damage. Births at around 28 weeks of gestation and evidence of intraventricular haemorrhage are both more likely, in males than in females, to result in white-matter abnormalities and delayed cortical development (Kapellou et al., 2006). The neuropsychological effects of early brain damage are also, and correspondingly, moderately raised in males by comparison with females. Cerebral palsy is 30% more likely to develop in males, whether or not they are born at term (Jarvis et al., 2005). In other early brain disorders, the incremental risk imposed by male gender is similar. The emotional and behavioural consequences are still very significant in females, but greater in males—albeit usually less than doubled.

Damage later in childhood is more complicated. Boys are more likely than girls to suffer traumatic brain injury, essentially because they are more likely to be exposed to it. The more adventurous nature of typical male play is more likely to expose them to all kinds of accidental injury. The brain results of damage are then more likely in males and, possibly, more damaging. Verbal learning was a little worse after head injury in boys than in girls (Donders & Hoffman, 2002).

In some contrast, it might be a different story for injury after puberty. Female steroids, such as progesterone and their metabolites, would be expected to act as neuroprotective factors. They probably inhibit proinflammatory cytokines. Nevertheless, a study reporting severity of injury and mortality in adults after brain injury indicated worse outcomes for females than for males (Farace & Alves, 2000). The evidence is not unequivocal and perhaps adult females suffer worse injuries.

7.11.2 Epilepsy and masculinity

Epilepsy shows fairly equal gender ratios overall (Christensen et al., 2005). Focal epilepsies were a little more common in adult males in a Danish clinical register (55% versus 45%). By contrast, generalized idiopathic epilepsies were more common in females. Perhaps the difference reflected greater male vulnerability to damage from seizures.

A systematic review by Pericall and Taylor (2013) found that females with epilepsy were still less likely than males with epilepsy to show ASD and/or ADHD—but their *relative* protection (1.49 for ADHD, 1.67 for ASD) was much less raised than in the general population (for whom the gender ratio is about 3 for ADHD, 5 for ASD).

7.11.3 ADHD and ASD and masculinity

A much greater male vulnerability seems to apply to those neurodevelopmental disorders in early life that are not secondary to obvious neurological conditions (Hanamsagar & Bilbo, 2016). Rates of about four to five males to every female are widely reported for children with autism, three males to every female for children with ADHD; and more males in chronic tic disorders (varying figures). The gender difference is typically smaller in adult-onset cases. One concludes that other processes are likely to be involved as well as a general factor of early male brain vulnerability (Hanamsagar, 2015). There may well be:

- Female protection against typical features of ADHD such as motor overactivity and impulsiveness. This is not only protection against pathogenic influences but represents a difference in whole populations.
- Female protection against certain features of ASD such as social isolation and vulnerability to anxiety.
- Bias against recognizing ADHD in females because of stereotyped perceptions of them as compliant and studious.
- Bias against recognizing ASD in females because of stereotyped perceptions of them as socially competent.
- Greater female vulnerability to anxiety and depression (after puberty) modifying the symptom profiles.
- Stronger female immune responses making inflammatory disorders less likely (and autoimmune ones more likely).

In adult life, it is very often a different story. In late-onset cases of ADHD, the male:female ratio was much closer to 1:1 (Agnew–Blais et al., 2016). This was not because of higher persistence of symptoms in females. Rather, females tended to have an absence of symptoms in childhood altogether. ADHD symptoms may be less likely to come to the attention of parents and teachers early because of lower rates of externalizing-type behaviours. Alternatively, late-onset cases could represent a different disorder and aetiology. Alternatively again, sex differences might reflect microglial and inflammatory differences between the genders, reducing female protection in adulthood (Hanamsagar & Bilbo, 2016).

In most studies, autism, too, has a later age of first diagnosis in girls than in boys, though exact results vary (Rutherford et al., 2016). The gender ratio appears to be more equal in later-onset cases than in early. If indeed any part of female protection in early life is due to an unduly male-centric definition of the diagnoses, then more knowledge would become important. It would be needed to counteract any tendency in clinicians to neglect the less gender-typical features of the diagnoses.

REFERENCES

Abel, E. L. (1998). Fetal alcohol syndrome: the 'American Paradox'. *Alcohol and Alcoholism*, *33*(3), 195–201.

Abel, M. H., Caspersen, I. H., Meltzer, H. M., Haugen, M., Brandlistuen, R. E., Aase, H., Alexander, J., Torheim, L. E., & Brantsæter, A. L. (2017). Suboptimal maternal iodine intake is associated with impaired child neurodevelopment at 3 years of age in the Norwegian Mother and Child Cohort Study. *Journal of Nutrition*, *147*(7), 1314–1324.

Agnew–Blais, J. C., Polanczyk, G. V., Danese, A., Wertz, J., Moffitt, T. E., & Arseneault, L. (2016). Evaluation of the persistence, remission, and emergence of attention-deficit/hyperactivity disorder in young adulthood. *Journal of the American Medical Association: Psychiatry*, *73*(7), 713–720.

Ahn, K. H., Park, Y. J., Hong, S. C., Lee, E. H., Lee, J. S., Oh, M. J., & Kim, H. J. (2016). Congenital varicella syndrome: a systematic review. *Journal of Obstetrics and Gynaecology*, *36*(5), 563–566.

Andersson, M., Karumbunathan, V., & Zimmermann, M. B. (2012). Global iodine status in 2011 and trends over the past decade. *Journal of Nutrition*, *142*(4), 744–750.

Bashash, M., Thomas, D., Hu, H., Martinez–Mier, E. A., Sanchez, B. N., Basu, N., Peterson, K. E., Ettinger, A. S., Wright, R., Zhang, Z., Liu, Y., Schnaas, L., Mercado–Garcia, A., Téllez–Rojo, M. M., & Hernández–Avila, M. (2017). Prenatal fluoride exposure and cognitive outcomes in children at 4 and 6–12 years of age in Mexico. *Environmental Health Perspectives*, *125*(9), 097017. https://doi.org/10.1289/EHP655

Bassell, G. J., & Warren, S. T. (2008). Fragile X syndrome: loss of local mRNA regulation alters synaptic development and function. *Neuron*, **60** (2), 201–14. https://doi.org/10.1016/j.neuron.2008.10.004

Bateman, B., Warner, J. O., Hutchinson, E., Dean, T., Rowlandson, P., Gant, C., Grundy, J., Fitzgerald, C., & Stevenson, J. (2004). The effects of a double blind, placebo controlled, artificial food colourings and benzoate preservative challenge on hyperactivity in a general population sample of preschool children. *Archives of Disease in Childhood*, *89*(6), 506–511.

Belsky, J., & Pluess, M. (2009). Beyond diathesis stress: differential susceptibility to environmental influences. *Psychological Bulletin*, *135*(6), 885.

Bernard, S., Enayati, A., Redwood, L., Roger, H., & Binstock, T. (2001). Autism: a novel form of mercury poisoning. *Medical Hypotheses*, *56*(4), 462–471.

Bernstein, D. I. (2017). Congenital cytomegalovirus: a 'now' problem—no really, now. *Clinical and Vaccine Immunology*, *24*(1), e00491–16.

Black, M. M., Baqui, A. H., Zaman, K., Ake Persson, L., El Arifeen, S., Le, K., McNary, S. W., Parveen, M., Hamadani, J. D., & Black, R. E. (2004). Iron and zinc supplementation promote motor development and exploratory behavior among Bangladeshi infants. *American Journal of Clinical Nutrition, 80*(4), 903–910.

Boivin, M. J., Bangirana, P., Byarugaba, J., Opoka, R. O., Idro, R., Jurek, A. M., & John, C. C. (2007). Cognitive impairment after cerebral malaria in children: a prospective study. *Pediatrics, 119*(2), e360.

Brown A. S. (2006). Prenatal infection as a risk factor for schizophrenia. *Schizophrenia Bulletin, 32*(2), 200–202. https://doi.org/10.1093/schbul/sbj052

Brunson, K. L., Kramár, E., Lin, B., Chen, Y., Colgin, L. L., Yanagihara, T. K., Lynch, G., & Baram, T. Z. (2005). Mechanisms of late-onset cognitive decline after early-life stress. *Journal of Neuroscience, 25*(41), 9328–38.

Budimirovic, D. B., & Kaufmann, W. E. (2011). What can we learn about autism from studying fragile X syndrome? *Developmental Neuroscience, 33* (5), 379–94.

Bull, M. J., & the Committee on Genetics. (2011). Health supervision for children with Down syndrome. *Pediatrics, 128*, 393–406.

Cahalan, S. (2018). *Brain on fire: my month of madness*. Simon & Shuster.

Caldwell, P. D., & Smith, D. W. (1972). The XXY (Klinefelter's) syndrome in childhood: detection and treatment. *Journal of Pediatrics, 80*(2), 250–258.

Carothers, A. D., Hecht, C. A., & Hook, E. B. (1999). International variation in reported livebirth prevalence rates of Down syndrome, adjusted for maternal age. *Journal of Medical Genetics, 36*(5), 386–393.

Caspi, A., Moffitt, T. E., Cannon, M., McClay, J., Murray, R., Harrington, H., Taylor, A., Arseneault, L., Williams, B., Braithwaite, A., Poulton, R., & Craig, I. W. (2005). Moderation of the effect of adolescent-onset cannabis use on adult psychosis by a functional polymorphism in the catechol-O-methyltransferase gene: longitudinal evidence of a gene X environment interaction. *Biological Psychiatry, 57*(10), 1117–1127.

Chin, J. H., & Mateen, F. J. (2013). Central nervous system tuberculosis: challenges and advances in diagnosis and treatment. *Current Infectious Disease Reports, 15*(6), 631–635.

Christensen, J., Kjeldsen, M. J., Andersen, H., Friis, M. L., & Sidenius, P. (2005). Gender differences in epilepsy. *Epilepsia, 46*(6), 956–960.

Class, Q. A., Abel, K. M., Khashan, A. S., Rickert, M. E., Dalman, C., Larsson, H., Hultman, C. M., Långström, N., Lichtenstein, P., & D'Onofrio, B. M. (2014). Offspring psychopathology following preconception, prenatal and postnatal maternal bereavement stress. *Psychological Medicine, 44*(1), 71–84.

Crombie, I. K., Todman, J., Kennedy, R. A., McNeill, G., & Menzies, I. (1990). Effect of vitamin and mineral supplementation on verbal and non-verbal reasoning of schoolchildren. *Lancet, 335*(8692), 744–747.

Danese, A., Caspi, A., Williams, B., Ambler, A., Sugden, K., Mika, J., Werts, H., Freeman, J., Pariante, C. M., Moffitt, T. E., & Arseneault, L. (2011). Biological embedding of stress through inflammation processes in childhood. *Molcular Psychiatry, 16*(3), 244–246.

Danese, A., & McCrory, E. (2015). Child maltreatment. In A. Thapar, D. S. Pine, J. F. Leckman, S. Scott, M. J. Snowling, & E. Taylor (Eds.), *Rutter's child and adolescent psychiatry* (pp. 364–375). Wiley–Blackwell.

Danese, A., & McEwen, B. S. (2012). Adverse childhood experiences, allostasis, allostatic load, and age-related disease. *Physiology & Behavior, 106*(1), 29–39.

Danese, A., Pariante, C. M., Caspi, A., Taylor, A., & Poulton, R. (2007). Childhood maltreatment predicts adult inflammation in a life-course study. *Proceedings of the National Academy of Sciences*, 104(4), 1319–1324.

Dillon, D. G., Holmes, A. J., Birk, J. L., Brooks, N., Lyons-Ruth, K., & Pizzagalli, D. A. (2009). Childhood adversity is associated with left basal ganglia dysfunction during reward anticipation in adulthood. *Biological Psychiatry*, 66(3), 206–213.

Donders, J., & Hoffman, N. M. (2002). Gender differences in learning and memory after pediatric traumatic brain injury. *Neuropsychology*, 16(4), 491.

Farace, E., & Alves, W. M. (2000). Do women fare worse: a meta-analysis of gender differences in traumatic brain injury outcome. *Journal of Neurosurgery*, 93(4), 539–545.

Feyrer, J., Politi, D., & Weil, D. N. (2017). The cognitive effects of micronutrient deficiency: evidence from salt iodization in the United States. *Journal of the European Economic Association*, 15(2), 355–387.

Flak, A. L., Su, S., Bertrand, J., Denny, C. H., Kesmodel, U. S., & Cogswell, M. E. (2014). The association of mild, moderate, and binge prenatal alcohol exposure and child neuropsychological outcomes: a meta-analysis. *Alcoholism: Clinical and Experimental Research*, 38(1), 214–226.

Frank, D. A., Augustyn, M., Knight, W. G., Pell, T., & Zuckerman, B. (2001). Growth, development, and behavior in early childhood following prenatal cocaine exposure: a systematic review. *Journal of the American Medical Association*, 285(12), 1613–1625.

Genetic and Rare Diseases Information Center: https://rarediseases.info.nih.gov/

Green, R. F., & Stoler, J. M. (2007). Alcohol dehydrogenase 1B genotype and fetal alcohol syndrome: a HuGE minireview. *American Journal of Obstetrics and Gynecology*, 197(1), 12–25.

Griffiths, P. D., & Walter, S.(2005) Cytomegalovirus. *Current Opinion in Infectious Diseases*, 18(3), 241–245.

Grizenko, N., Fortier, M. E., Zadorozny, C., Thakur, G., Schmitz, N., Duval, R., & Joober, R. (2012). Maternal stress during pregnancy, ADHD symptomatology in children and genotype: gene–environment interaction. *Journal of the Canadian Academy of Child and Adolescent Psychiatry*, 21(1), 9.

Han, J. Y., Kwon, H. J., Ha, M., Paik, K. C., Lim, M. H., Lee, S. G., Yu, S. J., & Kim, E. J. (2015). The effects of prenatal exposure to alcohol and environmental tobacco smoke on risk for ADHD: a large population-based study. *Psychiatry Research*, 225(1–2), 164–168.

Hanamsagar, R. (2015). Sex differences in neurodevelopmental and neurodegenerative disorders: a largely ignored aspect of research. *Current Neurobiology*, 6, 15–16.

Hanamsagar, R., & Bilbo, S. D. (2016). Sex differences in neurodevelopmental and neurodegenerative disorders: focus on microglial function and neuroinflammation during development. *Journal of Steroid Biochemistry and Molecular Biology*, 160, 127–133.

Hantsoo, L., Kornfield, S., Anguera, M. C., & Epperson, C. N. (2018). Inflammation: a proposed intermediary between maternal stress and offspring neuropsychiatric risk. *Biological Psychiatry*, 85. 97–106.

Harada, M., Akagi, H., Tsuda, T., Kizaki, T., & Ohno, H. (1999). Methylmercury level in umbilical cords from patients with congenital Minamata disease. *Science of the Total Environment*, 234(1–3), 59–62.

Henn, B. C., Ettinger, A. S., Schwartz, J., Téllez-Rojo, M. M., Lamadrid-Figueroa, H., Hernández-Avila, M., Schnaas, L., Amarasiriwardena, C., Bellinger, D., Hu, H., & Wright, R. O. (2010). Early postnatal blood manganese levels and children's neurodevelopment. *Epidemiology*, 21(4), 433.

Hilker, R., Helenius, D., Fagerlund, B., Skytthe, A., Christensen, K., Werge, T. M., Nordentoft, M., & Glenthøj, B. (2018). Heritability of schizophrenia and schizophrenia spectrum based on the nationwide Danish twin register. *Biological Psychiatry*, 83(6), 492–498.

Hsu, S. T., Ma, C. I., Hsu, S. K. H., Wu, S. S., Hsu, N. H. M., Yeh, C. C., & Wu, S. B. (1985). Discovery and epidemiology of PCB poisoning in Taiwan—a 4-year follow-up. *Environmental Health Perspectives*, 59, 5–10.

Hurst, J. A., Baraitser, M., Auger, E., Graham, F., & Norell, S. (1990). An extended family with a dominantly inherited speech disorder. *Developmental Medicine & Child Neurology*, 32(4), 352–355.

Institute of Medicine (US): Committee to Review Adverse Effects of Vaccines, Stratton, K. R., & Clayton, E. W. (2012). *Adverse effects of vaccines: evidence and causality.* National Academies Press.

Jarvis, S., Glinianaia, S. V., Arnaud, C., Fauconnier, J., Johnson, A., McManus, V., Topp, M., Uvebrant, P., Cans, C., Krägeloh–Mann, I. (2005). Case gender and severity in cerebral palsy varies with intrauterine growth. *Archives of Disease in Childhood*, 90, 474–479.

Johnson, M., Fernell, E., Preda, I., Wallin, L., Fasth, A., Gillberg, C., & Gillberg, C. (2019). Paediatric acute-onset neuropsychiatric syndrome in children and adolescents: an observational cohort study. *The Lancet Child & Adolescent Health*, 3(3), 175–180.

Johnston, M. V., & Hagberg, H. (2007). Sex and the pathogenesis of cerebral palsy. *Developmental Medicine & Child Neurology*, 49(1), 74–78.

Kapellou, O., Counsell, S. J., Kennea, N., Dyet, L., Saeed, N., Stark, J., Maalouf, E., Duggan, P., Ajayi–Obe, M., Hajinal, J., Allsop, J. M., Boardman, J., Rutherford, M. A., Cowan, F., & Edwards, A. D. (2006). Abnormal cortical development after premature birth shown by altered allometric scaling of brain growth. *PLoS Medicine*, 3(8), e265. https://doi.org/10.1371/journal.pmed.0030265

Kennedy, M., Kreppner, J., Knights, N., Kumsta, R., Maughan, B., Golm, D., Rutter, M., Schlotz, W., & Sonuga–Barke, E. J. (2016). Early severe institutional deprivation is associated with a persistent variant of adult attention-deficit/hyperactivity disorder: clinical presentation, developmental continuities and life circumstances in the English and Romanian Adoptees study. *Journal of Child Psychology and Psychiatry*, 57(10), 1113–1125.

Kern, J. K., Geier, D. A., Sykes, L. K., Haley, B. E., & Geier, M. R. (2016). The relationship between mercury and autism: a comprehensive review and discussion. *Journal of Trace Elements in Medicine and Biology*, 37, 8–24.

Khandaker, G. M., Zimbron, J., Dalman, C., Lewis, G., & Jones, P. B. (2012). Childhood infection and adult schizophrenia: a meta-analysis of population-based studies. *Schizophrenia Research*, 139(1–3), 161–168.

Knopik, V. S. (2009). Maternal smoking during pregnancy and child outcomes: real or spurious effect?. *Developmental Neuropsychology*, 34(1), 1–36.

Knopik, V. S., Heath, A. C., Jacob, T., Slutske, W. S., Bucholz, K. K., Madden, P. A., Waldron, M., & Martin, N. G. (2006). Maternal alcohol use disorder and offspring ADHD: disentangling genetic and environmental effects using a children-of-twins design. *Psychological Medicine*, 36(10), 1461–1471.

Köhler–Forsberg, O., Petersen, L., Gasse, C., Mortensen, P. B., Dalsgaard, S., Yolken, R. H., Mors, O., & Benros, M. E. (2019). A nationwide study in Denmark of the association between treated infections and the subsequent risk of treated mental disorders in children and adolescents. *Journal of the American Medical Association: Psychiatry*, 76(3), 271–279.

Larsson, H., Chang, Z., D'Onofrio, B. M., & Lichtenstein, P. (2014a). The heritability of clinically diagnosed attention deficit hyperactivity disorder across the lifespan. *Psychological Medicine*, 44(10), 2223–2229.

Larsson, H., Sariaslan, A., Långström, N., D'Onofrio, B., & Lichtenstein, P. (2014b). Family income in early childhood and subsequent attention deficit/hyperactivity disorder: a quasi-experimental study. *Journal of Child Psychology and Psychiatry*, 55(5), 428–435.

Liu, J., & Schelar, E. (2012). Pesticide exposure and child neurodevelopment: summary and implications. *Workplace Health & Safety*, 60(5), 235–242.

Lindblad, F., & Hjern, A. (2010). ADHD after fetal exposure to maternal smoking. *Nicotine & Tobacco Research*, 12(4), 408–415.

Loeber, J. G., Burgard, P., Cornel, M. C., Rigter, T., Weinreich, S. S., Rupp, K., Hoffmann, G. F., & Vittozzi, L. (2012). Newborn screening programmes in Europe: arguments and efforts regarding harmonization. Part 1–From blood spot to screening result. *Journal of Inherited Metabolic Disease*, 35(4), 603–611.

Lozoff, B., Clark, K. M., Jing, Y., Armony–Sivan, R., Angelilli, M. L., & Jacobson, S. W. (2008). Dose–response relationships between iron deficiency with or without anemia and infant social-emotional behavior. *Journal of Pediatrics*, 152(5), 696–702.

Lozoff, B. (2007). Iron deficiency and child development. *Food and Nutrition Bulletin*, 28(4 Suppl), S560–S571.

Lubman, D. I., Cheetham, A., & Yücel, M. (2015). Cannabis and adolescent brain development. *Pharmacology & Therapeutics*, 148, 1–16.

Lumey, L. H., Stein, A. D., & Susser, E. (2011). Prenatal famine and adult health. *Annual Review of Public Health*, 32, 237–262.

Lussier, A. A., Morin, A. M., MacIsaac, J. L., Salmon, J., Weinberg, J., Reynolds, J. N., Pavlidis, P., Chudley, A. E., & Kobor, M. S. (2018). DNA methylation as a predictor of fetal alcohol spectrum disorder. *Clinical Epigenetics*, 10(1), 5.

MacKinnon, N., Kingsbury, M., Mahedy, L., Evans, J., & Colman, I. (2018). The association between prenatal stress and externalising symptoms in childhood: evidence from the Avon Longitudinal Study of Parents and Children. *Biological Psychiatry*, 83(2), 100–108.

Manzardo, A. M., Weisensel, N., Ayala, S., Hossain, W., & Butler, M. G. (2018). Prader–Willi syndrome genetic subtypes and clinical neuropsychiatric diagnoses in residential care adults. *Clinical Genetics*, 93(3), 622–631.

Mariussen, E., & Fonnum, F. (2006). Neurochemical targets and behavioral effects of organohalogen compounds: an update. *Critical Reviews in Toxicology*, 36(3), 253–289.

Martin, N. D., Snodgrass, G. J., & Cohen, R. D. (1984). Idiopathic infantile hypercalcaemia—a continuing enigma. *Archives of Disease in Childhood*, 59(7), 605–613.

McAuley, J. B. (2014). Congenital toxoplasmosis. *Journal of the Pediatric Infectious Diseases Society*, 3(Suppl 1), S30–S35. https://doi.org/10.1093/jpids/piu077

McLaughlin, K. A., Sheridan, M. A., Winter, W., Fox, N. A., Zeanah, C. H., & Nelson, C. A. (2014). Widespread reductions in cortical thickness following severe early-life deprivation: a neurodevelopmental pathway to attention-deficit/hyperactivity disorder. *Biological Psychiatry*, 76(8), 629–638.

Meyer–Lindenberg, A., Hariri, A. R., Munoz, K. E., Mervis, C. B., Mattay, V. S., Morriss, C. A., & Berman, K. F. (2005). Neural correlates of genetically abnormal social cognition in Williams syndrome *Nature Neuroscience*, 8, 991–993.

Miike, T., Ogata, T., Ohtani, Y., Yamaguchi, H., & Yokoyama, Y. (1988). Atypical Prader–Willi syndrome with severe developmental delay and emaciation. *Brain and Development*, 10(3), 186–188.

Morales, D. R., Slattery, J., Evans, S., & Kurz, X. (2018). Antidepressant use during pregnancy and risk of autism spectrum disorder and attention deficit hyperactivity disorder: systematic review of observational studies and methodological considerations. *BMC Medicine*, 16(1), 6.

Newman, L., Judd, F., & Komiti, A. (2017). Developmental implications of maternal ante-natal anxiety mechanisms and approaches to intervention. *Translational Developmental Psychiatry*, 5(1), 1309879.

Nguyen, T. H., Day, N. P., Ly, V. C., Waller, D., Mai, N. T., Bethell, D. B., Tran, T. H., & White, N. J. (1996). Post-malaria neurological syndrome. *Lancet*, 348(9032), 917–921.

Niesink, R. J., & van Laar, M. W. (2013). Does cannabidiol protect against adverse psychological effects of THC? *Frontiers in Psychiatry*, 4, 130.

Nyhan, W. L. (1976). Behavior in the Lesch–Nyhan syndrome. *Journal of Autism and Childhood Schizophrenia*, 6(3), 235–252.

O'Connor, T. G., Heron, J., Golding, J., Glover, V., & ALSPAC Study Team. (2003). Maternal antenatal anxiety and behavioural/emotional problems in children: a test of a programming hypothesis. *Journal of Child Psychology and Psychiatry*, 44(7), 1025–1036.

Oliver, B. R., Trzaskowski, M., & Plomin, R. (2014). Genetics of parenting: the power of the dark side. *Developmental Psychology*, 50(4), 1233–1240. https://doi.org/10.1037/a0035388

Pechtel, P., & Pizzagalli, D. A. (2011). Effects of early life stress on cognitive and affective function: an integrated review of human literature. *Psychopharmacology*, 214(1), 55–70.

Piña-Garza, J. E. (2013). *Fenichel's clinical pediatric neurology: a signs and symptoms approach.* Elsevier Health Sciences.

Pober, B. R. (2010). Williams–Beuren syndrome. *New England Journal of Medicine*, 362(3), 239–252.

Qian, M., Wang, D., Watkins, W. E., Gebski, V., Yan, Y. Q., Li, M., & Chen, Z. P. (2005). The effects of iodine on intelligence in children: a meta-analysis of studies conducted in China. *Asia Pacific Journal of Clinical Nutrition*, 14(1), 32–42.

Ramchandani, P. G., Richter, L. M., Norris, S. A., & Stein, A. (2010). Maternal prenatal stress and later child behavioral problems in an urban South African setting. *Journal of the American Academy of Child & Adolescent Psychiatry*, 49(3), 239–247.

Reiss, F. (2013). Socioeconomic inequalities and mental health problems in children and adolescents: a systematic review. *Social Science and Medicine*, 90, 24–31.

Richardson, G. A., Goldschmidt, L., Larkby, C., & Day, N. L. (2015). Effects of prenatal cocaine exposure on adolescent development. *Neurotoxicology and Teratology*, 49, 41–48.

Rossignol, D. A., Genuis, S. J., & Frye, R. E. (2014). Environmental toxicants and autism spectrum disorders: a systematic review. *Translational Psychiatry*, 4(2), e360.

Roza, S. J., Verhulst, F. C., Jaddoe, V. W., Steegers, E. A., Mackenbach, J. P., Hofman, A., & Tiemeier, H. (2009). Maternal smoking during pregnancy and child behaviour problems: the Generation R Study. *International Journal of Epidemiology*, 38(3), 680–689.

Russell, A. E., Ford, T., Williams, R., & Russell, G. (2016). The association between socioeconomic disadvantage and attention deficit/hyperactivity disorder (ADHD): a systematic review. *Child Psychiatry & Human Development*, 47(3), 440–458.

Rutherford, M., McKenzie, K., Johnson, T., Catchpole, C., O'Hare, A., McClure, I., Forsyth, K., McCartney, D., & Murray, A. (2016). Gender ratio in a clinical population sample: age of diagnosis and duration of assessment in children and adults with autism spectrum disorder. *Autism*, 20(5), 628–634.

Sampson, P. D., Streissguth, A. P., Bookstein, F. L., Little, R. E., Clarren, S. K., Dehaene, P., Hanson, J. W., & Graham Jr, J. M. (1997). Incidence of fetal alcohol syndrome and prevalence of alcohol-related neurodevelopmental disorder. *Teratology*, 56(5), 317–326.

Schedlowski, M., Engler, H., & Grigoleit, J. S. (2014). Endotoxin-induced experimental systemic inflammation in humans: a model to disentangle immune-to-brain communication. *Brain, Behavior, and Immunity*, 35, 1–8.

Selten, J. P., & Termorshuizen, F. (2017). The serological evidence for maternal influenza as risk factor for psychosis in offspring is insufficient: critical review and meta-analysis. *Schizophrenia Research, 183,* 2–9.

Sonuga–Barke, E. J., Brandeis, D., Cortese, S., Daley, D., Ferrin, M., Holtmann, M., Stevenson, J., Danckaerts, M., van der Oord, S., Döpfner, M., Dittmann, R. W., Simonoff, E., Zuddas, A., Banaschewski, T., Buitelaar, J., Coghill, D., Hollis, C., Konofal, E., Lecendreux, M. … & European ADHD Guidelines Group. (2013). Nonpharmacological interventions for ADHD: systematic review and meta-analyses of randomized controlled trials of dietary and psychological treatments. *American Journal of Psychiatry, 170*(3), 275–289.

Sugrue, L. P., & Desikan, R. S. (2019). What are polygenic scores and why are they important? *Journal of the American Medical Association, 321*(18), 1820–1821.

Swedo, S. E., Leckman, J. F., & Rose, N. R. (2012). From research subgroup to clinical syndrome: modifying the PANDAS criteria to describe PANS (pediatric acute-onset neuropsychiatric syndrome). *Pediatrics & Therapeutics, 2*(2), 1000113, 1–8. https://doi.org/10.4172/2161-0665.1000113

Swedo, S. E., Leonard, H. L., Garvey, M., Mittleman, B., Allen, A. J., Perlmutter, S., Lougee, L., Dow, S., Zamhoff, J., & Dubbert, B. K. (1998). Pediatric autoimmune neuropsychiatric disorders associated with streptococcal infections: clinical description of the first 50 cases. *American Journal of Psychiatry, 155,* 264–271.

Telias, M. (2019). Molecular mechanisms of synaptic dysregulation in fragile X syndrome and autism spectrum disorders. *Frontiers in Molecular Neuroscience, 12,* 51.

Tick, B., Bolton, P., Happé, F., Rutter, M., & Rijsdijk, F. (2016). Heritability of autism spectrum disorders: a meta-analysis of twin studies. *Journal of Child Psychology and Psychiatry, 57*(5), 585–595.

Tobi, E. W., Goeman, J. J., Monajemi, R., Gu, H., Putter, H., Zhang, Y., Slieker, R. C., Stok, A. P., Thijssen, P. E., Müller, F., van Zwet, E. W., Bock, C., Meissner, A., Lumey, L. H., Slagboom, P. E., & Heijmans, B. T. (2014). DNA methylation signatures link prenatal famine exposure to growth and metabolism. *Nature Communications, 5,* 5592.

Torrey, E. F., Bartko, J. J., Lun, Z. R., & Yolken, R. H. (2006). Antibodies to toxoplasma gondii in patients with schizophrenia: a meta-analysis. *Schizophrenia Bulletin, 33*(3), 729–736.

Udwin, O., Yule, W., & Martin, N. (1987). Cognitive abilities and behavioural characteristics of children with idiopathic infantile hypercalcaemia. *Journal of Child Psychology and Psychiatry, 28*(2), 297–309.

van Harmelen, A–L, van Tol, M–J, Demenescu, L. R., van der Wee, N. J. A., Veltman, D. J., Aleman, A., van Buchem, M. A., Spinhoven, P., Penninx, B. W. J. H., & Elzinga, B. M. (2013). Enhanced amygdala reactivity to emotional faces in adults reporting childhood emotional maltreatment. *Social, Cognitive and Affective Neuroscience, 8*(4), 362–369.

Villoria, J. G., Pajares, S., López, R. M., Marin, J. L., & Ribes, A. (2016). Neonatal screening for inherited metabolic diseases in 2016. In J. Campistol (Ed.), *Seminars in pediatric neurology* (Vol. 23, No. 4, pp. 257–272). W. B. Saunders.

Wapner, R. J., Martin, C. L., Levy, B., Ballif, B. C., Eng, C. M., Zachary, J. M.,Savage, M., Platt., L. D., Saltzman, D., Grobman, W. A., Klugman, S., Scholl, T., Simpson, J. L., McCall, K., Aggarwal, V. S., Bunke, B., Nahum, O., Patel, A., Lamb, A. N. … & Jackson, L. N. (2012). Chromosomal microarray versus karyotyping for prenatal diagnosis. *New England Journal of Medicine, 367*(23), 2175–2184.

Wani, A. L., Ara, A., & Usmani, J. A. (2015). Lead toxicity: a review. *Interdisciplinary Toxicology, 8*(2), 55–64.

Whitley, R. J., & Kimberlin, D. W. (2005). Herpes simplex: encephalitis children and adolescents. In R. Feigin (Ed.), *Seminars in pediatric infectious diseases* (Vol. 16, No. 1, pp. 17–23). W. B. Saunders.

Winter, R. M., & Baraitser, M. (2013). *Multiple congenital anomalies: a diagnostic compendium.* Springer.

World Health Organization & United Nations Children's Fund. (2009). *WHO child growth standards and the identification of severe acute malnutrition in infants and children: a joint statement.*

Zwicker, A., MacKenzie, L. E., Drobinin, V., Bagher, A. M., Howes Vallis, E., Propper, L., Bagnell, A., Abidi, S., Pavlova, B., Alda, M., Denovan-Wright, E. M. (2020). Neurodevelopmental and genetic determinants of exposure to adversity among youth at risk for mental illness. *Journal of Child Psychology and Psychiatry, 61*(5), 536–544.

CHAPTER 8

PSYCHOLOGICAL INTERVENTIONS

THERE have been many attempts to provide and evaluate systematic interventions for children and young people with neurodevelopmental disorders. They will be described, like psychopharmacological interventions, according to their purposes and transdiagnostically. Some interventions address the core problems of a disorder and seek to alleviate them. Examples include motor problems such as tics, defining features of impulsiveness and inattentive behaviour in attention deficit hyperactivity disorder (ADHD), communication disabilities of autism spectrum disorder (ASD), and psychotic phenomena such as hallucinations.

Other interventions aim primarily to reduce associated problems and promote adjustment. Examples of these kinds of intervention targets include emotional changes such as anxiety and depression, behavioural changes such as aggression and self-injury, and cognitive alterations such as weaknesses of memory. These changes are not usually different in kind from those arising in children who are otherwise developing typically, but usually differ in detail. This latter group of interventions will often be based on considerations of how to adapt widely used techniques, such as the cognitive and behavioural therapies for otherwise typically developing young people, to the needs of those with difficulties in communication or learning.

Yet other interventions seek to reduce, or alleviate the effects of, the unfriendly environments that act as mediators of disability. They are considered in Chapter 10.

Methods of intervention also vary, some being delivered within an existing community setting (such as school or home), others in clinic, laboratory, or residential settings. There is a grey line between what constitutes a psychosocial intervention and what is an educational process. Speech and language therapists, occupational therapists, counsellors, physical therapists, specialist nurses, and family and creative therapists: all have valued roles alongside educators, medical specialists, and psychologists. In an ideal world, they would work in effective multidisciplinary teams—and even in this world, they often do.

8.1 Explanation and support

Families come for help already possessed with resources of knowledge, beliefs, and values. Explanation and advice will need to be understandable in the light of existing health beliefs, but also to come from an overall professional formulation.

Diagnostic labels can be a useful start. They should have been constructed to convey a simple, accurate, and useful message. They may be the only information that a family carries securely away from an initial consultation. They will be incomplete; further information sharing should follow and move on to a formulation and developmental account (see 'Encounters with diagnosis', Chapter 10, Section 10.13). The conveying of a diagnosis to a family should combine sensitivity and responsive discussion with authority and an atmosphere of calm. Professionals who prefer not to use diagnostic labels should still aim for succinct summaries, backed up by written information, that can set the scene for fuller understanding. Psychoeducation should add:

- key problems to address
- plans for intervention
- likely outcomes with and without treatment
- what is known about influences on course for this child or young person
- indications of what is not yet known
- genetic counselling, which is often provided separately and by experts but is often asked about at an early stage of contact. Where a provisional risk of recurrence in the family can be given at this early stage, it is usually appreciated.

Families should be put in touch with community support agencies. Voluntary advocacy and service user groups can be knowledgeable and valuable about the range of services that is available. Multiple needs often entail a bewildering range of physical and mental health, education, and social service agencies. Primary healthcare resources ought to be able to guide and coordinate. Volunteers from the affected community are often the most knowledgeable helpers around.

8.2 Counselling and advice

It would be not only wrong but discriminatory to assume that children with impairments cannot understand their predicament. To the contrary, many will feel a need to communicate about themselves but hesitate to start it. Intelligent listening is the hallmark of humanistic counselling and is not the sole province of any one discipline.

Children may face problems of emotional adjustment as they compare themselves with their peers and siblings, or see their parents struggling. Reactions of other children are prominent sources of puzzlement and distress. Adolescents face conflicts between the need for independence and requirements for assistance. Families will struggle with implications for long-term care and the emotional consequences for different family members.

How far clinicians involve themselves in general advice will depend on what other services are available. Social skills and emotional literacy may well be taught more effectively by teachers and caregivers than in a clinic. When clinicians are involved in developing skills in the young people—such as independence, relaxation training, and anger management—they may well find it better to situate their work in schools and colleges than in mental health settings.

Widely available community interventions based on psychological understanding include:

Portage, a home-visiting educational service for preschool children who are showing developmental delays (www.portage.org.uk).
EarlyBird (for preschoolers) and *EarlyBirdPlus* (for children 4 to 9 years), giving support to parents when their child is first diagnosed with ASD, and providing continuing advice (www.autism.org.uk/earlybird).
Hanen aims at teaching effective communication skills to parents of young people at risk of developing problems (www.hanen.org).

8.3 COGNITIVE BEHAVIOURAL THERAPIES

There is now a substantial scientific literature on the evaluation of behavioural and cognitive approaches to therapy. Antagonism between behaviourally and cognitively orientated therapists is now mostly a thing of the past. Cognitive behavioural therapy (CBT) draws on both types of interventions, in different balances according to the individual and the nature of their problems. Systematic trials to evaluate outcomes are usually based on detailed sets of procedures that can be taught and monitored. The techniques used have very wide applicability and need to be adapted to individuals' strengths and weaknesses. Courses of treatment are therefore even harder to standardize than is the case for drugs.

Most interventions are based on a selection of a limited set of techniques, briefly outlined here, combined into different packages. Controlled trials of therapy packages are difficult to mount and correspondingly scanty. A good deal depends not only on the effectiveness of the particular methods but also on the fidelity with which they are given (e.g. closely following the way they were applied in a successful research evaluation) and on the skill of the therapist in involving and maintaining the cooperation of the subjects and their families.

8.3.1 Behavioural methods

Target identification: there should be clear and explicit definition of a behaviour that it is intended either to increase or reduce. A goal will often be specified in advance (e.g. 10-minute periods free of spitting).

Monitoring: the target should be monitored (e.g. for how closely the goal is being approached). Raters will be given charts or other means of recording the changes. Ideally, the raters will include the subjects themselves.

Functional analysis: the purpose of the behaviours for the individual should be understood. A good approach is through A–B–C analysis: Antecedents–Behaviours–Consequences. Close description of the situation in which a behaviour is shown, as well as what happens afterwards, often clarifies the causal processes involved.

8.3.1.1 *Reinforcers and contingency management*

Reinforcers are events after a behaviour that increase its frequency in the future. They are not necessarily desirable: for example, self-injuring behaviours may be being maintained by social attention following contingently on injury. Both this adverse process and the inculcation of prosocial behaviour by social reward are examples of reinforcement. Behavioural therapists make extensive use of schedules of reinforcement that are delivered after the desired behaviour—*contingency management.*

Negative reinforcers are events that increase a behaviour's frequency when they stop.

Differential reinforcement can shape behaviours when desired ones are followed by a reinforcer and unwanted ones are not. It can also be used to encourage behaviours that are incompatible with those that are problematic, or to encourage problematic behaviours to be emitted at a lower rate.

Token economies are forms of contingency management in which the reinforcers are symbols or tokens that can be exchanged for other reinforcers that are valued in themselves. For example, points, stickers, or counters can be exchanged later for privileges or treats.

Extinction is the withdrawal of a reinforcer in order to reduce the target behaviour. (It can also produce a transient increase, about which caregivers will need to be warned.)

Exposure with response prevention (ERP) allows 'exposure' to anxiety-inducing situations, so that avoiding them is no longer subject to maintenance by the negative reinforcement of anxiety being reduced. 'Response prevention' includes refraining from ritualized thoughts that act as avoidance.

Graded change is used to help people whose fixed habits or fears are restricting their lives. Very small changes in a situation or stimulus may allow exposure (e.g. to a picture or a small part of a phobic stimulus), with successive small approximations to the real thing.

8.3.2 Cognitive methods

Some cognitive techniques used to be regarded as out of reach for people with intellectual deficits or in the spectrum of autism. Increasingly, however, it is being recognized that many people with neurodevelopmental disorders can indeed be capable of the essential steps of identifying and linking thoughts with emotions.

> *Examining evidence* (e.g. through Socratic questioning) can be used to identify cognitive errors and generate alternatives; for example, to realize that name calling by other young people might not be based on personal hatred but rather on ignorance and following the herd.
>
> *Metaphors* (e.g. of oneself as a scientist) can be helpful as vivid ways of learning how to explore feelings.
>
> *Mood monitoring* is a key part of learning to cope with anger, misery. and anxiety.

Both behavioural and cognitive techniques typically involve homework, motivational procedures, coping and relaxation skills, and problem-solving skills (e.g. in organization). Relatives, other caregivers, and teachers are often drawn in as collaborators with the therapists. Social modelling is a kind of vicarious learning in which the learner can see or hear a therapist, a relative, or a peer performing valuable skills such as fearless interaction with a potentially anxiety-inducing situation, effective communication of needs, or helpfulness to others. The goal of these behavioural and cognitive strategies is more than achieving behavioural change in isolation. It is to enhance personal choice, community participation, communication, and respect.

Applied behaviour analysis (ABA) and *positive behavioural support* (PBS) are comprehensive systems of intervention with many applications and purposes. They are reviewed in Section 8.10.

8.3.3 Acceptance and commitment therapy (ACT)

ACT developed from cognitive approaches but takes a different line. It is not primarily based on symptom reduction but on developing a better quality of life and psychological flexibility. It is not seeking to eliminate unpleasant feelings but to promote acceptance of them, avoid overreacting, and a move towards valuing life as it is. Key concepts are the reduction of avoidance and increase in the ability to reflect about feelings—for instance, to experience a negative thought such as 'I am disabled' as a thought about disability, not an experience of it. This should make it less necessary to avoid situations that emphasize the presence of disability. More positive behaviours could then follow.

Empirical investigation of ACT is in its infancy. Swain et al. (2015) provide a systematic review of studies in childhood, but small samples, and lack of comparator interventions or randomization, mean that ACT cannot yet be advocated as an evidence-based therapy. The best evidence from that review was for the treatment of tic disorders, depressive symptoms, and high-risk sexual behaviour by adolescents.

8.3.4 Psychodynamic approaches

Psychodynamic approaches have often been taken to ASD (Haag et al., 2005) but have not lent themselves to systematic trials evidence. Practitioners often address themselves to developing and sharing with the team their understanding of the patient's subjective world.

8.4 INTERVENTIONS TO REDUCE MOTOR PROBLEMS

8.4.1 Chronic tics

Support should include both counselling and explanation to other people (e.g. teachers and friends), and encouragement to reduce victimization and punishment. Support and advocacy groups are usually available in the voluntary sector.

Habit reversal training begins with enhancing the understanding of the children and young people about their tics. The circumstances likely to evoke them are identified. Awareness of the premonitory signs (urges) is developed. The therapist and patient then develop a competing response that cannot be performed at the same time as the tic, and practise it when the urge arrives. For instance, a blinking tic might be replaced by a forced eye widening; a coughing tic might be replaced by a swallow. The patient is then encouraged and supported to incorporate the procedure into everyday life.

Even if it is not feasible to do this all the time, it can be a real source of reassurance for the ticqueur to know that there is a means available of suppressing the tic at times when it would be particularly embarrassing (e.g. an interview or a date). The goal is not usually to get rid of the tics completely, but rather to reduce their frequency and increase controllability.

Other behavioural approaches include an extension of habit reversal into the comprehensive behavioural tntervention for tics (CBIT), which adds relaxation training and behavioural rewards.

Massed negative practice requires the forced and voluntary repetition of the tic (which can help, but occasionally makes matters worse).

Exposure with response prevention differs from CBIT in expecting voluntary suppression of the tic rather than learning an incompatible movement.

Randomized trials of behavioural treatment for tics have received a systematic review by McGuire et al. (2015). The effect sizes, by comparison with waiting lists or standard supportive therapy, are moderate to large (about 0.6 to 0.9 SD). Habit reversal and CBIT are the treatments of choice. Predicted adverse effects—worsening of anxiety, rebound of tics after suppression, excessive focus on the tics—do not seem to have materialized. They are established therapies and are often recommended by guidelines as the first choice, unless the tics are so severe, or have such impact, that medication is required from the start. A simplified programme of four sessions of psychoeducation, habit reversal training, relaxation training, and education on tic relapse prevention has been trialled against usual treatment with education and pyridoxine only (Chen et al., 2019). The intervention reduced the frequency and severity of tics in young people aged 6 to 18 years.

Psychological treatment for the mental problems associated with tics and Tourette will usually be based on identification of those problems, and then on application of CBT or other psychotherapy, as for children who do not tic. ADHD is a very frequent concomitant; obsessive-compulsive disorders only a little less so. Both, like the anxiety disorders, can be the major indications for therapy, rather than the tics themselves.

A complexity, however, appears in the presence of unacceptable actions, such as poking other children, which may or may not be involuntary. Coprophenomena and aggression, for instance, may be either tics or learned behaviours that are rewarded by attention. A behavioural approach such as differential reinforcement does not depend upon a clear formulation of whether the behaviour was voluntary or not. The attitudes of adults, however, may be very strongly conditioned by whether the young person is perceived as responsible for the actions. Discussion between involved adults and therapist or physician can usually defuse toxic attitudes.

8.4.2 Complex stereotypies

Stereotyped, repetitive behaviours can require intervention if they are interfering with constructive activities or becoming damaging to self or others. Behavioural interventions will use functional analysis and differential reinforcement of alternative behaviours. This can be effective, at least in non-autistic children, even when given remotely via a DVD watched at home (Specht et al., 2017). Cognitive approaches can also be helpful for those whose stereotypies appear when they are anxious or distressed. The primary target is then the distress rather than the motor change.

8.5 Interventions to promote compliant behaviours and appropriate discipline

Cognitive and behavioural methods are widely used, both within and outside the clinical category of ADHD, to control behaviour problems such as disruptive non-compliance. Disobedient and destructive behaviours in children often arise from causes other than neurodevelopmental delays. Oppositional and conduct disorders may be based on family disadvantage and dysfunction. Such disorders and their psychosocial causes can also be an important part of the full complex of symptoms of ADHD, intellectual disability (ID), and chronic tics.

Several disciplines use similar behavioural and cognitive methods, often in ways that are individual to the case. Unregulated professions such as coaching, unspecified psychotherapy, personal tutoring, and family counselling rely on recommendations and informal marketing rather than a systematic evidence base. Such practitioners vary greatly in training and skill. Many draw on lessons from the systematized programmes and randomized trials of defined interventions for their knowledge and confidence.

8.5.1 Parent training in behavioural methods

Young children are often helped through modifying their parents' reactions to hard-to-manage behaviours. This is not just to make life easier for parents. The outcome for oppositional and conduct problems is all too often one of increasing cycles of coercion that limit life opportunities and lead on to emotional problems. Early intervention is recommended by guidelines in the hope that it can prevent hostile and coercive cycles of interaction before they become ingrained into family life.

Several programmes have an evidence base for their efficacy in promoting effective handling of problem behaviours. 'Parent training' is not an acceptable term if it is taken to imply that the parents are deficient in love and care. It is best presented as a set of learnable but non-intuitive skills in specifying the behaviours to change, effective guidance, and altering the rules of what is and is not rewarded. Some widely used and evaluated interventions are:

Incredible Years Parent Training Programme (Webster Stratton et al., 2011) is often given as a group-based intervention over 12–20 weekly sessions, with adaptation for ADHD, including directive coaching for caregivers. Trials indicate that mothers (not necessarily fathers) change to use more appropriate discipline, less physical punishment, and more monitoring for children with ADHD. The children improve on parental ratings of hyperactivity, inattentive and oppositional behaviours, and emotion regulation. At school, teachers' ratings report improvements in disruptive behaviours. A version designed especially for children with other developmental disabilities, as well as ADHD, covered developmentally appropriate play, praise, rewards, limit setting, and handling challenging behaviour. It had positive effects on parenting and child behaviour (McIntyre, 2008).

Triple P—Positive Parenting Programme (Bor et al., 2002) is a well-known system of modifying antisocial behaviour and emotional distress through 'parent training'. It has been developed in children who present behaviour problems but are not disabled, for whom it has positive effects on child and parental behaviour. It takes several forms, including one for children with mixed disabilities that had helpful effects on parental behaviour even when presented online (Hinton et al., 2017).

It has been modified for children with disabilities into *Stepping Stones Triple P* (SSTP). In randomized controlled trials (RCTs) it has been superior to standard care for several populations. For instance, SSTP and ACT were evaluated in a trial that targeted behaviour problems in children with cerebral palsy (Whittingham et al., 2014). Sixty-seven families of children at a mean age of 5.3 years reported results significantly superior to being placed on a waiting list.

Parent–child interaction therapy was originally introduced to improve parenting of preschool children with conduct problems (Eyberg et al., 1995). This parent training programme has now been used in many settings. A systematic meta-analysis of 23 studies has indicated a substantial effect size (SMD = 0.87) for reduction of disruptive behaviour and parental stress (Thomas et al., 2017).

Helping the non-compliant child (Abikoff et al., 2015) uses similar methods to the above, both in specialized and generic settings. Its effects, like the other programmes described here, appear to be on the behaviours rather than on any hypothesized underlying psychopathology.

New Forest Parenting Programme (Lange et al., 2018) is provided on an individual rather than a group basis, so as to be more accessible for hard-to-reach families of young children with ADHD. It has a sound evidence base in several countries.

8.5.2 CBT for older children and adolescents

As children develop outside their families, methods for promoting non-aggressive and compliant interactions with others become less dependent on parents to provide and make more use of individual or group sessions for the young people themselves. Behavioural parent training is still relevant. It is advised by guidelines, such as those from the National Institute for Health and Care Excellence (NICE), as the first line of treatment for mild or moderate ADHD (NICE, 2018b). Its value, however, does not depend upon helping the core features of ADHD. Rather, it helps to reduce the oppositional or antisocial features that are associated with ADHD.

The details of therapy include procedures derived from the theory and practice of operant conditioning. Token economy systems, response cost, time out from positive reinforcement, shaping and fading out response sequences are all in use. Some interventions target schoolchildren via their classrooms rather than their families.

- Instructing teachers about the difficulties attendant on ADHD. A short brochure explaining ADHD, given to elementary class teachers, had an effect size around 0.3 SD in reducing ADHD as rated by teachers by comparison with those in schools where brochures were not given (Tymms & Merrell, 2006).
- Training teachers in behavioural management, along the lines of that provided for parents, can have good results for young schoolchildren (Plueck et al., 2015). Techniques include contingent praise, planned ignoring, explicit behaviour targets, daily report cards, points systems, and time out from positive reinforcement.
- Modifying the structure of the classroom (e.g. with individual, separated desks rather than communal tables, for at least some topics) can reduce the distractions that students with ADHD may both suffer and inflict on others.
- Rule-governed rather than teacher-governed discipline, which operates when the classroom walls display visual information about the rules of discipline and expectations for behaviour—rather than relying on the teacher's individual use of authority, threats, or charm.

Many trials and systematic reviews have contributed to current practice. Evans et al. (2014), NICE (2018b), and Fabiano et al. (2015) review them and provide guides on psychosocial interventions. They often need to be supplemented with measures to enhance young people's cooperativeness with the process: motivational interviewing (Sibley et al., 2016), to help them to clarify and remember their purposes; self-reinforcement, to be more in control of their learning; and family therapy, to communicate more clearly with other family members (Robin, 2014).

> The *Challenging Horizons Programme* (CHP) is a package of many techniques given in different formats (e.g. as after-school sessions, 3 days a week for 22 weeks), targeting academic and social functioning, to help young people succeed independently (Evans et al., 2011; Molina et al., 2008). The skills taught include social skills for relating to peers, taking notes and using them, self-organization, and problem solving.
>
> *HOPS (homework, organization, and planning skills)* is another combination of multiple techniques which has received systematic testing. Langberg et al. (2012) reported a randomized comparison with a waiting-list control group. The procedures, delivered both by parents and teachers, yielded significantly improved outcomes according to accounts by parents, but not according to those from teachers.
>
> The *Multimodal Treatment Study of Children with ADHD* (MTA) assembled the techniques that had been used in several different successful programmes. The idea was to give the best opportunity for psychological interventions to show their potential for improving the psychosocial outcomes of ADHD, and to compare

their effects with those of carefully given medication, as described in Chapter 9, Section 9.4 and by Molina et al. (2009). The package included individual and group work in classrooms, families, and recreational camps. They were given either with or without careful medication, and contrasted with groups randomized to receive medication only or to routine treatment only—the last involving the usual level of medication and psychosocial interventions that applied in the community. Results unequivocally favoured the careful medication, at the 14-month outcome, over the treatments given in routine care. There was no untreated group. Psychosocial management added little to medication in the group receiving both, but the combination was more effective than psychosocial intervention alone.

Observational follow-up over the next few years indicated that after two years, the difference between groups was smaller, and after three years, all had equivalent outcomes: the reasons are considered in Chapter 9, Section 9.4.

8.6 INTERVENTIONS TO REDUCE IMPULSIVENESS AND INATTENTIVENESS

The positive account of effects on problems of oppositional behaviour, as described here, is not, according to current knowledge, matched by strong evidence about effects on the core ADHD problems of impulsiveness, inattentiveness, and lack of controlled attention. They sound similar, but differ in associations and course (see 'Coexistent problems of conduct', Chapter 3, Section 3.5).

Many behavioural and cognitive methods have indeed been developed for the problems of dysregulated impulse control that are at the core of ADHD. Inattentive and disorganized behaviours have also been addressed, often in combination with a focus on impulsive overactivity, and often using similar interventions to those described here to promote compliant behaviours and appropriate discipline.

A systematic review and meta-analysis by Daley et al. (2014) focused on those RCTs that have reported outcomes on the full set of ADHD criteria in rating scales (a smaller group of trials than those in the review by Fabiano et al. (2015) cited earlier). Daley et al. went on to analyse according to who the raters of outcome were and whether they were (probably) blind to the treatment being given. This agreed, in part, with the conclusion from the account of behavioural parent training referred to earlier. The procedures were efficacious when judged by those giving them. When, however, the raters had not administered the treatment, and so were probably blind to which treatment was given, there was no effect on ADHD scores, or only vanishingly small effect sizes.

This does not mean that the interventions were useless. It is likely that much of the positive gain in non-blinded ratings was due to the non-specific aspects of raters judging the results of their own actions. Cognitive dissonance and good morale may well be responsible—but if these reflect more positive attitudes towards the children, they may well be welcomed. Furthermore, the same analyses also found statistically significant effects on the probably blinded ratings of oppositional and conduct problems, and on parents' reactions to them. These are developmentally important problems in leading on to the 'antisocial trap' of hostile behaviour and hostile reactions by others.

8.7 Interventions to reduce disorganization

Cognitive and behavioural methods are often applied to the tasks of teaching self-organization (Evans et al., 2014). They are very relevant to children in secondary education who have developed difficulties in academic learning because of attention problems. Impairments of executive function can be addressed by cognitive training; incompetent approaches to study, by problem-solving techniques; and emotional avoidance of challenging tasks, by reframing harmful cognitive distortions.

Behavioural techniques have been adapted to the treatment of disorganized children who are often, but not always, given a diagnosis of ADHD.

The *Child Life and Attention Skills (CLAS) Programme* (Pfiffner et al., 2014) works with parents and teachers to focus on strategies for improving homework, home routines, organization, independence in self-care, time management, friendship-making, and social assertion (with less emphasis on improving impulse management than in the programmes described previously). A randomized trial against treatment as usual (TAU), in children aged 7 to 11 years, found that receiving CLAS was associated with significantly fewer inattention symptoms, greater organizational skills, and greater overall improvement than in the TAU group. Both parents and teachers participated in the therapies, and both reported positive results.

Several training approaches incorporate cognitive therapy.

Problem-solving techniques include cueing procedures to reduce distractibility. For instance, students can set the alarms on their mobile phones or watches to go off every 20 minutes. The alarm should then lead the students to check on whether they have been distracted from the main task on which they should be engaged.

Challenging distorted cognitions may involve reality testing about depressive thinking. 'I can't do maths' may become self-fulfilling unless it is identified as an invasive thought rather than a scientific fact.

Simplifying by breaking forbiddingly complex tasks into simple components can also be taught as a study skill. Rewarding students getting started on them, and setting priorities among them, can help to overcome the anticipatory anxiety that deters many people with cognitive impairments from tackling activities that are difficult for them.

Discouraging avoidance and procrastination can be tackled by learning to list the different alternative solutions to a problem and to choose the best possible solution. This skill can assist with impulsivity as well as procrastination.

Direct training of performance on laboratory tests of cognition has been attempted, for several tests that are impaired in ADHD or ID. Working memory is the function most targeted, since an initial, positive report came from Klingberg et al. (2005) on children with ADHD.

Adaptive thinking instructs adolescents to observe and modify their own style of focusing attention, and to develop the most effective ways for them to learn. The idea is to avoid downward spirals of intensifying emotions and avoidance of circumstances (e.g. homework) that are perceived as overwhelming (Brown, 2000).

Evaluation of all these cognitive training approaches has not yielded strong enough evidence for any of them to be generally and routinely recommended. Systematic review and meta-analysis of cognitive training trials for young people with ADHD have been reported by Cortese et al. (2015). They could find evidence only of small (usually absent) effect sizes. The trials have often been compromised by using outcome measures rated by people who are not blind to the interventions being assessed. The meta-analysis by Cortese et al. was based on 15 trials meeting the analysts' criteria. Where a single function—usually working memory—was being trained, there was no evidence of benefit for ADHD as a whole. It seems possible that young people were admitted to the trials on the basis of showing ADHD, and the assumption may have been invalid that they would all have been disabled by the dysfunction identified as a group property of people with ADHD. Further advance may require more precise identification of the cognitive function to be trained in the individuals for whom it is recommended.

Neurofeedback has also been regarded as a means of promoting self-organization, executive function, attention, and learning. There is great variation in the technologies used, and no one technique has dominated the field. Most published trials have focused on ADHD, and trained either more power in fast rhythmical EEG activity over the frontal lobes or greater amplitude in slow EEG potentials. It is plain that these physiological goals can be achieved, at least on a temporary basis, but not that they have effects on mental life, test performance, or behaviour.

Cortese et al. (2016) have systematically reviewed 13 RCTs of feedback. None has yet survived the rigorous demands of having a sham or active control procedure and raters who are probably blind to the procedure being offered. Other reviewers note disparity between the methods of feeding back physiological changes and find that standard protocols yield small to medium effect sizes (Arns et al., 2020). Statistical significance is (just) achieved, but with wide limits of confidence Trials with statistically significant results, according to non-blind raters of the young people's performance, could well be vulnerable to artefacts of expectation and suggestion.

A systematic review of trials in ASD has been reported by Holtmann et al. (2011), but for this purpose, too, the results are not yet scientifically persuasive or sufficient to recommend its use.

Neurofeedback approaches are taking in other techniques, such as electromyography and magnetic resonance imaging. They continue to be interesting but not widely available. So far, the theoretical basis of the approaches has been to reverse the changes that are linked with ADHD in group-association studies, rather than to be informed by deep neurophysiological understanding. Further interest from researchers and commerce can be confidently expected.

8.8 INTERVENTIONS TO PROMOTE PEER RELATIONSHIPS

Evaluations of training in social skills have not been unanimous. Storebo et al. (2011), in a Cochrane review, found no justifying evidence for either supporting or refuting skills training for young people with ADHD. There were small effects (SMD −0.26) on teacher ratings of ADHD, but no evidence for good or bad effects on teacher ratings of social skills, or on emotional competencies.

The learning of skills, however, may not be a key problem for peer relationships in ADHD: application of them in practice may be closer to the issue. Unpopularity and isolation often result from impulsive and tactless conduct or from not taking the time to learn the rules by which their peers conduct themselves. When these are addressed in real-life situations (e.g. recreational camps, which are widely used in the USA), then behavioural approaches have a beneficial effect. A meta-analysis indicated that behavioural interventions using points systems for cooperation and acceptable conduct were consistently more effective than other approaches, with effect sizes round about 0.44 (Pelham & Fabiano, 2008). These programmes have not, however, been evaluated or widely used in cultures other than North America.

Contingency management in real-life settings has much to recommend it. Even if no particular programme is being followed, it still makes sense to encourage play-based strategies (with involvement of parents, other carers, and teachers) to increase joint attention, engagement, and reciprocal communication.

8.9 INTERVENTIONS TO AID COMMUNICATION AND LANGUAGE

Communication difficulties are a core part of the autism spectrum, language disability, and ID. They also need attention for many children with ADHD and specific learning disorders. Involvement of parents and teachers in play-based strategies can increase reciprocal communication. Clinical strategies, chosen according to the child or young person's developmental level, should include encouraging parents' and/or teachers' recognition of children's patterns of communication and interaction and encouragement of them.

Speech and language therapists have developed many ways of helping impaired children to communicate. Many of the approaches start with learning to imitate sounds. Those with unusual difficulties in sound production or reception may well be educated to use alternative communication systems, such as sign language or a simplified system of signs such as Paget Gorman. Picture communication systems are also used. In cases of ASD and some receptive language disorders, the early goal is to instil the basic skills of communication.

There are also comprehensive interventions to accelerate social and cognitive development and communication in autistic children and language disorders.

Treatment and Education of Autistic and Related Communication Handicapped Children (TEACCH) is extensively used as a community-delivered system to develop social and language function. It has received a meta-analysis of 13 trials (Virues-Ortega et al., 2013). Only small or negligible effects were found for communication, or indeed for verbal and cognitive skills. Moderate social gains did appear, but overall it should be seen as a promising approach, not a scientifically established one. Nevertheless, the system is well received by families and teachers.

The *Picture Exchange Communication System* (PECS) was developed with early communication as a key aspect. Children begin by being trained to exchange a single picture for a desired item and to make requests. When teaching communicative initiation, the system typically separates the function of a communicative partner (to interact socially with the child) from that of a guide (to provide physical prompting from behind the child without interacting with the child socially). Prompting is then faded out in the interests of developing spontaneity. In later stages, children learn to construct picture-based sentences and use a variety of attributes in their requests. A picture with a meaning such as 'I need a break' can be used for many purposes—including providing an alternative to challenging behaviours that have the function of escape from imposed tasks. Within-case studies have been reported to indicate that children can use this kind of pictorial system to develop spoken language (Charlop–Christy et al., 2002).

Parent-mediated social communication therapy (PACT) involves collaboration between professionals and carers. Green et al. (2010) found encouraging results in a randomized trial of an approach in which experienced speech and language therapists joined parents in joint sessions with the individual child, at ages 2 to 4 years, over a period of a year. The intervention consisted of one-to-one clinic sessions between therapist and parent, with the child present. The idea was, first, to increase parents' sensitivity and responsiveness to child communication and reduce mistimed parental responses, using video-feedback methods. Later, a wider range of tactics to promote simple communication skills was introduced—familiar, repetitive language and routines, and pauses. The outcome was a significant increase in child–parent communication. At 5-year follow-up, there was an effect size of 0.55 for reduction of symptom severity (Pickles et al., 2016).

Pivotal response treatment (PRT) is described in Section 8.10.2 as a general approach to training abilities on which a whole range of other skills depend. In the example of developing communication and language, motivation and initiation of social contact can be considered as fundamental abilities. Gengoux et al. (2019) have described an effect size of 0.61, by comparison with routine support, for a 24-week behavioural programme for 2- to 5-year-olds along the lines of PRT. In this application, there was a combination of parent training and clinician-delivered in-home intervention. The key was to increase child motivation to interact by focusing on their interests, and noticing and rewarding their spontaneous efforts to communicate with language. Parents successfully learned the approach and the children came to communicate more frequently. The longer-term results on language development are awaited.

Interventions such as these have shown a real opportunity for modifying the course of communication development in autistic children by collaboration between specialists and parents in the preschool period.

Other approaches include animal-assisted therapy, floor time, sensory integration therapy, and several parent-training models. They have not received enough support from trials to be regarded as established therapy. NICE advised that auditory integration training and neurofeedback should not be used to manage speech and language problems in children and young people with autism (NICE, 2013).

8.10 INTERVENTIONS TO COMBAT CORE PROBLEMS IN AUTISTIC PEOPLE

Several ambitious and expensive approaches have been taken over the years to improve quality of life in autistic young people, and some have become controversial. They are not exclusively focused on reducing behaviour problems, but include promotion of pro-social and cognitive skills. Applied behaviour analysis, positive behavioural support, and pivotal response treatment are widely used in affluent parts of the USA, and in some other regions.

8.10.1 Applied behavioural analysis (ABA)

ABA was initially developed following Skinnerian behavioural principles. It aimed to develop behavioural control to the point where affected people could lead ordinary lives (Lovaas, 2003). Operant conditioning over long periods was the rule, often using tangible reinforcers such as food and sometimes using aversive consequences. Initial publications reported therapy lasting up to 40 hours a week. Families sometimes reported very good educational outcomes—but only for a few, and systematic research evaluations have not been convincing or extensive enough to establish a credible evidence base.

Both the use of punishment and the goal of curing autism have been rejected, often passionately, by many in the community of autism. The historical importance has nevertheless been to emphasize that many of the skill deficiencies and unacceptable behaviours can be remedied. ABA has come to take on a somewhat different meaning for some, describing a broader approach of functional analysis and behavioural development of skills. There is still much controversy about how rigorously the original techniques should be applied.

8.10.2 Pivotal response treatment (PRT)

PRT developed, as an alternative to the ABA approach of intensive training of single behaviours, into a focus on those behaviours and abilities that could be seen as critical for a whole range of learning. These 'pivots' include motivation, initiating social contacts, self-management, and responsiveness to multiple cues. Whether improving them does in fact lead on to generalized progress is not yet fully established. Meta-analysis of 43 trials, involving some 420 children, has concluded that increases in self-initiations, as a result of PRT or related procedures such as NLP (neurolinguistic programming), do indeed tend to be accompanied by collateral improvements (Verschuur et al., 2014). The improvements extended to increases in communication and language skills, play skills, and affect and reductions in maladaptive behaviour.

8.10.3 Positive behaviour support (PBS)

PBS has developed out of ABA, but differs in important respects: the goal of behavioural strategies is to achieve enhanced community presence, choice, personal competence, respect, and community participation, rather than simply behavioural change in isolation. It, too, is founded on functional analysis of behaviour, but with the further purpose of understanding it from the person's point of view. Behavioural methods aim to develop a wide range of skills, including those of coping and tolerance, using environmental change and differential reinforcement. Furthermore, and importantly, it avoids punishment-based procedures except in the most extreme circumstances.

A systematic review was based on the reported outcomes of 12 trials (423 cases), some of them single-case. It concluded that there are positive effects, even for severe problems, and that it is not exorbitantly expensive (LaVigna & Willis, 2012). A systematic review of training staff, both in residential institutions and community settings, has described positive impacts (MacDonald & McGill, 2013). After training, staff improved in knowledge, attitudes, and emotional responding. There was even some evidence of reduction in levels of challenging behaviour from service users. For the important outcome of quality of life, however, service users did not show improvement. More development and fuller evaluation both seem to be called for.

8.11 INTERVENTIONS TO REDUCE BEHAVIOUR THAT CHALLENGES

'Behaviour that challenges' refers especially to some dangerous behaviours that have proved very problematic in that they often lead to restrictive environments in the interests of people's safety (see 'Behaviour problems in autism', Chapter 4, Section 4.1.5.3). They are mostly encountered in children or young people with an (often severe) learning disability, autism spectrum condition, or both. Self-mutilation, violent and threatening aggression, and destruction of property are very often the targets for intervention. Some would expand the concept to include sleeplessness, poor eating, and non-compliance with medical requirements. The 'challenge' is therefore particularly to caregivers. There can accordingly be a conflict between respecting the autonomy of the individual and advancing the quality of life.

A careful trial by Aman et al. (2009) addressed problems of frequent tantrums, self-injury, and aggression in ASD children, with 24 weeks of training for parents in PBS. There were statistically significant and positive effects on the behaviour problems, even larger ($d = 0.34$) than those for medication with risperidone. Those who received PBS in addition to medication did better than those given medication alone.

General advice for therapy is to be guided by a careful functional assessment. As in other applications of behavioural approaches, it should identify antecedents, triggers, and consequences of the behaviour, and consider especially the needs that the child or young person is attempting to meet by performing the behaviour. The target behaviour(s) in such an approach will be measured and tracked, and there will be a clear schedule of reinforcement, and an ability to offer it promptly and contingently on demonstration of the desired behaviour.

Quality statement 8 of the UK National Institute of Clinical Excellence guidelines (2013) also recommends:

- *a specified timescale* to meet intervention goals (and, therefore, a change of intervention strategies if they have not led to change within a reasonably expected time)
- *consistent application* in all areas of the child or young person's environment (e.g. at home and at school, or by all the professional staff in a residential setting).

Disagreement among parents, carers, and professionals is very common unless explicit instruction and rationale, sometimes even involving videos, is provided.

Behaviours that challenge can sometimes be reduced by alleviating triggers such as painful conditions, insomnia, or stimuli to which people have become unduly sensitive. Sleep problems are managed with a combination of environmental change, behavioural analysis, and medical advice.

8.11.1 Interventions to promote good sleep patterns

Once it is clear that there is no medical cause such as badly timed stimulant medication, sleep apnoea, genetic syndromes such as Smith–Magenis, phobic avoidance of nightmares, painful or irritating illnesses such as eczema, or severe worries and fears at night, the next step is usually to develop a sleep plan.

The sleep environment may need to be modified to achieve a comfortable bedroom with a low level of background noise and illumination. Consistency of bedtimes should be attempted. Screen time should be adjusted—preferably banned from places for sleeping because of the action of light emitted from screens in inhibiting melatonin. Physical activity in the day should promote sleep at night. Family rows and ineffective nagging about bedtime should be discouraged in favour of calm and pleasant bedtime routines and relaxation.

All these laudable approaches are often more easily advised than carried out. Behavioural analysis will specify when the sleep problem occurs (delay falling asleep, frequent waking, unusual behaviours such as night terrors, or sleepiness during the day). Sleep routines will be encouraged, sometimes with rewards. Limit setting may be needed, and reduction of positive reinforcers of wakefulness. Extinction procedures for waking in the night may replace prolonged comforting and conversation with a calm and speedy return to the place of sleeping. (Alternatively, the behavioural goal may not be to sleep for longer periods but rather to engage in constructive activities that do not disturb other people.) If diurnal rhythm has been disrupted, gradual change can be used to accelerate time of settling or of rising. (If there is an extreme pattern of late hours, as for some adolescents, sleep times may be brought forward to synchronize with hours of darkness.) Cognitive techniques may include thought stopping of worries and ruminations at bedtime, and rehearsal in imagination of banishing night fears.

A proportion of young people with ASD or severe ADHD may be in chronic states of overarousal and over-reactiveness to sensory stimulation. Methods that have been advocated for reducing hyper-reactiveness include muscular relaxation, breathing exercises, mindfulness, yoga, and manipulation of various kinds of object. Robust evidence about their effects is lacking.

Autistic people at all ages have very high rates of sleep disorders. Their insomnia is disruptive to family life as well as to their own development. A lack of trial evidence on how to treat led to a systematic review of experience and expert development of a pathway of therapy (Malow et al., 2012). It includes suggestions similar to those just mentioned and might also be relevant to helping the sleep problems of ADHD.

Psychological interventions may make hypnotic medication unnecessary; but the very wide use of medication, especially melatonin, testifies to the limitations of their effectiveness.

8.12 Interventions to reduce hallucinations and other features of psychosis

Most current applications of CBT to the positive signs of schizophrenia follow the conceptualizations about adults' auditory hallucinations that were set out by Chadwick and Birchwood (1994). These emphasized the importance, not only of the presence of hallucinations, but of beliefs about them. Attitudes to the experiences could be fear of malevolent ones, or reassurance if they were perceived as benign. Either engagement with voices or resistance to them followed. Key actions by therapists were therefore to challenge and test beliefs about the voices' omnipotence, identity, and purpose. A systematic review and meta-analysis (Jauhar et al., 2014) has confirmed statistically significant effects of CBT in reducing positive symptoms of schizophrenia in adults, but found them to be small, with an effect size around 0.25.

Similar approaches, often delivered in groups, were soon taken for young people (Newton et al., 2005). CBT is widely offered in the UK for adolescents with schizophrenia spectrum disorders. The evidence base is less convincing than for adults (Stafford et al., 2015). The trials have often focused on the difficult goal of preventing a first episode of psychosis by treating those at high risk because of psychosis-like symptoms. Results are somewhat conflicting. Ising et al. (2017) found a lower rate of transition into psychosis for those treated with CBT than for those randomized to receiving routine care. Stain et al. (2016) compared CBT with a counselling approach (non-directive receptive listening) for young people considered to be at ultra-high risk for schizophrenia. Neither approach was superior to the other for reducing the presence of positive symptoms such as hallucinations; the control condition was, however, superior to CBT for reducing distress from hallucinations.

The effects of individual psychological treatment with CBT approaches have not yet been shown to modify the course of schizophrenia. Adding CBT to standard care appears to have no effect on long-term risk of relapse (Jones et al., 2018). A very small proportion of the available evidence in the Jones et al. (2018) meta-analysis indicated that CBT plus standard care may improve long-term global state and may reduce the risk of adverse events. Whether adding CBT to standard care for schizophrenia leads to clinically important improvement in patients' long-term mental state, quality of life, and social function remains unclear. Satisfaction with care (measured as the number of people leaving the study early) was no higher for participants receiving CBT compared to participants receiving standard care. It should be noted that although much research has been carried out in this area, the quality of evidence available is poor (mostly low or very low quality) and we still cannot make firm conclusions until more high-quality data are available.

8.12.1 Family interventions for psychosis

By contrast with attempts to treat individual patients with CBT, family interventions have been widely recommended and adopted for adult service users in recovery from psychosis. For young people and their families, family interventions aim to promote general functioning and reduce relapses, rather than to cure. The interventions are not directive and focussed, but promote communication between family members and knowledge about psychoses and coping with them.

Systematic review and meta-analysis of 14 trials of intervention was carried out by Claxton et al. (2017). The findings were for a significant effect in reducing the frequency of relapse, but not for a short-term effect on the number of symptoms. Relapse frequency is important in reducing the disruptive effects of loss of education and employment on recovery. Carers learned how to recognize the signs of imminent relapse and gained information about the services to use and how to engage effectively with them. Furthermore, carers developed lower levels of critical expressed emotion which is emphasized in Chapter 10, Section 10.6 as a significant source of disability.

Family psychoeducational sessions should, therefore, be included in the management of psychotic conditions in young people to promote recovery, coping, and social inclusion.

8.13 INTERVENTIONS TO TREAT EMOTIONAL AND RELATED DISORDERS IN PEOPLE WITH NEURODEVELOPMENTAL IMPAIRMENTS

Cognitive behavioural therapies have an evidence base that has established them as treatments of first choice for anxiety and depression in children and young people who are free of neurodevelopmental disorders (Cartwright–Hatton et al., 2004) and for minimizing psychological harm after trauma (Wethington et al., 2008). There are several ways in which they have been modified to be acceptable and useful to those whose ASD, ID, ADHD, or tic disorder is complicated by anxiety, obsessions, depression, or eating disorder. The modifications required are substantial. The general principles are described in the following sections.

8.13.1   For anxiety in ADHD

CBT is widely used for children and young people whose ADHD coexists with high levels of anxiety. Formal trials have mostly been small-scale and combine individual therapy with family interventions to reduce dysfunctional parenting strategies such as overcontrol and rejection. For the most part, they show small and inconstant effects on anxiety in this group.

The Multimodal Treatment Study of Children with ADHD (MTA) provided and compared intensive psychosocial and stimulant drug treatment approaches (described by Molina et al. (2009) and in Section 8.5.2). In this instance, psychosocial and stimulant approaches both reduced emotional problems, separately or in combination, even though neither contained elements directly targeting anxiety. Neither could be compared with an untreated group. It may well be that ADHD problems have direct and indirect effects on anxiety, and that the effect of intensive therapies is dependent on their reduction of ADHD rather than directly on anxiety.

A potentially positive finding came from Gould et al. (2018). They described a large series of treated young people with a primary problem of anxiety. Cognitive behavioural therapies directed at anxiety were given. Those who also showed features of ADHD were no more and no less likely to respond in their anxiety to CBT than those without. The ADHD features, however, were not the primary problems and were mostly mild.

When the ADHD features are severe, they may compromise the effectiveness of CBT for anxiety. Halldorsdottir et al. (2015) reported a RCT of CBT and/or medication in anxious young people aged 7 to 17 years who did or did not have ADHD as a primary problem. For those receiving only CBT, ADHD predicted a less satisfactory response of anxiety symptoms than was the case for those without. For those receiving both CBT and medication strategies, there was no such decrement of response in ADHD. The authors of the trial emphasized the possibility that 'anxious youth with comorbid ADHD are less likely to benefit from CBT strategies alone'. A related conclusion might be that research should examine what is responsible for the decrement in relieving anxiety and whether it might be overcome by interventions other than medication.

8.13.2   For anxiety in ASD

Ten trials received a systematic analysis by Walters et al. (2016). Parent and teacher ratings consistently found 'large' effect sizes. The authors had clear recommendations from the trial evidence: 'CBT should be offered as an intervention for young people with ASD and comorbid mental health problems including anxiety disorders, OCD and depression.' The review is correct to acknowledge the presence of additional mental health problems including depression and obsessive-compulsive disorder (OCD). However, rather than referring to problem-specific modifications for any of these disorders, the recommendation is for (unspecified) CBT.

8.13.3 For depression in ADHD, ASD, and ID

CBT is considered second only to antidepressant drugs for the treatment of major depressive disorders (March et al., 2004). As with drug treatments, good practice includes the provision of therapies such as psychoeducation, somatic management, problem solving, and cognitive restructuring for children and young people whose neuropsychiatric conditions are associated with major depression. There is rather little by way of systematic evidence to support or disconfirm the widespread practice. In one randomized trial against a waiting-list control, CBT displayed only a small effect size on depressive symptoms (McGillivray & Evert, 2012).

Clinicians are advised to follow recommendations for typically developing young people. The same advice applies to body dysmorphic disorder and post-traumatic stress disorder.

8.13.4 For obsessive-compulsive behaviour in ASD

It can be hard to distinguish obsessive-compulsive behaviour from the repetitive behaviours of ASD. A treatment manual designed specifically for people with ASD included four components of CBT: psychoeducation about anxiety and the cognitive cycle; problem solving; cognitive restructuring; and ERP (Russell et al., 2013). The intervention was compared with a control 'anxiety management' procedure providing psychoeducation about anxiety and relaxation strategies. Findings suggested a reduction in obsessive-compulsive symptoms and a greater number of treatment responders in the CBT group compared to those receiving only advice, but differences were not statistically significant.

8.13.5 For irritability

The emotional changes of excessive anger (irritability) (see Chapter 2, Section 2.9) have been addressed with anger control therapies. They are also relevant to the issues of behaviour that challenges, discussed earlier. Techniques used are, typically, learning to recognize the early triggers for, and signs of, anger and responding with countermeasures (e.g. of relaxation and positive imagery). Meta-analysis of trials in children and adolescents by Sukhodolsky et al. (2004) indicated them to be effective, subject to a lack of independent raters of their effect. Effect sizes for the therapy types reviewed were in the moderate range (0.36 to 0.79). Methods using feedback, modelling, and homework assignments were superior to those based on relaxation or attempts to modify internal constructs. These trials did not include children with ID. The study by Aman et al. (2009), referred to earlier, included positive changes in ratings of irritability as well as of hyperactivity and non-compliance.

8.13.6 Modification of CBT for emotional disorders in ID, ASD, and ADHD

The National Institute for Clinical Excellence (2013) recommends several ways in which CBT can be adjusted to be helpful to people with altered understanding.

8.13.6.1 *Modification for ID*

A wide range of methods has been used in published studies of adapting techniques to the needs of children with mild ID, and adolescents with mild to moderate ID. They are described in more detail by Hronis et al. (2017). Simplified and structured learning programmes can be achieved, taking into account the individual's abilities. They will often be given with breaks. Sessions in a programme should be concrete, practical, and creative. Structured worksheets will take the students through explicit stages, for instance of a desensitization programme. Information about a programme will often be presented in a factual style, perhaps using interactive multiple-choice formats. Therapists will model desired behaviours (e.g. fearless interaction), video the child practising them, and give positive feedback for success. Even more than for most people being treated, parents and carers will be included as much as possible in the delivery of therapy.

Children with ID are often said to be more visual than auditory learners, and more 'person-orientated' than 'task-orientated'. It is wise, however, to recognize the great range of ways in which people at all levels of development organize themselves, and to be guided by what works best for the individual rather than by prediction from the group.

8.13.6.2 *Modification for ASD*

Rigidity in thinking and pacing sessions appropriately are major challenges. Most therapists will need guidance and mentoring as they learn how to work with this group. Over-literal understanding of advice can be met by increasing the structure and clarity of written instructions. Modification of fears and worries is likely to include emotion recognition training. Therapists may be able to incorporate the child or young person's special interests into therapy (e.g. with an animated on-screen robot as the guide through a programme). Generalization into everyday life will call for explicit rehearsal of what has been learned in naturalistic settings. Difficulty with generalizing what has been learned can be met with prompting and reminding between sessions (perhaps with notes and a relative's involvement) of what has been taught.

A fuller range of the adaptations that have been used in published trials for autistic people is provided by Walters et al. (2016).

8.13.6.3 *Modification for ADHD*

Maintaining attention on a learning programme may mean offering not only regular breaks but also tangible rewards for participation. Sessions should be kept fairly short and activities should use a variety of modalities, colours, and pictures. Rewards will probably be offered with extra clarity and short delays to overcome difficulties in linking actions with consequences. Tasks and reinforcers will often need to be varied to prevent boredom.

REFERENCES

Abikoff, H. B., Thompson, M., Laver–Bradbury, C., Long, N., Forehand, R. L., Miller Brotman, L., Klein, R. G., Reiss, P., Huo, L., & Sonuga–Barke, E. (2015). Parent training for preschool ADHD: a randomized controlled trial of specialized and generic programs. *Journal of Child Psychology and Psychiatry*, 56(6), 618–631.

Aman, M. G., Mcdougle, C. J., Scahill, L., Handen, B., Arnold, L. E., Johnson, C., Stigler, K. A., Bearss, K., Butter, E., Swiezy, N. B., Sukhodolsky, D. D., Ramadan, Y., Pozdol, S. L., Nikolov, R., Lecavalier, L., Kohn, A. E., Koenig, K., Hollway, J. A., Korzekwa, P., Gavaletz, A., Mulick, J. A., Hall, K. L., Dziura, J., Ritz, L., Trollinger, S., . . . & Research Units on Pediatric Psychopharmacology Autism Network. (2009). Medication and parent training in children with pervasive developmental disorders and serious behavior problems: results from a randomized clinical trial. *Journal of the American Academy of Child & Adolescent Psychiatry*, 48(12), 1143–1154.

Arns, M., Clark, C. R., Trullinger, M., deBeus, R., Mack, M., & Aniftos, M. (2020). Neurofeedback and attention-deficit/hyperactivity-disorder (ADHD) in children: rating the evidence and proposed guidelines. *Applied Psychophysiology and Biofeedback*, 1–10.

Bor, W., Sanders, M. R., & Markie–Dadds, C. (2002). The effects of the Triple P–Positive Parenting Program on preschool children with co-occurring disruptive behavior and attentional/hyperactive difficulties. *Journal of Abnormal Child Psychology*, 30(6), 571–587.

Brown, T. E. (2000). *Attention-deficit disorders and comorbidities in children, adolescents, and adults*. American Psychiatric Publishing.

Chadwick, P., & Birchwood, M. (1994). The omnipotence of voices: a cognitive approach to auditory hallucinations. *British Journal of Psychiatry*, 164(2), 190–201.

Charlop–Christy, M. H., Carpenter, M., Le L., LeBlanc, L. A., & Kellet, K. (2002). Using the picture exchange communication system (PECS) with children with autism: assessment of PECS acquisition, speech, social-communicative behavior, and problem behavior. *Journal of Applied Behavior Analysis*, 35(3), 213–231.

Cartwright-Hatton, S., Roberts, C., Chitsabesan, P., Fothergill, C., & Harrington, R. (2004). Systematic review of the efficacy of cognitive behaviour therapies for childhood and adolescent anxiety disorders. *British Journal of Clinical Psychology*, 43(4), 421–436.

Chen, C. W., Wang, H. S., Chang, H. J., & Hsueh, C. W. (2019). Effectiveness of a modified comprehensive behavioral intervention for tics for children and adolescents with Tourette's syndrome: a randomized controlled trial. *Journal of Advanced Nursing*, 76(3), 903–915.

Claxton, M., Onwumere, J., & Fornells–Ambrojo, M. (2017). Do family interventions improve outcomes in early psychosis? A systematic review and meta-analysis. *Frontiers in Psychology*, 8, 371.

Cortese, S., Ferrin, M., Brandeis, D., Buitelaar, J., Daley, D., Dittmann, R. W., Holtmann, M., Santosh, P., Stevenson, J., Stringaris, A., Zuddas, A., Sonuga–Barke, E. J., & European ADHD Guidelines Group (EAGG). (2015). Cognitive training for attention-deficit/hyperactivity disorder: meta-analysis of clinical and neuropsychological outcomes from randomized controlled trials. *Journal of the American Academy of Child & Adolescent Psychiatry*, 54(3), 164–174.

Cortese, S., Ferrin, M., Brandeis, D., Holtmann, M., Aggensteiner, P., Daley, D., Santosh, P., Simonoff, E., Stevenson, J., Stringaris, A., Sonuga–Barke, E. J., & European ADHD Guidelines Group (EAGG). (2016). Neurofeedback for attention-deficit/hyperactivity disorder: meta-analysis of clinical and neuropsychological outcomes from randomized controlled trials. *Journal of the American Academy of Child & Adolescent Psychiatry*, 55(6), 444–455.

Daley, D., Van der Oord, S., Ferrin, M., Danckaerts, M., Doepfner, M., Cortese, S., Sonuga–Barke, E. J. S., & European ADHD Guidelines Group. (2014). Behavioral interventions in attention-deficit/hyperactivity disorder: a meta-analysis of randomized controlled trials across multiple outcome domains. *Journal of the American Academy of Child & Adolescent Psychiatry*, 53(8), 835–847.

Evans, S. W., Owens, J. S., & Bunford, N. (2014). Evidence-based psychosocial treatments for children and adolescents with attention-deficit/hyperactivity disorder. *Journal of Clinical Child & Adolescent Psychology*, 43(4), 527–551.

Evans, S. W., Schultz, B. K., DeMars, C. E., & Davis, H. (2011). Effectiveness of the Challenging Horizons after-school program for young adolescents with ADHD. *Behavior Therapy*, 42(3), 462–474.

Eyberg, S. M., Boggs, S. R., & Algina, J. (1995). Parent–child interaction therapy: a psychosocial model for the treatment of young children with conduct problem behavior and their families. *Psychopharmacology Bulletin*, 31(1), 83–91.

Fabiano, G. A., Schatz, N. K., Aloe, A. M., Chacko, A., & Chronis–Tuscano, A. (2015). A systematic review of meta-analyses of psychosocial treatment for attention-deficit/hyperactivity disorder. *Clinical Child and Family Psychology Review*, 18(1), 77–97.

Gengoux, G. W., Abrams, D. A., Schuck, R., Millan, M. E., Libove, R., Ardel, C. M., ... & Hardan, A. Y. (2019). A pivotal response treatment package for children with autism spectrum disorder: an RCT. *Pediatrics*, 144(3).

Gould, K. L., Porter, M., Lyneham, H. J., & Hudson, J. L. (2018). Cognitive-behavioral therapy for children with anxiety and comorbid attention-deficit/hyperactivity disorder. *Journal of the American Academy of Child & Adolescent Psychiatry*, 57(7), 481–490.

Green, J., Charman, T., McConachie, H., Aldred, C., Slonims, V., Howlin, P., ... & PACT Consortium. (2010). Parent-mediated communication-focused treatment in children with autism (PACT): a randomised controlled trial. *The Lancet*, 375(9732), 2152–2160.

Haag, G., Tordjman, S., Duprat, A., Urwand, S., Jardin, F., Cukierman, A., Druon, C., Du Chatellier, A. M., Tricaud, J., & Dumont, A. M. (2005). Psychodynamic assessment of changes in children with autism under psychoanalytic treatment. *International Journal of Psychoanalysis*, 86(2), 335–352.

Halldorsdottir, T., Ollendick, T. H., Ginsburg, G., Sherrill, J., Kendall, P. C., Walkup, J., Sakolsky, D. J., & Piacentini, J. (2015). Treatment outcomes in anxious youth with and without comorbid ADHD in the CAMS. *Journal of Clinical Child & Adolescent Psychology*, 44(6), 985–991.

Hinton, S., Sheffield, J., Sanders, M. R., & Sofronoff, K. (2017). A randomized controlled trial of a telehealth parenting intervention: a mixed-disability trial. *Research in Developmental Disabilities*, 65, 74–85.

Holtmann, M., Steiner, S., Hohmann, S., Poustka, L., Banaschewski, T., & Bölte, S. (2011). Neurofeedback in autism spectrum disorders. *Developmental Medicine & Child Neurology*, 53(11), 986–993.

Hronis, A., Roberts, L., & Kneebone, I. I. (2017). A review of cognitive impairments in children with intellectual disabilities: implications for cognitive behaviour therapy. *British Journal of Clinical Psychology*, 56(2), 189–207.

Ising, H. K., Lokkerbol, J., Rietdijk, J., Dragt, S., Klaassen, R. M., Kraan, T., Boonstra, N., Nieman, D. H., van den Berg, D. P. G., Linszen, D. H., Wunderink, L., Veling, W., Smit, F., & van der Gaag, M. (2017). Cost-effectiveness of cognitive behavior therapy for preventing first-episode psychosis in people with ultra-high risk. *Journal of Mental Health Policy and Economics*, *20*, S17–S17.

Jauhar, S., McKenna, P. J., Radua, J., Fung, E., Salvador, R., & Laws, K. R. (2014). Cognitive–behavioural therapy for the symptoms of schizophrenia: systematic review and meta-analysis with examination of potential bias. *British Journal of Psychiatry*, *204*(1), 20–29.

Jones, C., Hacker, D., Xia, J., Meaden, A., Irving, C. B., Zhao, S., Chen, J., & Shi, C. (2018). Cognitive behavioural therapy plus standard care versus standard care for people with schizophrenia. *Cochrane Database of Systematic Reviews*, *12*, CD007964. https://doi.org/10.1002/14651858.CD007964.pub

Klingberg, T., Fernell, E., Olesen, P. J., Johnson, M., Gustafsson, P., Dahlström, K., Gillberg, C., Forssberg, H., & Westerberg, H. (2005). Computerized training of working memory in children with ADHD—a randomized, controlled trial. *Journal of the American Academy of Child & Adolescent Psychiatry*, *44*(2), 177–186.

Langberg, J. M., Epstein, J. N., Becker, S. P., Girio-Herrera, E., & Vaughn, A. J. (2012). Evaluation of the Homework, Organization, and Planning Skills (HOPS) intervention for middle school students with ADHD as implemented by school mental health providers. *School Psychology Review*, *41*(3), 342.

Lange, A. M., Daley, D., Frydenberg, M., Houmann, T., Kristensen, L. J., Rask, C., Sonuga–Barke, E., Søndergaard–Baden, S., Udupi, A., & Thomsen, P. H. (2018). Parent training for preschool ADHD in routine, specialist care: a randomized controlled trial. *Journal of the American Academy of Child & Adolescent Psychiatry*, *57*(8), 593–602.

LaVigna, G. W., & Willis, T. J. (2012). The efficacy of positive behavioural support with the most challenging behaviour: the evidence and its implications. *Journal of Intellectual and Developmental Disability*, *37*(3), 185–195.

Lovaas, O. I. (2003). *Teaching individuals with developmental delays: basic intervention techniques*. Pro-ed.

MacDonald, A., & McGill, P. (2013). Outcomes of staff training in positive behaviour support: a systematic review. *Journal of Developmental and Physical Disabilities*, *25*(1), 17–33.

Malow, B. A., Byars, K., Johnson, K., Weiss, S., Bernal, P., Goldman, S. E., Panzer, R., Coury, D. L., Glaze, D. G., & Sleep Committee of the Autism Treatment Network. (2012). A practice pathway for the identification, evaluation, and management of insomnia in children and adolescents with autism spectrum disorders. *Pediatrics*, *130*(Suppl 2), S106–S124.

March, J., Silva, S., Petrycki, S., Curry, J., Wells, K., Fairbank, J., Burns, B., Domino, M., McNulty, S., Vitiello, B., Severe, J., & Treatment for Adolescents with Depression Study (TADS) Team. (2004). Fluoxetine, cognitive-behavioral therapy, and their combination for adolescents with depression: Treatment for Adolescents with Depression Study (TADS) randomized controlled trial. *Journal of the American Medical Association*, *292*(7), 807–820.

McGillivray, J. A., & Evert, H. T. (2014). Group cognitive behavioural therapy program shows potential in reducing symptoms of depression and stress among young people with ASD. *Journal of Autism and Developmental Disorders*, *44*(8), 2041–2051.

McGuire, J. F., Ricketts, E. J., Piacentini, J., Murphy, T. K., Storch, E. A., & Lewin, A. B. (2015). Behavior therapy for tic disorders: an evidenced-based review and new directions for treatment research. *Current Developmental Disorders Reports*, *2*(4), 309–317.

McIntyre, L. L. (2008). Adapting Webster–Stratton's incredible years parent training for children with developmental delay: findings from a treatment group only study. *Journal of Intellectual Disability Research*, 52(12), 1176–1192.

Molina, B. S., Flory, K., Bukstein, O. G., Greiner, A. R., Baker, J. L., Krug, V., & Evans, S. W. (2008). Feasibility and preliminary efficacy of an after-school program for middle schoolers with ADHD: a randomized trial in a large public middle school. *Journal of Attention Disorders*, 12(3), 207–217.

Molina, B. S., Hinshaw, S. P., Swanson, J. M., Arnold, L. E., Vitiello, B., Jensen, P. S., Epstein, J. N., Hoza, B., Hechtman, L., Abikoff, H. B., Elliott, G. R., Greenhill, L. L., Newcorn, J. H., Wells, K. C., Wigal, T., Gibbons, R. D., Hur, K., Houck, P. R., & MTA Cooperative Group. (2009). The MTA at 8 years: prospective follow-up of children treated for combined-type ADHD in a multisite study. *Journal of the American Academy of Child & Adolescent Psychiatry*, 48(5), 484–500.

National Institute for Clinical Excellence. (2013). *Autism spectrum disorder in under 19s: support and management*. NICE guideline [CG170]. https://www. nice. org. uk/guidance/cg170

National Institute for Health and Care Excellence (NICE). (2018a). *Learning disabilities and behaviour that challenges: service design and delivery*. NICE guideline [NG 9]. https://www.nice.org.uk/guidance/ng93

National Institute for Health and Care Excellence (NICE). (2018b). *Attention deficit hyperactivity disorder: diagnosis and management*. NICE guideline [NG87]. https://www. nice. org. uk/guidance/cg87

Newton, E., Landau, S., Smith, P., Monks, P., Shergill, S., & Wykes, T. (2005). Early psychological intervention for auditory hallucinations: an exploratory study of young people's voices groups. *Journal of Nervous and Mental Disease*, 193(1), 58–61.

Pelham Jr, W. E., & Fabiano, G. A. (2008). Evidence-based psychosocial treatments for attention-deficit/hyperactivity disorder. *Journal of Clinical Child & Adolescent Psychology*, 37(1), 184–214.

Pfiffner, L. J., Hinshaw, S. P., Owens, E., Zalecki, C., Kaiser, N. M., Villodas, M., & McBurnett, K. (2014). A two-site randomized clinical trial of integrated psychosocial treatment for ADHD-inattentive type. *Journal of Consulting and Clinical Psychology*, 82(6), 1115.

Pickles, A., Le Couteur, A., Leadbitter, K., Salomone, E., Cole-Fletcher, R., Tobin, H., ... & Green, J. (2016). Parent-mediated social communication therapy for young children with autism (PACT): long-term follow-up of a randomised controlled trial. *The Lancet*, 388(10059), 2501–2509.

Plueck, J., Eichelberger, I., Hautmann, C., Hanisch, C., Jaenen, N., & Doepfner, M. (2015). Effectiveness of a teacher-based indicated prevention program for preschool children with externalizing problem behavior. *Prevention Science*, 16(2), 233–241.

Robin, A. L. (2014). Family therapy for adolescents with ADHD. *Child and Adolescent Psychiatric Clinics*, 23(4), 747–756.

Russell, A. J., Jassi, A., Fullana, M. A., Mack, H., Johnston, K., Heyman, I., & Mataix–Cols, D. (2013). Cognitive behaviour therapy for comorbid obsessive-compulsive disorder in high-functioning autism spectrum disorders: a randomised controlled trial. *Depression and Anxiety*, 30, 679–708.

Sibley, M. H., Graziano, P. A., Kuriyan, A. B., Coxe, S., Pelham, W. E., Rodriguez, L., Sanchez, F., Derefinko, K., Helseth, S., & Ward, A. (2016). Parent–teen behavior therapy + motivational interviewing for adolescents with ADHD. *Journal of Consulting and Clinical Psychology*, *84*(8), 699.

Specht, M. W., Mahone, E. M., Kline, T., Waranch, R., Brabson, L., Thompson, C. B., & Singer, H. S. (2017). Efficacy of parent-delivered behavioral therapy for primary complex motor stereotypies. *Developmental Medicine & Child Neurology*, *59*(2), 168–173.

Stafford, M. R., Mayo–Wilson, E., Loucas, C. E., James, A., Hollis, C., Birchwood, M., & Kendall, T. (2015). Efficacy and safety of pharmacological and psychological interventions for the treatment of psychosis and schizophrenia in children, adolescents and young adults: a systematic review and meta-analysis. *PloS One*, *10*(2), e0117166.

Stain, H. J., Bucci, S., Baker, A. L., Carr, V., Emsley, R., Halpin, S., Lewin, T., Schall, U., Clarke, V., Crittenden, K., & Startup, M. (2016). A randomised controlled trial of cognitive behaviour therapy versus non-directive reflective listening for young people at ultra high risk of developing psychosis: the detection and evaluation of psychological therapy (DEPTh) trial. *Schizophrenia Research*, *176*(2–3), 212–219.

Storebø, O. J., Skoog, M., Damm, D., Thomsen, P. H., Simonsen, E., & Gluud, C. (2011). Social skills training for attention deficit hyperactivity disorder (ADHD) in children aged 5 to 18 years. *Cochrane Database of Systematic Reviews*, 12, CD008223. https://doi.org/10.1002/14651858.CD008223.pub2

Sukhodolsky, D. G., Kassinove, H., & Gorman, B. S. (2004). Cognitive-behavioral therapy for anger in children and adolescents: a meta-analysis. *Aggression and Violent Behavior, 9*(3), 247–269.

Swain, J., Hancock, K., Dixon, A., & Bowman, J. (2015). Acceptance and commitment therapy for children: a systematic review of intervention studies. *Journal of Contextual Behavioral Science, 4*(2), 73–85.

Thomas, N., Hayward, M., Peters, E., van der Gaag, M., Bentall, R. P., Jenner, J., Strauss, C., Sommer, I. E., Johns, L. C., Varese, F., García–Montes, J. M., Waters, F., Dodgson, G., McCarthy–Jones, S. (2014). Psychological therapies for auditory hallucinations (voices): current status and key directions for future research. *Schizophrenia Bulletin, 40*(Suppl 4), S202–S212.

Thomas, R., Abell, B., Webb, H. J., Avdagic, E., & Zimmer–Gembeck, M. J. (2017). Parent–child interaction therapy: a meta-analysis. *Pediatrics, 140*(3), e20170352.

Tymms, P., & Merrell, C. (2006). The impact of screening and advice on inattentive, hyperactive and impulsive children. *European Journal of Special Needs Education, 21*(3), 321–337.

Verschuur, R., Didden, R., Lang, R., Sigafoos, J., & Huskens, B. (2014). Pivotal response treatment for children with autism spectrum disorders: a systematic review. *Review Journal of Autism and Developmental Disorders, 1*(1), 34–61.

Virues–Ortega, J., Julio, F. M., & Pastor–Barriuso, R. (2013). The TEACCH program for children and adults with autism: a meta-analysis of intervention studies. *Clinical Psychology Review, 33*(8), 940–953.

Walters, S., Loades, M., & Russell, A. (2016). A systematic review of effective modifications to cognitive behavioural therapy for young people with autism spectrum disorders. *Review Journal of Autism and Developmental Disorders, 3*(2), 137–153.

Webster–Stratton, C. H., Reid, M. J., & Beauchaine, T. (2011). Combining parent and child training for young children with ADHD. *Journal of Clinical Child & Adolescent Psychology, 40*(2), 191–203.

Wethington, H. R., Hahn, R. A., Fuqua–Whitley, D. S., Sipe, T. A., Crosby, A. E., Johnson, R. L., Liberman, A. M., Moscicki, E., Price, L. N., Tuma, F. K., Kalra, G., Chattopadhyay, S. K., & Task Force on Community Preventive Services. (2008). The effectiveness of interventions to reduce psychological harm from traumatic events among children and adolescents: a systematic review. *American Journal of Preventive Medicine*, *35*(3), 287–313.

Whittingham, K., Sanders, M., McKinlay, L., & Boyd, R. N. (2014). Interventions to reduce behavioral problems in children with cerebral palsy: an RCT. *Pediatrics*, *133*(5), e1249–e1257.

CHAPTER 9

··

DRUG TREATMENTS

··

THIS chapter describes the use of medication in alleviating the problems of young people with neurodevelopmental disorders. It gives special emphasis to its use in multiple overlapping conditions, the long-term impact on functioning, and the avoidance of harm from unwanted drug effects.

9.1 CLASSIFICATION

Psychotropic drugs are mostly classified by the indications for which they were originally introduced into adult psychiatry: antidepressant, antimanic, mood-stabilizing, antipsychotic, antianxiety (anxiolytic), hypnotic, and so on. Stimulant and other antihyperactivity drugs are the exception, since they were introduced and developed specifically for children with attentional deficit hyperactivity disorder (ADHD).

This functional way of describing drugs is useful in guiding clinicians to practical decisions about what to prescribe for whom. It also carries some disadvantages. It oversimplifies the range of indications and drug actions. Communication with patients and families can be made awkward. If, for instance, the prescription of an antipsychotic to control severe anxiety is taken by the family to imply that the prescriber thinks that the patient has schizophrenia, the impact can be confusion. Confused communication is not necessarily an overwhelming objection. It does mean that advice, to patients and families, needs to be clear and explicit—in other words, to follow good practice.

Another potential difficulty is that the traditional terminology by indications says little about the type of action and, therefore, confounds together many different types of drug. Combinations of drugs are so common in the treatment of complex cases that prescribers need to keep clarity about whether they are combining different modes of action or using multiple drugs with similar pharmacological actions. The latter may in effect be increasing dosage and can invite toxicity.

A shift to a neuroscience-based classification of drug therapies is well under way in general adult psychiatry (Caraci et al., 2017). It is based on the pharmacological targets and the modes of action. It reflects the massive growth in knowledge about brain chemistry and function. At the time of writing, however, it has not been extended to a paediatric system and so is not recommended for general use in children. It may be a helpful tool for thought when considering the choice of drugs for adolescents and young adults. It is always useful to bear in mind the pharmacological targets and intended modes of action of drugs to be prescribed. Psychotropic drugs work through interactions with the neurotransmitters and receptors in the brain.

> *Pharmacological targets* include levels of acetylcholine, dopamine, GABA, glutamate, histamine, ion channels, melatonin, noradrenaline (norepinephrine), opioids, serotonin, and an uncertain number of substances considered as possible targets in incomplete knowledge (e.g. inositol for lithium-mimetic drugs).
>
> *Pharmacological modes of action*: A drug may act as a receptor agonist, receptor partial agonist, receptor antagonist, or a reuptake inhibitor or releaser. Other actions include: activating or inhibiting enzymes that regulate intracellular pathways; blocking or opening ion channels that influence sodium, potassium, or calcium entry into neurons; regulating the release of other neuromodulators; and positive allosteric modulation (binding to part of a receptor or enzyme that is different from the part of the molecule that constitutes its principal binding site).

An individual drug may well have several targets and modes of action. Classification on this neuroscience basis would do better justice to the complexity of action than traditional descriptions such as 'antidepressant'. By the same token, it would be harder to understand and could hinder communication with the public and other professionals. This chapter is organized by the effects likely to be desired in clinical practice.

9.2 SPECIAL CONSIDERATIONS IN NEUROPSYCHIATRY

In the treatment of neurodevelopmental disorders, special considerations apply.

9.2.1 Multiple diagnoses

Several diagnoses are very often present in the same person. It can therefore be difficult to apply official guidelines, which often focus on one diagnosis considered in the absence of others. Similarly, the trials of drugs usually focus on one diagnosis considered singly. This limitation comes mostly from the requirement of many national drug regulators that the introduction of a new drug should be for a specified diagnosis. The evidence base of drug trials is therefore only a partial guide to practice in complex neuropsychiatric conditions. Nevertheless, clinicians need to bear it very much in mind.

9.2.2 Off-label prescribing

Governmental rules can sometimes make it impossible, or at least difficult, to prescribe for 'off-label' indications. The licence issued by national and supranational regulators is not to the prescriber, but to the company distributing the medicine. It gives permission for marketing. It is restricted to the disorder, the approved dosage, the approved age range, and the duration of treatment. In most countries, it is still possible to prescribe outside the approved use (i.e. 'off label'). It is not the same as contraindication. The lack of approval may simply mean that it has not been formally considered. Use in childhood is very often outside the licensed indications even for well-established drugs. Until recent years, approval for children was often simply not sought by the marketing company, for economic reasons.

Off-label use can be entirely appropriate. Nevertheless, if a drug is being prescribed outside the licensed indications, there may well not be enough evidence, for instance about adverse effects, to guide confident practice. The young people and/or those consenting on their behalf should be explicitly informed as part of the process of obtaining informed consent.

9.2.3 Adverse effects

Adverse effects are usually more frequent in people with compromised brains than in typically developing people. They may limit the dosage and the value of the treatment. They create difficult clinical choices between benefits and harms. Ethical issues arise if people without the capacity to consent are given medication that will mostly benefit the carers looking after them, yet the adverse effects of which are borne by themselves.

9.2.4 Multiple indications and actions

The multiplicity of drug actions also makes it difficult to translate the official and pharmacological classifications into practice. Antipsychotic drugs that block dopaminergic transmission, for example, are useful not only for psychotic conditions but also for emotional dysregulation, obsessive-compulsive disorders, severe anxiety, tics and Tourette, and states of high agitation and aggression.

This chapter will therefore include both a general account of approaches to drug management and a description of the use of selected drugs, organized by the behavioural targets that clinicians are likely to want to modify, rather than by the diagnoses or the pharmacological actions on receptors. The targets are, for the most part, to remove or reduce obstacles to healthy development and independence.

9.3 APPROACHES TO DRUG MANAGEMENT

9.3.1 The first trial of medication

When first considering drug use for an individual patient, clinicians organize their analysis by the following set of questions and factors.

9.3.1.1 *Is medication appropriate?*

This will involve consideration of the likely natural course and the possibility of non-drug intervention (see Chapter 8). For some conditions—notably ADHD of at least moderate severity, schizophrenia, and bipolar disorder—medication will be a first line of treatment. For others—such as mild to moderate aggression, tics, and anxiety– it will make sense to begin with supportive measures or psychological treatment, but include sufficient monitoring of outcome that it is possible to decide reasonably quickly whether or not it will be enough in the longer term. For depression, most guidelines advocate beginning with a psychotherapy such as cognitive behavioural therapy (CBT). The guidelines have not, however, been elaborated for people in whom depression coexists with conditions such as ADHD, autism spectrum disorder (ASD), or the presence of neurological abnormalities. Nor have they fully digested the evidence that a combination of CBT and a selective serotonin reuptake inhibitor (SSRI) from the start will result in fewer suicidal thoughts and self-harming actions for most children with moderate to severe depression (National Collaborating Centre for Mental Health, 2005).

9.3.1.2 *Choice of target(s)*

Many young people have multiple disorders. Most disorders have many components. Successful prescribing therefore needs clear formulation about the targets for treatment in the individual case. Which components of the overall presentation are responsible for the impact, and which are most likely to respond to medication?

If diagnosis alone is the target, there is a risk of missing therapeutic possibilities that do not involve all aspects of the diagnosis. In ASD, for instance, there is usually no overall effect of drug treatment on the diagnosis. Nevertheless, there can be useful reduction of single components, such as irritability, that have a major effect on quality of life. Similarly, in the spectrum of schizophrenia, dopamine-blocking drugs can have a very helpful effect on the positive features of hallucinations and delusions without much benefit on the negative symptoms of flattened affect and social withdrawal. If there is little benefit on the latter, it does not mean that the drug is ineffective.

A target is partly a hypothesis about the nature of a young person's condition, and any change with a drug is a test of the hypothesis.

9.3.1.3 *Monitoring targets*

The selection of the most promising target(s) for the individual needs to be written down in the case records, the rationale recorded, and a suitable scheme of monitoring devised. This may be a brief rating scale of the severity of the usual features of the disorder, but one should add the key target if it is not on the checklist already. Adverse effects should also be monitored—with a standard scale if possible. Relying on spontaneous accounts may well miss unobtrusive early signs of danger such as muscle stiffness in people taking antidopaminergic drugs. Patients and their families may be reluctant to reveal some types of problem, such as sexual dysfunction, unless they are directly asked for.

Monitoring should be started before treatment so that the initial impact can be documented. If there are serious possible hazards of a drug—for instance, of movement disorders appearing in the course of treatment with dopamine-blocking drugs—then there should be a detailed assessment of the pre-treatment status. In this example, it is common for young people developing schizophrenia to have minor, and unnoticed, extrapyramidal motor signs that are later misattributed to an adverse drug effect.

The broad picture needs to be born in mind, as well as the details of impact on targets. The clinician's overall impression should be recorded as part of the evaluation of drug effectiveness.

9.3.1.4 *Choice of drug*

Nowadays, there are many drugs available for the indications of ADHD, depression, anxiety, and disruptive behaviour. These are summarized in the tables in this chapter. They are too numerous for any but the most expert practitioners to command full knowledge. Accordingly, most practitioners are advised to know their limits and to master just one drug in each class. It should be selected on the basis of availability, acceptability, and (for most societies) cost. This personal favourite will be the 'P drug'—'P' for personal (recommendation from the World Health Organization (WHO) manual by DeVries et al. (1994)). It will be the one usually given and the one for which the prescriber has good recent knowledge about doses, indications, adverse effects, prices, and drug interactions. Naturally, there will be occasions when it is not appropriate for an individual patient. However, in choosing a drug with which one is unfamiliar, it is sensible to consult with others with expertise and/or with an authoritative manual for the important details of timing of action, dose schedules, and interactions. It should be kept readily available, on the desk or computer. The *British National Formulary* has the important benefit of detailed cover for paediatric practice (BNFC, 2019). It is available free on the NICE (National Institute for Health and Care Excellence) website. (There are more drugs available in the USA.)

Sometimes, the choice is easy. Fluoxetine is the only antidepressant drug with robust evidence for value in depressed children; from a careful network analysis by Cipriani et al. (2016). With other indications (e.g. the antipsychotics and antidepressants), the choice is much wider and one's 'P drug' may need to be reviewed as new ones come into the market, new evaluations appear, and costs vary with expiry of patents. Some clinicians dislike any idea of using price as a criterion for drug choice. Is it not more ethical, they may say, to base the choice purely on the best interest of the individual patient? Most clinicians, however, recognize a duty to society as well as the individual patient. In a cash-limited service, unnecessary cost reduces the chance of other potential patients being properly treated.

Community services may well be resistant to off-label or unusually expensive prescriptions. The need for them would have to be made explicit from an early stage. Specialist teams might need to take on routine monitoring and prescription. If this becomes frequent, commissioners of the service will need to be informed of the implications for the risk of specialist services becoming overwhelmed by an accumulation of long-term cases.

9.3.1.5 *What medications are they already taking?*

Most drug trials are not conducted on patients who are naïve to medication. For ethical reasons, many trials exclude subjects who have had a poor response already. Conversely, for reasons of practicality and recruitment, they also exclude those who are faring exceptionally well with their prescribed drug. This selection process will limit the confidence in the application of trial results to the individual.

By contrast, the first clinical decision to prescribe is, by definition, taken for patients who are new to drug therapy. In the case of stimulants for ADHD, the initial prescription may well be taken by a non-specialist. Methylphenidate is a first-line treatment for which severe adverse effects are uncommon and it is so quick in its action that titration is simple. It is therefore not unreasonable, albeit not ideal, for the drug to be an early recourse for general practitioners, generalist paediatricians, and general psychiatrists. When this is the case, referral to a specialist in neurodevelopmental disorders may well come only after failure of the first-line treatment. A careful drug history of the individual patient should be taken.

Polypharmacy is often decried. Certainly, at the outset of drug treatment, it should be avoided unless the key drug also requires an antidote to its adverse effects. Combinations of drugs may seem to increase the chance of a good drug response right away, but the price is uncertainty about which drug is helping. In the long haul of prescribing for a chronic disorder (see Section 9.3.2), effective therapy needs to be based on a strategy and clear knowledge of what has been helpful or unhelpful in the past.

9.3.1.6 *Explanation*

The choice of what and how to treat will not only be that of the individual prescriber. The young person and their caregivers need to be involved. In a multidisciplinary service, other professionals in the therapeutic team should be encouraged to contribute. Other specialist services need to know what is being proposed, not least because of the possibility that they prescribe drugs for other conditions that will interact.

Young people and their families will come to discussions about medication with attitudes, hopes, and fears. Their trust in the advice they get is crucial. It will determine their adherence to therapy plans. That adherence will sometimes have to be maintained by them in the face of conflicting advice from friends, family, estranged partners, teachers, or social workers with different beliefs about what should help. The clinician's advice about drugs will therefore need to be subsequent to, and founded on, the careful formulation of the patient's problems, strengths, weaknesses, and likely future. Consent and assent should be unforced and founded on good information. Ideally, this should be given in person, and in ways that are understandable to the individual, backed up with written information that can be more comprehensive. The information that they will need includes:

- The condition to be treated and the targets chosen
- The nature of the drug being proposed
- The time the drug may need to work
- The strength of evidence for benefits
- The likelihood and nature of significant adverse events (bearing in mind that a comprehensive list of all reported harms would be valueless to most people and scary to many)
- The risks and potential benefits of alternative treatments, including withholding medication.

Standard fact sheets are usually available from pharmacies. For people with literacy problems, easy-reading versions should be provided. For people with wider communication problems, extra time is probably necessary to convey information with added clarity and simplicity, and for checks that it has been understood. Even then, miscommunication is easy.

The final responsibility for medication lies with the prescriber. Accordingly, if the routine prescription after initial assessment is to be handed over, perhaps to the general practitioner, then that person should be consulted from the start.

9.3.1.7 *Dosage and administration*

The pharmacokinetics of young people are more complex than the simple recognition that they are smaller and weigh less. The special considerations can be summarized as:

Will the drugs be swallowed? Many neurodevelopmental conditions involve compromised motor function, making swallowing uncoordinated. Strong aversion to the taste or texture or colour of medication may limit the chance of medication reaching the gut. Hostility towards medication by the wider range of caregivers (e.g. grandparents, estranged partners, care workers, class teachers) may mean that the drug is not given at all or given only intermittently. Liquid preparations are often available (though not for controlled drugs); granular preparations can be sprinkled on food. Unpleasant tastes can be dispersed with chewing gum or with cold drinks (e.g. sour ones such as lemonade). Other drugs may be more acceptable.

Will they be absorbed from the gut? The stomach in children is a less acid environment than in adults, so acidic drugs may be less well absorbed.

Will they survive hepatic metabolism? Children's livers, after the first years, are large and very effective at conjugation and oxidization, so blood levels may be lower than would be the case in adult life.

Will they be more diluted in the extracellular fluid? Before adolescence, this fluid comprises a greater proportion of the body.

All these influences tend to reduce bioavailability in childhood. None of them is fully compensated by the usual advice to prescribe on a mg/kg basis. Dilution in the extracellular fluid could, in principle, be allowed for by calculation on the basis of surface area, but an unfamiliar calculation invites prescribing errors. Furthermore, other influences may act in opposition, to increase bioavailability. The blood–brain barrier is more permeable in children than adults (reflected by higher levels of protein in the cerebrospinal fluid), so more drug may enter the brain to interact with receptors.

These uncertainties combine to make fixed doses impractical. Accordingly, many of the doses in the following sections are given as ranges. Within them, the prescriber should titrate according to the behavioural response. The general advice is to expect adverse events, begin with a dose at the bottom of the range, and work up slowly to a level that is either effective or producing adverse effects. This general advice to 'start low and go slow' is easy to apply for short-acting drugs. It may need to be modified for drugs, such as dopamine blockers, that take weeks for a full response to appear. A very long schedule of introduction risks persuading caregivers that the drugs are not working and should be stopped. Pragmatic choices should be made.

9.3.1.8 *Methods of monitoring*

Ideal monitoring will be more detailed than an overall impression as the treatment proceeds. Drugs whose full action appears only over a course of some weeks may still show the beginning of helpful action earlier. If the subtler signs of action start to appear, then it may be important to detect them so as to sustain the morale of those who are giving them or taking them. At the time of writing, a number of apps are appearing with the purpose of monitoring doses and actions. This may be on the basis of self-report (e.g. of mood state for rapidly changing emotional states) or of objective findings (e.g. of accelerometer-measured activity for drugs modifying hyperactivity). It is too soon to be clear whether their reliability and sensitivity to change is up to the mark, but they are popular as adjuncts to the full clinical review.

9.3.2 Considerations after the first episode of treatment is completed

After the initial decisions, explanations, and trial of medication, there will be various further needs for good prescribing.

9.3.2.1 *Evaluation*

Were the effects as hoped? Was the treatment acceptable and taken as intended? Has the attitude towards the disorder changed?

The initial setting of targets and goals will have been created jointly with the patient and their family. The initial trial should lead on to a joint decision about the extent to which the goals have been achieved, and any harms that have been incurred. The published trials will have led prescribers to an expectation about the effect size on (for instance) symptom reduction, and they will want to review whether it has been achieved. For patients and their families, they will be able to revise their expectations after they have seen and discussed the effects of the first period of treatment.

In the long term, it will be very helpful to make a record of the evaluation. Perhaps patients and families will have been encouraged to document before and after states, possibly with a recording on their smartphones. Future uncertainty about whether the drug is really helping can be resolved with a contemporary record. An initially good response may have led to a recalibration of family expectations and, thereby, to later dissatisfaction with the treatment.

9.3.2.2 *Case review*

If the response has been less than satisfactory, the review will need to ask why. In retrospect, was the target appropriate? Was the dose too low (or too high)? Did adverse effects limit how much could be given? Did a good initial response wane, suggesting a need for a higher dose? Does the diagnosis need to be revised? Was adherence compromised by avoidable problems? Is the patient being scapegoated for a poor response—'it shows that your bad behaviour is not an illness, it is your own fault'? Alternatively, after a very good response, would a lower dose have some value and less toxicity? Initial delight from parents may lead to different inferences about the problem. Sometimes this is liberating—'now we know that your problems have answers'. Sometimes it is oppressive, if a premature and overoptimistic decision is made about the kind of education or employment they can cope with.

A good response to stimulants in ADHD or to anti-tic medication can be very educational. It differentiates the problem from the person. It will help the young people to review themselves with and without the problem that has been treated. It sometimes leads to their setting differing goals for themselves. This self-understanding is so important to people living with a disability that it is worth extended discussion. The young people will often say that they want more time to discuss the implications of their response with the prescriber. The time is worth taking in helping them to become intelligent consumers of their medicine.

Consent and explanation are not a one-off matter. They usually need repeating as time goes by, as the concerns of young people and their families change, and often as more complex aspects can be understood.

9.3.2.3 *Adherence*

Continuing use of medication can be challenged in several ways. Adverse effects may not have been successfully dealt with. Control of dosage may not have been close enough. An efficacious medication may have been discontinued even though it is still having the intended effects. (See 'Effectiveness in the long term', Section 9.4.7).

9.3.2.4 *Strategic planning*

In the long term, there will be many changes. The disorder itself may change, as one or another of its components becomes more important in limiting adjustment. The environmental challenges will be changing, too. Sometimes, the changes will be predictable, for instance with secondary-school entry or taking an apprenticeship. Sometimes, they will be unpredictable, for instance in encountering the justice system or family turbulence. In either case, the young person's resources and understanding will condition the impact.

Some of the implications for drug treatment will, therefore, change over time. As young people get older and their bodies change and they encounter more difficult topics in education, stimulant drugs (for example) may need as much or more adjustment as would insulin administration in diabetes. Accordingly, successive decisions about treatment will need a strategic approach. Suggested principles for long-term thinking are:

- Ensuring that the patient and caregivers are part of decision making and understand the rationale for changes.
- Making one change at a time.
- Optimizing one drug before changing to another.
- Encouraging intelligent adherence.
- Keeping medicines safe.
- Consulting with other professionals when introducing an unfamiliar drug.
- Applying caution about polypharmacy and consulting references about drug interactions. Polypharmacy, however, should not be avoided altogether. When two indications are present (e.g. depression and ADHD), it may be better to use separate drugs for each (e.g. methylphenidate and fluoxetine) rather than one drug with combined actions (e.g. sertraline). The dual-action drug may be suboptimal for either condition and harder to adjust. Furthermore, drug combinations may be intended to have an adjuvant effect, for instance when a mood stabilizer is added to an antidepressant. When a change of medication is planned (e.g. from a stimulant to a nonstimulant, to reduce inattention/impulsiveness), then it may well be justified to give both together for a period. It is all too easy, however, to drift into a prolonged period of drug combination. The original rationale should be recorded and respected.

The young people may well wish to have continuity of care from their clinician(s) but it is not always possible to provide it. A new prescriber will have to take over a complex history. The clearer the documentation of treatment changes, the easier handover will be. The frequent situation of multiple drug changes over the years is greatly helped if there is a continuing record of changes of drug, the reasons for them, and the effects on symptoms and overall adjustment. Graphical representations of progress for the individual case over time are usually a better communication than a search of the case notes. Unfortunately, many current electronic case records do not allow simple presentations of course in relation to treatment. Prescribers then need to develop their personal systems.

People with complex genetic or neurological conditions will often have several providers of service. They should be kept informed. Sometimes drugs that can interact with each other are being prescribed by different teams. Clearly, this can create problems. An important and frequent example comes from the coexistence of needs for psychotropics and drugs to control epilepsy—which is considered separately in Sections in Chapter 6, on iatrogenic problems, 6.2.6.5, and treatment of mental disorders in epilepsy, 6.2.7. Cooperation between services can also be very helpful, for instance when a mental health service can call on a learning disability service for assistance with monitoring and swallowing. When a specialist service is sharing care with general practice, the monitoring of adverse physical effects can be made in the general practice, to be convenient for the family. There must, however be clear arrangements in place for who does what.

9.4 Pharmacology of drugs to reduce inattention and hyperactivity-impulsiveness

The treatment of people with ADHD is the most frequently researched topic in the whole of developmental neuropsychiatry. It has attracted systematic reviews and meta-analyses. There is much agreement: for instance, virtually all trials of stimulant medication show significant reduction of core features of ADHD. There is also scope for controversy. The quality of trials is not high by modern standards and attracts different ratings by different reviewers. The correct balance of psychological versus pharmacological interventions is arguable and varies between individuals. The limitations of current therapies, including stimulant drugs, are not always fully appreciated. The use of medication varies greatly from place to place and from time to time.

Most trials are funded by companies and, correspondingly, their designs follow registration and marketing purposes. Subjects in the trials are most often school-age children and adolescents selected, in part, for the absence of intellectual disability (ID) and autism.

9.4.1 Central nervous system (CNS) stimulants

9.4.1.1 *Effects*

Stimulants—methylphenidate and amphetamines—are the most widely used drugs. Methylphenidate is the usual first choice in children (outside the USA, where amphetamines predominate). It acts primarily as an inhibitor of the reuptake of dopamine and noradrenaline (NDRI) by inhibiting the transporter. It also has some agonist activity at the serotonin type 1A receptor and inhibits the vesicular monoamine transporter. Amphetamine actions also include dopamine and noradrenaline transporter inhibition and, additionally, monoamine oxidase inhibition. It contributes to the release of monoamines via inhibition of the vesicular monoamine transporter 2 (VMAT-2). The difference in mechanism of action between methylphenidate and amphetamine results in methylphenidate inhibiting amphetamine's effects on releasing monoamines if they are given at the same time.

About 70% of the children with uncomplicated ADHD respond to the first stimulant tried—usually methylphenidate or lisdexamfetamine. If the first drug tried fails, replacement with a second stimulant increases the response rate in trials to about 90%.

Meta-analysis by Faraone and Buitelaar (2010) drew on 23 randomized controlled trials, involving 3,760 patients. It indicated large effect sizes for stimulants in reducing rated severity of hyperactivity/impulsiveness and inattention. Effect sizes for methylphenidate were 0.9 SD; for amphetamines, 1.2 SD—corresponding to figures for numbers needed to treat (NNT) of 2.6 for methylphenidate and 2.0 for amphetamines. The stimulants also have more beneficial effects than placebo on a variety of tests of cognitive performance. A systematic review by Coghill et al. (2014) indicated significant effect sizes on executive memory (0.26), non-executive memory (0.60), reaction time (0.24), reaction time variability (0.62), and response inhibition (0.41).

9.4.1.2 *Time course*

The various preparations of methylphenidate differ mostly in their duration of action, as set out in Table 9.1. The choice of preparation should reflect the time course of activities during the day. Deterioration of attention in the afternoon ('postprandial dip') will be familiar to most teachers. More, the difference between methylphenidate and placebo tends to be smaller in the afternoons. This was the rationale for the formulation of Concerta™, designed to give a rising blood level as the day wears on. Other extended-release preparations typically aim to mimic the blood levels achieved by twice-daily doses of immediate-release methylphenidate. There are advantages to choosing extended-release preparations. A single daily dose is more likely to be remembered and taken regularly. A dose that can be taken before school maintains privacy and is less likely to attract disapproving attention from teachers and peers. Some clinicians, however, prefer to use immediate-release medication from the start. This can provide an obvious guide to the size of effect and helps to give a clear idea of changing need during the day and, therefore, to the timing of doses.

Table 9.1 Widely available drugs for hyperactivity–impulsiveness

Drug Legal status	Preparations	Dose (per day)	Duration	Principal action
Methylphenidate Controlled drug	Immediate-release	5–60 mg in divided doses	2–4 hours	Noradrenaline–dopamine reuptake inhibitor
Extended-release methylphenidate (proprietary names given) Controlled drugs	OROS (osmotic-release): Concerta™ Equasym-XL™ (beaded); Medikinet–retard™ (beaded)	18–72 mg single dose 10–60 mg single dose	up to 12 hours up to 8 hours	As MPH; release controlled by capsule shell As MPH; release controlled by graded beads
Dexamphetamine Lisdexamphetamine (LDX) Controlled drugs	Immediate-release Extended-release (conjugated with lysine)	2.5–40 mg 20–70 mg	3–6 hours 10–13 hours	Noradrenaline–dopamine reuptake inhibitors and release agents LDX release controlled by metabolism
Atomoxetine Not controlled	Prolonged-action	0.5 mg/kg for first week, then 1.2 mg/kg; max. 1.8 mg/kg	Varies with individual metabolism (P450 (CYP) 2D6)	Noradrenaline reuptake inhibitor in the prefrontal cortex and elsewhere

Continued

Table 9.1 Continued

Alternative ADHD Drugs, not controlled

Drug	Special notes	Dose (per day)	Duration	Principal action
Bupropion	Not licensed in UK; caution re. seizures	50–200 mg divided doses (or single dose of XL formulation)	c. 6 hours	Nicotinic antagonism
Clonidine	Not licensed for children in most countries	0.05–0.4 mg divided doses (or single dose of XL formulation)	c. 4 hours	Alpha2-A,-B, & -C agonists, reducing NA release
Guanfacine	Licensed in Europe for children, not adults, not in combination with a stimulant	1–4 mg single dose	Prolonged (extended-release formulation)	Selective alpha2-A agonist
Modafinil	Licensed in Europe for narcolepsy in adults	200–425 mg single dose	Prolonged	Unknown; induces wakefulness

Doses for children aged 6 years or more. They should be regarded as indicative only; individual titration against response is required, and some children may need higher doses after appropriate review. Financial costs are not included as they vary between countries. The table does not include drugs considered too hazardous for this purpose (e.g. pemoline and desipramine) or refused a European licence (Adderall™, a mixture of amphetamine salts).

MPH = methylphenidate; LDX = lisdexamphetamine

Adapted from Sonuga-Barke E, Taylor E, Chapter 55: ADHD and hyperkinetic disorder. In: Thapar A, Pine DS, Leckman JF, et al., [Eds.], *Rutter's Child and Adolescent Psychiatry*, Sixth edition, pp. 738–756, Copyright (2015), with permission from John Wiley and Sons.

One reason for an apparent initial failure of medication is a mismatch between the timing and duration of doses given and the changing needs. If the medication has worn off in the evening, the parents may see less change than the teachers. If the prescriber is guided only by parent reports, the dose arrived at may then be too high for optimal action as seen by teachers, and cause undue subduing. Alternatively, a longer-acting medication may interfere more than a shorter-acting one with settling to sleep. Ideally, therefore, monitoring of action will take account of fluctuation through the day. It may well be that an extended-release preparation will need to be supplemented with immediate-release at certain times of the day. This should be regarded as dosage adjustment, not as polypharmacy.

9.4.1.3 *Effects in complex neurodevelopmental conditions*

Valuable changes in inattentive and impulsive behaviours can still be achieved in young people who show not only ADHD but also ASD and/or ID. The evidence base in this indication is useful but not complete, and there are differences between trials. Simonoff et al. (2013) compared stimulant and placebo in a randomized trial on 122 drug-free children aged 7–15 years with hyperkinetic disorder (severe ADHD) and an IQ of 30–69. Stimulant was favoured over placebo for ratings of impulsiveness and inattention. Effect sizes were somewhat smaller than for children with an ordinary IQ: 0.39 for the parent-rated Conners ADHD index; 0.52 for teacher ratings. Concerningly, adverse effects were substantially more common than in those without ASD or ID, and often restricted the dosage that could be given. A clinical implication is that dosage in those with complex disorders should be titrated against adverse events rather than size of beneficial effect.

Milder levels of familial ID may not, by themselves, raise quite the same concerns. Pearson et al. (2003) reported on the effects of methylphenidate in a group of 24 children with ADHD and 'mental retardation' but free of ASD and other psychiatric diagnoses (mean age 10.9 years and mean IQ 56.5). There were positive effects on teacher (not parent) ratings of hyperactivity by comparison with placebo. A higher dose (0.60 mg/kg twice a day) was more effective than a lower one (0.15 mg/kg), but came at a price of more problems in appetite and sleep suppression.

9.4.2 Atomoxetine

Atomoxetine is thought to act primarily as a selective inhibitor of the noradrenaline transporter. In the prefrontal cortex, therefore, it increases both noradrenaline (NA) and dopamine, since they are both removed by the NA transporter at that site. In the striatum and accumbens, however, atomoxetine has little effect on dopamine levels. Adverse events due to striatal stimulation, such as tics, are therefore less marked than with amphetamines, and atomoxetine is referred to as a non-stimulant. By the same token, it is less effective on the core features of ADHD. (Atomoxetine also binds to the serotonin transporter and blocks the N-methyl-d-aspartate (NMDA) receptor.)

The selectiveness of atomoxetine actions has theoretical potential for the safe reduction of ADHD features when they occur in people with ASD or other developmental disabilities. The available research, however, suggests only that it can reduce the core features, albeit to an uncertain extent (Aman et al., 2014). Increased irritability limits its value for complex cases, as is the case for stimulants.

The time course of action of atomoxetine is different from that of the stimulants. It takes weeks for the full effect to become apparent. For that reason, a dosage recommendation is given in Table 9.1, rather than a period of titration. Careful observation, however, will often detect the beginning of improvement in activity control and attention after a shorter period, perhaps a fortnight. This can speed up the period of initial trial.

The cytochrome enzyme that metabolizes atomoxetine has variations of structure that determine its speed of action. 'Rapid' or 'ultra rapid' time courses of action may allow a swifter increase of dose and, therefore, a shorter time to definitive dosage.

9.4.3   Other non-stimulants

Clonidine and *guanfacine* activate NA alpha-2 receptors and, thereby, reduce NA release. Consequently, they reduce both blood pressure and hyperactive behaviours, sometimes (not always) at the cost of sedation. They do not increase the severity of tics and may reduce them. There is a caution: the fluctuating course of tics in ADHD makes the value of NA agonists in the presence of Tourette disorder hard to assess in individual cases. Titration should be slow and monitoring careful. *Bupropion* is an aminoketone antidepressant and a non-competitive antagonist of nicotinic acetylcholine receptors. In its long-acting preparation, there is some evidence for anti-ADHD activity in adults. It can be considered off-label in young people refractory to better-established therapies.

A meta-analysis and network analysis by Cortese et al. (2018) was able to draw on efficacy and safety data for 10,068 children and adolescents, and 8,131 adults, from a range of trials. Out of the drugs mentioned in Table 9.1, methylphenidate emerged as first-choice medication for the short-term treatment of ADHD in children and adolescents. For adults, amphetamines took the first place. For both age groups, the likely balance of beneficial and adverse effects needs to be considered individually, as in Table 9.1.

9.4.4   Adverse effects of stimulants

To set against these positive findings, adverse events on stimulants are frequent but mostly mild: anorexia, headache, anxiety, tachycardia, possible growth reduction, and minor increases in blood pressure. They can usually be managed by symptomatic measures, or by modifying the dose or the drug (see Table 9.2). Severe adverse events are rare. In particular, sudden death is too rare to have figured even in large database searches, and cardiovascular changes are mostly mild and manageable (Hennissen et al., 2017).

Table 9.2 Management of adverse effects of stimulants

Symptom	Monitoring	Symptomatic	Second line
Appetite loss and growth reduction	Growth charts	Altering intake through day Modifying times of doses Dose reduction Drug holiday	Alternative antihyperkinetics or non-drug therapy
Sleep problems	Parent report pre- and post-medication	Altering dose regime (either reducing or increasing evening cover) Sleep hygiene Melatonin	Replace with atomoxetine Alternative antihyperkinetics Non-drug therapy
Blood pressure increase	Measurement and plotting on age charts: every 6 months when treatment is stable	Dose reduction Clonidine	24-hour recording Specialist referral if over 95th centile
Tachycardia	Pre-treatment history and examination Measurement when BP recorded	ECG evaluation Dose reduction	Specialist referral
Substance misuse	Tablet count Enquiry at psychiatric review	Psychoeducation Extended-release Motivational interview	Replace with atomoxetine
Mood change, irritability in ASD and ID	Psychiatric review Dose reduction	Consider alternative antihyperkinetic	Add fluoxetine or mood stabilizer
Tics	Monitor frequency and impact	Review dose	Supplement or replace with clonidine, guanfacine or atomoxetine

Misuse of medication is often feared, but dependence and unprescribed use almost never appear in those given therapeutic doses by mouth. Stimulants are capable of inducing dependent use, but only if the time course of action is short enough to be equivalent to that of another dopamine stimulant, cocaine. Intravenous injection and intranasal snorting of amphetamines produce a very rapid initiation of action, a quick 'high', and a depressed craving during the rapid offset of action. Neither of these dangerous reactions is seen when methylphenidate is taken orally. Illicit users, by contrast, typically take huge doses via rapid-action routes. This should be seen as a contraindication to prescribing.

There is also a pattern of misuse not related to dependency. Unprescribed use of stimulants in attempts to improve academic and cognitive performance is widespread among college students and other young people in cognitively demanding settings (Benson et al., 2015). Anecdotally, the main effect they are seeking is resistance to fatigue.

Modafinil, a wakefulness-inducing drug, is more popular than methylphenidate among students at elite UK universities.

There are also some unresolved questions about the correct use of stimulants. Clinicians should appreciate the issues and follow the scientific findings as they emerge.

9.4.5   Are stimulants overprescribed?

The great international differences in diagnoses of ADHD were highlighted in 'Prevalence of ADHD', Chapter 3, Section 3.6. They are matched by differences in the use of drugs. Raman et al. (2018) used population registers covering 154.5 million individuals to define the prevalence of prescribed medication for ADHD (mostly methylphenidate) in various parts of the world. For people aged 3 to 18 years, rates varied greatly, as shown in Table 9.3. There were increases in all regions and all age groups between 2010 and 2015.

How this relates to the ideal level of prescription is harder to define. Applying the assumptions about prevalence of ADHD considered in Chapter 3, Section 3.6, the rates of prescription should be similar across regions. Applying recommendations from NICE in Europe and Practice Parameters in North America and Australia, medication would be expected to be offered to all with severe ADHD (hyperkinetic disorder)—about 1.5% of school-age children—and also to those with less severe ADHD who do not respond well to psychological therapy alone (around 2% of children) (National Collaborating Centre for Mental Health, 2018; Pliszka et al., 2007). This would suggest the possibility of substantial undermedication outside North America, especially in France and the UK, but overmedication in some parts of the USA. In North Carolina, at an extreme, 7.3% of young people received medication (Angold et al., 2000). Most of those with a DSM-III-R diagnosis of ADHD did get medication, but most of those given medication did not have the DSM diagnosis. Male gender and a diagnosis of oppositional-defiant disorder were the key drivers.

Table 9.3 Prescribing rates of medication for ADHD by region and age group

Region	Age 3 to 18 years	Age 9 years and over
North America	4.48%	1.42%
Northern Europe	1.95%	0.47%
Asia/Australia	0.95%	0.05%
Western Europe	0.70%	0.03%

Rates of medication for ADHD from population registers

Data from *Lancet Psychiatry*, 5(10), Raman, S. R., Man, K. K., Bahmanyar, S., et al., Trends in attention-deficit hyperactivity disorder medication use: a retrospective observational study using population-based databases, pp. 824–835. Copyright (2018), Elsevier Ltd.

9.4.6   What is the place of drugs when psychotherapies are available?

Drugs and psychotherapies have somewhat different benefits and harms. In summary, stimulants have larger benefits on ratings of hyperactivity-impulsivity and inattention than any psychological treatment. When these are the key targets, drug treatment should always be offered if a psychotherapy is not working well, and should be at least considered as the first-line treatment. Other outcomes, such as social behaviour, oppositional symptoms, and academic functioning should show more improvement if psychological interventions are provided as well as medication.

9.4.7   Effectiveness in the long term

Long-term value is still argued about. Only two randomized controlled trials have continued for as long as a year, while the disadvantages attributable to ADHD features continue into adult life.

The course of drug therapy over periods of about one year were closely observed in a large trial comparing drug therapy with behavioural interventions (but not with placebo)—the MTA (Multimodal Treatment of ADHD) study (MTA Cooperative Group, 2004). Carefully crafted medication was superior both to community treatment and to intensive behavioural therapy. Those with the severe form of ADHD (described as 'hyperkinetic disorder') showed strong relative advantage over those with milder forms of ADHD. Over longer periods than a year, rigorous placebo control has not proved realistic. The follow-up of the MTA study indicated that the initial real benefits of drug therapy on symptom severity were still there 1 year after treatment, present but diminished at 2 years, yet absent at 3 years and thereafter (Molina et al., 2009). Not even the subgroup of hyperkinetic disorder showed continuing superiority to psychological approaches (Arnold et al., 2019). The reasons for this apparent waning of drug effect can be multiple and should be watched for during the supervision of therapy:

- *The pharmacological actions of medication might wear off over time.* It is not that stimulants are ineffective in adult life: to the contrary, both controlled trials in adults and case-register recordings of outcomes on and off medication indicate their effectiveness in the short term. Rather, the concern is that prolonged administration, at any age, could lead to the development of pharmacological tolerance. Mechanisms such as the multiplication of dopamine transporter molecules after long-term exposure to stimulants could be responsible (Fusar–Poli et al., 2012). We do not yet know how to overcome this, and it does not apply to everyone, but good monitoring should detect it and drug holidays might reduce it.
- *The medication is often discontinued prematurely.* The use of medication falls off quickly as young people get older. In a national (UK) survey by McCarthy et al.

(2009), the key age for discontinuing was 16 years, which is also the age at which compulsory schooling ends. The reasons include: the presence of adverse effects; the adolescent desire for autonomy; stigma and hostile cultural attitudes to medication; simple forgetfulness; and development of a despondent attitude to the condition and its treatment.

To overcome these obstacles, clinicians will need to create a climate of communication that allows understanding of the obstacles in the individual case. Respect for autonomy may mean encouraging teenagers to take responsibility for reassessment periods in which they evaluate the effects of drug-free periods on themselves and on the reports from other people. Again, a clinical implication would be that those with ADHD will need good long-term monitoring and advice.

- *Continuing effectiveness of treatment might require more than routine monitoring.* Enhanced care would include careful attention to reviewing the changing needs for dosage and drug type over time (Coghill & Seth, 2015); the symptomatic management of adverse effects (Graham & Coghill, 2008); and the responsive discussion of attitudes, beliefs, and the experience of taking medication (Ferrin & Taylor, 2011).

- *Self-selection might equalize the outcomes between treatments in trials.* Most people receive several interventions during their lives and choose the one that suits them best. Those who perceive benefit from medication may well be those who choose to continue it; those who benefit from an alternative approach, such as behavioural therapy, might also choose to continue that. There might then be little long-term difference between medical and non-medical interventions for those with access to both. The clinical implication would be that those with ADHD will need good long-term monitoring to give them the knowledge on which to base rational choices.

9.5 PHARMACOLOGY OF DRUGS TO REDUCE AGITATION, AGGRESSION, AND PSYCHOTIC SYMPTOMS

Antipsychotic drugs (neuroleptics) have proved to be necessary for young people with schizophrenia or bipolar disorder. They can also be helpful in a wider range of conditions involving excitement and severe disturbances of behaviour and emotions. Most are considered to work by blocking dopamine and serotonin receptors, especially the dopamine-2 (D2) receptor. Neuroimaging studies in adults, with positron emission tomography, indicate that 60–70% blockade is the optimum level to aim for.

The distinction between 'first-generation' and 'second-generation' antipsychotics can be confusing. It is based mostly on historical and marketing considerations. The key pharmacological distinction is between those antipsychotics that do, and those that do not, carry strong risks for extrapyramidal problems. In this sense, many drugs that are low in extrapyramidal effects (e.g. thioridazine) were introduced a long time ago and so are historically, but not pharmacologically, 'first-generation'. Some recently introduced antipsychotic drugs (e.g. aripiprazole) still carry risks for extrapyramidal effects that need to be borne in mind by prescribers.

The precise choice of drug is usually dominated by the balance of adverse effects. First-generation antipsychotics (FGAs) became notorious for their ability to cause unsightly and unpleasant effects on movement. Extrapyramidal signs such as parkinsonian slowness, muscular rigidity, posturing, and akathisia (extreme of restlessness) affected large numbers of patients. The extreme was the irreversible syndrome of tardive dyskinesia. Drugs of this kind are still available and used in adults and older adolescents with schizophrenia. They include chlorpromazine, flupenthixol, haloperidol, levomepromazine, pericyazine, perphenazine, prochlorperazine, promazine, sulpiride, trifluperazine, and zuclopenthixol. They are seldom indicated for children. Haloperidol is occasionally used, in cases refractory to everything else, on the basis of its high potency in antagonizing D2 receptors (dopamine type 2). It is often given in combination with an anticholinergic drug, to reduce its potency to cause extrapyramidal disorders.

Their replacement by second-generation antipsychotics (SGAs) was characterized by less extrapyramidal damage, but more of the scarcely less harmful abnormalities of disordered metabolism and obesity. Their pharmacology includes rapid dissociation from D2 receptors and blockade of serotonin type 2A receptors.

SGAs (atypical antipsychotics) are widely accepted for treating schizophrenia and bipolar disorder in young people. Early recourse to them has been encouraged by the finding that long periods of untreated psychosis predict poor long-term outcome (Penttila et al., 2014). The prediction is subtle, but consistent in meta-analysis. It has led to the development of early-treatment teams in many countries. They often use the approaches to medication set out in Box 9.1, together with vigorous applications of the

---

Box 9.1 Drug treatment of early–onset schizophrenia and mania

Drug treatment should be in the explicit spirit of a therapeutic trial (NICE, 2013). This involves:

- beginning with antipsychotic medication in combination with psychological interventions;
- choosing the initial drug after discussion of adverse effects with patient and family;
- switching, if the outcome is unsatisfactory at 4--6 weeks on optimum dosage, to another antipsychotic;
- and eventually switching to clozapine if the first and second choices have not been good enough;
- and, if there is still inadequate response, adding a second antipsychotic that is unlikely to add to the adverse effects of clozapine.

Source: data from NICE (National Institute for Care and Health Excellence), *Psychosis and schizophrenia in children and young people: recognition and management.* Clinical guideline [CG155], Copyright (2013), NICE. Available via https://www.nice.org.uk/guidance/cg155 (Accessed 19/06/2020).

psychosocial interventions described in 'Hallucinations and other features of psychosis', Chapter 8, Section 8.12.

Both FGAs and SGAs have some evidence in their favour. A Cochrane review in 2007 found little to choose between the antipsychotics for outcomes of very early-onset schizophrenia (Kennedy et al., 2007). Clozapine was superior to haloperidol, but carried too many hazards for routine use. Benefits are generally greater for the 'positive symptoms' of hallucinations and delusions than for the 'negative symptoms' of apathy and withdrawal. Choice of drug therefore depends mostly upon profiles of adverse effects. Among FGAs, *sedation* is highest with chlorpromazine and promazine, lowest with fluphenazine, perphenazine, trifluoperazine, haloperidol, and sulpiride. The opposite balance generally applies to *extrapyramidal syndromes*, which are at their worst for the less sedative drugs such as haloperidol.

In general, SGAs are usually preferred for treating young people in acute psychosis.

9.5.1   Indications for SGAs for other than psychosis

The usual uses of SGAs in young people are off-label: for aggression, agitation, irritability, and other behaviours that challenge. Risperidone has a reasonable safety record and is often the first choice in the class. It has a European licence for irritability as well as for psychotic illnesses. The profile of adverse effects, however, varies from drug to drug and is often the major factor in deciding which drug should be given. Whichever is chosen, monitoring should be careful and families closely involved.

Use is increasing in many countries. In the UK, the prescribing of antipsychotics for children aged 7–12 years of age in primary care almost tripled between 1992 and 2005; the prescribing of SGAs increased sixtyfold during this period. The vast majority of this increased prescribing was for the management of aggression and challenging behaviours rather than psychosis (Rani et al., 2008).

Psychological interventions are the key therapies for young people with antisocial behaviour who are otherwise developing typically. NICE (2014) advises against the use of drugs except in ADHD or if there are 'problems with explosive anger and severe emotional dysregulation … which … have not responded to psychosocial interventions'. These circumstances are considered in Section 9.6.

9.5.1.1   *Drugs to modify behaviours that challenge in ID and ASD*

'Behaviours that challenge' comprise severe behavioural problems of aggression to self and others, destructiveness, and extreme oppositionality. As described in Chapter 8, Section 8.11, they are rather different from the usual run of conduct problems in typically developing young people. They are seldom seen outside the spectra of ASD and ID. They are not separately mentioned in the main diagnostic classifications and have not received a large evidence base to guide intervention with drugs.

A thorough and systematic review by NICE was conducted for trials of antipsychotics in children aged 13 years and under (National Collaborating Centre for Mental Health, 2015). The number of trials was small, and their quality was low or very low. There was some evidence for effectiveness. Aripiprazole, by comparison with placebo, led to challenging behaviours being 0.64 standard deviations lower. Risperidone, by comparison with placebo, was associated with an effect size in reducing challenging behaviours of 1.09 standard deviations. To set against this positive conclusion, adverse events were substantially increased. Obesity, elevated prolactin levels, sedation, and hyperlipidaemia were all more common in treated groups than in those receiving placebo.

The specific problem of severe self-injury has a dearth of trials despite its difficulty in management in practice. Gormez et al. (2014) attempted a systematic review of placebo-controlled drug trials in adults with ID. They found only seven trials, which between them involved only 50 subjects. On this slender base, they could not draw any conclusions about the value of naltrexone or clomipramine.

The effects of the behaviours on the lives of young people and their caregivers are so severe that they have led to widespread use of medication. Psychological treatments have an important role (see Chapter 8, Section 8.11) but often need to be given by specialists who are in short supply in many countries, including the UK. One result can be an over-reliance on medication in such countries.

9.5.2 Adverse effects of antipsychotic drugs

The many and varying actions of antipsychotic drugs are set out in Table 9.4. Most of them share, with risperidone, a generic set of actions on receptors in nerve cells. Many are antagonists of the D2 family (D_2, D_3, and D_5) of dopamine receptors and of the D1 family (D_1, D_3). Most are either antagonists or inverse agonists of a range of serotonin receptors. The balance is part of the reason for differing profiles of adverse effects, indicated in Table 9.4.

Table 9.4 Actions and safety issues specific to individual second–generation antipsychotics (SGAs)

Drug	Receptor actions other than generic	Other approved indications	Safety issues other than generic
Risperidone, paliperidone	Generic; it is the reference drug in the class	Irritability in autism	Generic; lower risk for seizures than many other SGAs
Quetiapine	H1 blocker Alpha-1 adrenoreceptor blockade Low D2 binding	Adjunctive in major depression	Sedative Hypothyroidism Often ineffective for aggression Low rate of EPS Low rate of epilepsy Low rate of hyperprolactinaemia

Continued

Table 9.4 Continued

Drug	Receptor actions other than generic	Other approved indications	Safety issues other than generic
Amisulpride Low dose	Inhibits dopamine autoreceptors	Not approved in USA (possibly helpful for negative symptoms)	Agitation
High dose (>400 mg)	Inhibits postsynaptic receptors Antagonizes 5HT-7 Little 5HT–1A, 2A, C blockade	(Possibly helpful for depression)	Q-T interval prolonged
Aripiprazole	Partial dopamine agonist	Adjunctive in major depression Irritability in autism	Less metabolic and endocrine risks than most SGAs; somewhat more EPS
Olanzapine	Multiple receptor antagonism including muscarinic M3	Alternative to clozapine in refractory psychosis	High efficacy High rates of obesity, metabolic, and endocrine problems
Clozapine	Low D2 binding, high D4, multiple actions on cholinergic and histaminergic antagonism	Refractory psychosis (non-response to two SGAs)	High efficacy, low EPS hazards, but high rates of obesity, metabolic, and endocrine problems Liver enzymes raised Agranulocytosis, so blood counts mandated Seizures Constipation
Ziprasidone	D2 and 5-HT_{2A} receptors antagonized	No licence in Europe	Tachycardia Hypotension Sedation
Lurasidone	D2, 5-HT2A, 5-HT7, alpha2A-, & 2C-adrenoceptors antagonized, partial agonist at 5HT1a receptors	Some evidence for value in major depression	Q-T prolongation

Individual SGAs vary in profiles of adverse effects.

EPS = extrapyramidal symptoms, SGA= second-generation antipsychotic

Adapted from Sonuga-Barke E, Taylor E, Chapter 55: ADHD and hyperkinetic disorder. In: Thapar A, Pine DS, Leckman JF, et al., [Eds.], *Rutter's Child and Adolescent Psychiatry*, Sixth edition, pp. 738–756, Copyright (2015), with permission from John Wiley and Sons.

Weight gain is common and can be a serious health problem. Pringsheim et al. (2011) noted, from a review of trials and cohort studies, a body mass index (BMI) increase of 1.92 kg/m^2 and a mean increase in waist circumference of 5.1 cm. Weight and BMI continue to increase over time, at least up to 2 years of treatment. In 24 trials of 3,048 paediatric patients with varying ages and diagnoses, ziprasidone was associated with the lowest weight gain (−0.04 kg on average), followed by aripiprazole (0.79 kg), quetiapine (1.43 kg), and risperidone (1.76 kg) (De Hert et al., 2011). Olanzapine was associated with the most weight gain (3.45 kg).

Metabolic changes are associated with increase of weight. They are frequent in those with impaired glucose metabolism or a family history of diabetes. Increased appetite and consequent obesity are the major mediators. Insulin resistance can also play a part. The *metabolic syndrome* is a combination of abdominal obesity, dyslipidaemia, hypertension, insulin resistance, glucose intolerance, prothrombotic state, and proinflammatory state. The results are so serious for life and health that most guidelines recommend that SGAs for non-psychotic indications are given only for a period of, at most, a few months. Nevertheless, their beneficial results can be so pronounced that the initial trial is often prolonged, often for years. Prevention of obesity and metabolic problems involves encouragement of healthy eating and physical activity from the beginning of treatment. For children and young people who are already obese, either adjunctive metformin or a switch to aripiprazole should be considered (Correll et al., 2020).

Elevated prolactin levels are common at the 12-week endpoint of controlled trials. Genetic polymorphisms coding for D2 predict their occurrence. High levels, however, tend to reduce after the first months of treatment, so they can be managed expectantly in most cases. If they are symptomatic, they should be treated. Menstrual irregularity and polycystic ovaries in females, and osteoporosis and galactorrhoea in either sex should be watched for. If prolactin needs to be reduced, a lower dose of antipsychotic will often help. If dose reduction does not help, then a switch to an antipsychotic with less D2 binding (quetiapine, aripiprazole, or clozapine) should be sufficient. Use of dopamine agonists (amantadine, bromocriptine) risks worsening the symptoms for which the dopamine antagonist has been prescribed.

Children and adolescents have an even higher liability than adults to experience hyperprolactinaemia, antipsychotic-induced weight gain, and associated metabolic disturbances (De Hert et al., 2011). Routine monitoring should include regular measurement of height and weight, as well as blood levels of glucose, lipoproteins, triglycerides, prolactin, and any parameters recommended for the individual drug in Table 9.4. BMI above 85th centile, fasting plasma glucose levels of 7 mmol/L, or low-density lipoprotein/cholesterol levels above 4.15 mmol/L should all be warning signals, and lead to drug reduction or referral to specialist clinics.

9.5.2.1 *Cardiovascular adverse effects*

Rapid heart rate and low blood pressure are frequent complications, often resulting from anticholinergic effects. Abnormalities of rhythm should indicate an ECG, and this should in any case be done before treatment and after a stable dose has been achieved. Q-T prolongation above 450 msec after correction for heart rate should lead to referral to cardiology.

9.5.2.2 *Neurological adverse effects*

Sedation is possible and probably indicates that the dose is too high for the individual. Cognitive blunting can also occur without obvious lethargy. Reduction of dose usually helps; co-prescribed stimulants probably do not help much.

Movement problems are still seen even after the switch to SGAs.

Extrapyramidal symptoms (EPS) include both unwanted movements and deficiencies. There may be parkinsonian features: a coarse, rhythmic (3–6 cps) tremor at rest affecting head, mouth, or limbs is typical. Cogwheel or continuous 'lead pipe' rigidity occurs. A decrease in spontaneous facial expressions, gestures, speech, or body movements is termed akinesia.

Akithisia is the term used for a restless and involuntary excess of movement. It may take the form of continuous leg swinging, inability to sit or stand still for as long as a few minutes, rocking from foot to foot while standing, or relentless pacing around. In the context of treating people with hyperactivity, it can be mistaken for a return of the original symptoms.

Tardive dyskinesias are a variety of emerging movement problems typically appearing after long exposure to the drugs, and so are not often seen in young people. These involuntary movements of the tongue, jaw, trunk, or limbs can take many forms: choreiform or athetoid movements, or rhythmic stereotypies. They are not diminished by reduction of dose and are potentially irreversible. The first signs may be the appearance of 'vermiculation' (writhing movements of the tongue), or dyskinesias on reduction or discontinuation of drugs. They should be taken as a warning.

Seizures can appear for the first time.

For all these reasons, neurological examination—of alertness, history of episodic changes, and any movement changes—should be part of the evaluation of drug treatment. It should be carried out before treatment, after stable dose is achieved, and periodically (perhaps annually) if long-term medication has proved essential. Video recording is very helpful for complex pictures of involuntary movement.

9.5.2.3 *Neuroleptic malignant syndrome (NMS)*

All antipsychotics are capable of inducing NMS, which is a rare but very serious complication of exposure to them. It is considered to be a result of dopamine 2 receptor blockade, sometimes precipitated by dehydration or use of cocaine. Major signs are fever, fluctuating level of consciousness or confusion, muscle rigidity, and autonomic dysfunction (e.g. sweating). They can be accompanied by pallor, rapid heart rate and breathing, labile blood pressure, and urinary incontinence. The serum levels of creatine phosphokinase (like other enzymes released from muscles) are raised. This blood test is not a major sign; normal levels do not exclude NMS. Diagnosis requires a high level of suspicion and willingness to consider it, even at the stage of apparently minor symptoms.

The syndrome is a medical emergency: cooling and life support in an intensive care unit are needed. Treatment is mostly supportive and, even with intensive care, the death rate is around 20%. Dantrolene as a muscle relaxant, and bromocriptine or amantadine as dopaminergics, can also be used.

9.5.2.4 *Drug interactions*

Interactions *between* antipsychotics and other psychotropics can increase the blood levels and, therefore, their toxicity. The mechanisms include inhibition of cytochrome enzymes that usually metabolize drugs. Prominent examples include inhibition of CYP 2D6 by fluoxetine and paroxetine, increasing the blood levels of many antipsychotics, including risperidone and haloperidol; and inhibition of CYP 1A2 by fluvoxamine, affecting clozapine and olanzapine. Interactions between many psychotropics and antiepileptics are described below.

9.6 PHARMACOLOGY OF DRUGS TO MODIFY MOOD AND ANXIETY DISTURBANCES

People with neurodevelopmental disorders, such as ADHD, ID, ASD, and chronic tic disorders, can develop anxiety and mood disorders in the same way, and for the same reasons, as typically developing people. If this is the formulation, then drug treatments can follow the same lines (see Sonuga–Barke & Taylor, 2015; Walkup et al., 2008). Drugs would then be considered secondary to psychological approaches, adapted if necessary to the needs of people with communication difficulties (see Chapter 8, Section 8.13). When drugs are considered for anxiety or depression, then selective serotonin reuptake inhibitors (SSRIs), beta-blockers, antipsychotics, and occasionally benzodiazepines are all in use, on the basis essentially of trials in young people who are otherwise developing typically (e.g. as reported by March et al., 2004). Their value in complex neurodevelopmental situations is not supported by good quality evidence. They can all be considered, nevertheless—possibly in that order. In the case of benzodiazepines, however, the adverse effects are severe enough for cautions against their use for more than a few days. Dependence and sedation are common in extended use.

9.6.1 Drugs for anxiety in the presence of ASD

For those with ASD, the anxiety symptoms of phobias, compulsions, and obsessions can be confused with core autistic features of social disengagement and resistance to change. Recognition is considered under 'Autism Spectrum Disorders', Chapter 4, Section 4.1.5.4. The evidence base for anxiolytics in ASD is scanty, and they are not officially recommended for the usual forms of emotional problems in the presence of ASD.

Adverse effects of mood-altering drugs tend to be more common in young people with compromised brains.

Fluoxetine is the usual choice, but its capacity for harmful interactions with other drugs should give substantial pause. Citalopram and escitalopram are not safer, but they are more selective and less likely to interact with other drugs, so are often preferred in situations of polypharmacy.

Trials of SSRIs have not firmly established beneficial effects in people with anxiety who also have problems such as ASD and ID. Fluoxetine was (just) superior to placebo in a recent trial to reduce obsessive-compulsive features in children and adolescents diagnosed in the spectrum of autism (Reddihough et al., 2019). Citalopram and fluoxetine did not show good effect sizes for repetitive or obsessive-compulsive symptoms in the presence of ASD (Hollander et al., 2012). Clomipramine showed a significant improvement in obsessive-compulsive disorder (OCD) symptoms in an early trial on children with ASD—but only 10 children, and over only 12 weeks (Gordon et al., 1993).

The lack of a secure evidence base may be due to lack of trials and unsatisfactory measurement rather than lack of effect. Clinical experience supports the use of SSRIs for limited periods, even though there is little evidence for any specific action on anxiety in ASD. There is little to contraindicate them either. In the common situation of high anxiety being a distressing and impairing concomitant of ASD, it is still reasonable to follow the principles of drug treatment in young people without ASD.

9.6.1.1 *Second-generation antipsychotics*

SGAs (described earlier) for treating agitated and explosive behaviours, are also in use for anxiety conditions. They are only recommended in low doses and for short periods when other therapy has been insufficient. In the context of trials targeting irritability in young people with ASD/ID, risperidone (1.25–1.75 mg/day) had some limited evidence for reduction of OCD symptomatology (Kent et al., 2013). One measure of insecurity/anxiety improved in another randomized trial of risperidone by Shea et al. (2004) (in a trial focusing on irritability).

9.6.2 Drugs for anxiety in the presence of ADHD

Anxiety is not a contraindication to the use of stimulants in ADHD. To the contrary, it is plain from the many short-term trials of stimulants that they usually have beneficial effects on ratings of emotional problems in children treated for ADHD. If anxiety is still prominent after inattention and impulsiveness have been controlled, then the addition of antianxiety medication can be supported from clinical experience.

The choice of treatment should follow the clinical formulation. ADHD may be the primary problem, with anxiety being secondary to the frustrations, failures, and stigmatization that have followed. In such cases, reduction of ADHD will take priority, together with addressing educational and family problems. It may even allow the exhibition of psychological approaches that were not previously feasible. Behavioural desensitization, graded exposure, and relaxation techniques all rely on cooperation (see Chapter 8, Section 8.13). Sometimes, however, the reduction of anxiety needs to take pride of place in a therapeutic plan, and anxiolytic drugs should be considered.

9.6.3   Other anxiolytic drugs

Other drugs have anecdotal recommendations for young people with complex problems, including anxiety, but cannot yet be recommended for routine use. They include:

Propranolol, a non-selective blocker of beta-adrenergic receptors, has a long history of use for anxiety, especially when somatic symptoms of sympathetic system overactivation are prominent. The physical symptoms may themselves be exacerbating anxiety. It can be a helpful short-term method of reducing situational anxiety such as 'exam nerves' or 'stage fright' or a visit from a critical relative. (See also Section 9.6.7.)

Buspirone, a 5HT1a receptor partial agonist, has been used for anxious adults in the USA. Even though it is often given as a long-term treatment, it does not seem to give rise to withdrawal effects when it is stopped.

Pregabalin and *gabapentin* are antiseizure medications that act as voltage-gated calcium channel blockers to reduce the release of glutamate (an excitatory transmitter).

Hydroxyzine is a histamine receptor antagonist which has received several trials for generalized anxiety disorder in adults, but was not recommended by a Cochrane review (Guaiana et al., 2010).

Benzodiazepines and *barbiturates,* some of which are GABA positive allosteric modulator (GABA–PAM) drugs, are only advised for short-term use for adults.

9.6.4   Drugs for depression in the presence of neurodevelopmental disorders

As with anxiety, so with depression. Many people with ADHD, ASD, or Tourette conditions develop depressed mood in the context of functional deficits deriving from the conditions. The adverse environmental factors described in Chapter 10 play a part, and there are probably some shared familial influences (Daviss, 2008). Trials have not established the balance of risks and benefits of antidepressant drugs in this context. In one trial of citalopram conducted for young people with ASD, depression was not significantly improved (King et al., 2009).

As in the treatment of coexistent anxiety, it seems right to give disabled young people the same opportunity of successful therapy as their able peers. In the absence of secure information about hazards, however, one should proceed with all the caution needed for off-label treatments. Low doses and enhanced vigilance for adverse effects, including suicidality, should be the rule. In bipolar disorder, the danger of SSRIs precipitating a switch from depression into mania needs to be borne in mind.

9.6.5 Drugs for anger and irritability in the presence of neurodevelopmental disorders

Anger and irritability are also emotional states, and they often complicate neuro-developmental disorders. Excessive anger (irritability) is a defining part of *severe emotional dysregulation* (SED), described in Chapter 2, Section 2.9. In the DSM-5, it is considered as 'disruptive mood dysregulation disorder' (DMDD). The hallmarks are frequent temper outbursts and chronic states of anger/ resentment. DMDD is not a recognized indication for any medication. Irritability, however, considered transdiagnostically as a form of mood dysregulation, is a frequent reason for considering drug therapy.

9.6.6 Drugs for irritability in the presence of ADHD

In this circumstance, the control of ADHD should usually be the first step. It is often neglected because of a belief that stimulant medication is more likely to make emotional problems worse, rather than to improve them. The belief is not well founded in the case of ADHD. A review by Shaw et al. (2014) was able to address the issues from the results of randomized controlled trials of ADHD in which measures of behavioural and emotional adjustment were included as secondary outcomes. A stimulant or atomoxetine was preferable to placebo in five out of seven of the trials in young people, and four out of five of those in adults. It can be effective, but is not always necessary. Environmental adjustment is often the front line of management, to reduce the frustrations and humiliations that engender anger. A thorough functional analysis can follow, when necessary and available.

If neither such a psychological approach, nor a trial of stimulants, succeeds in promoting more regulated emotional reactions, then there is limited evidence for a trial of antiepileptic medication. Valproate in males, or lamotrigine in females, can be considered as mood stabilizers in this context. (Lithium, by contrast, does not seem to have a good balance of positive over adverse effects in children.) Blader et al. (2009) conducted a small randomized trial of valproate (mean daily dose of 567 mg) against placebo in 27 children and adolescents whose ADHD had been improved with stimulants but whose coexistent anger and aggression were continuing to be serious problems. The addition of valproate to the stimulant regime was efficacious. Those treated with it met the trial criteria for recovery (remission of aggression) more often than those who received placebo (in 8 out of 14 cases, compared with 2 out of 13 on placebo).

It may sometimes be necessary to use a combination of anti-ADHD drugs with a SGA or a SSRI for the control of irritability associated with severe episodes of aggression and/ or explosive outbursts. Clinical experience supports the use of combinations in severe cases that are not wholly attributable to environmental adversity. The combination can help to maintain young people in their communities—which is often better for their development than to be unmedicated but in residential care.

In short, stimulant medication and atomoxetine can be given in situations where both ADHD and emotional dysregulation are present and marked. They are not contraindicated and may well be helpful. Their adverse effects are usually minor and reversible by symptomatic treatment (Cortese et al., 2013). The contrast with the adverse effects of lithium, antiepileptic drugs, and the neuroleptics is striking enough to support the recommendation that the first line in drug management will be to control the ADHD, and then to review whether the irritability is severe enough to need further treatment. Treatment with stimulants should, nevertheless, be undertaken with enhanced monitoring and supervision in the combination of severe mood dysregulation and ADHD. The frequency and intensity of anger should be recorded as a baseline measure, and again during regular monitoring.

9.6.7 Drugs for irritability in the presence of ASD or ID

Excessive anger can be controlled by the SGAs that are used for excited aggression (Table 9.4), but with the same price to pay in adverse effects. Other drugs have scant evidence for their value in this indication.

Stimulants do not have a useful action in the absence of inattentive/impulsive features. N-acetylcysteine is a glutamatergic modulator which has a randomized trial (of 33 subjects aged between 3 and 11 years) in its favour (Hardan et al., 2012).

Antiepileptics are often used, but favourable trial evidence was not forthcoming from a systematic review by Hirota et al. (2014). Hollander et al. (2010) compared divalproex sodium with a placebo in 55 young people with ASD: 62.5% of divalproex subjects, versus 9% given placebo, responded well on a subscale of irritability from the aberrant behavior checklist. Single trials do not constitute enough of an evidence base to establish them as anything but occasional, alternative therapies. The dangers of valproate (especially on unborn children) contraindicate its use in females who might become pregnant.

Propranolol, as a beta-blocker, is also sometimes advocated for angry, explosive states in the context of high arousal. Emotional, behavioural, and autonomic dysregulation (EBAD) has been regarded as a distinct cluster of problems within ASD (Sagar–Ouriaghli et al., 2018). These authors reviewed case reports and case series of treatment with propranolol, but could conclude only that further study would be justified. For now, its use should be regarded as experimental.

9.6.7.1 *Adverse effects of SSRIs*

A key adverse effect to note is the appearance of activation—restlessness, irritability, insomnia, and maybe disinhibition—in a sizeable minority of those treated with SSRIs. It is more of an issue in children than in adults. It helps to raise the rate of suicidal thoughts and feelings—which is a serious concern for venlafaxine when given for depression, but probably not for fluoxetine. Other adverse effects of SSRIs are not usually very severe, but include agitation, gastrointestinal problems, nausea and loss of appetite, dry mouth, excessive sweating, and sexual difficulties. The last of these (especially problems in obtaining erections and orgasms) may not be mentioned spontaneously by adolescents.

Serotonin syndrome is a toxic effect of drugs raising serotonin levels—typically, a combination of SSRIs in high doses. It comprises high body temperature, agitation, increased reflexes, tremor, sweating, dilated pupils, and diarrhoea.

9.6.8 Interactions between psychotropic drugs and antiepileptics

Antiepileptics and psychotropic drugs have strong influences on each other (Patsalos & Perucca, 2003). Most of the clinically important interactions of antiepileptic drugs result from induction or inhibition of drug metabolism.

Carbamazepine, phenytoin, phenobarbital, and primidone are strong inducers of cytochrome P450 and glucuronizing enzymes. They will therefore accelerate the metabolism and reduce the effect of many antipsychotics (including risperidone, haloperidol, olanzapine, and clozapine), benzodiazepines, and some antidepressants (e.g. paroxetine). Valproate, by contrast, is an enzyme inhibitor and can raise the blood levels of lorazepam and paroxetine to worsen their adverse effects. Psychotropics, in their turn, can alter the metabolism of antiepileptics. Many antidepressants (fluoxetine, fluvoxamine, imipramine, sertraline, trazodone) can be expected to raise the blood levels of phenytoin and carbamazepine, and sertraline to have the same effect on levels of valproate and lamotrigine.

The picture of interactions is therefore complex. Detailed consultation with expert pharmacists is advised on individual cases. Newer antiepileptics such as gabapentin, levetiracetam, topiramate, and lamotrigine often do not enter the interactions at all. The picture becomes even more complicated if, as is often the case, separate teams are responsible for treating seizures and mental state. Poor communication can then be harmful to the individual patients and worrying for their families.

9.7 PHARMACOLOGY OF DRUGS TO TREAT ALTERED PATTERNS OF MOVEMENT

9.7.1 Tics

Not all people with chronic tics, or even Tourette disorder, need medication. Explanation and reassurance are often enough. Support can include encouragement to resist taunting from peers, and resilience against it. Some behavioural interventions, such as habit reversal, can also reduce tics and give the sufferer an added sense of control. If people with the condition, or their families, are overattached to the idea of medication, then it may be useful to point out that the effects of medication can be hard to assess because the condition fluctuates so much, and drugs are often started when it is at its worst. It is unwise to 'chase the symptom' by increasing the dose whenever tics are worsening.

When drug interventions are decided on, several types of drug are available.

Dopamine blockers used for this purpose include FGAs: haloperidol, fluphenazine, and pimozide. Their potency is in line with their ability to antagonize D2 receptors. Even so, there is a clinical impression that the dangers of dystonias, parkinsonism, akathisia, and tardive dyskinesia are less of a problem than when they are used for schizophrenia or bipolar disorder. This might simply be due to smaller doses. Some SGAs are also in use—risperidone has the most trial evidence, and aripiprazole has, in principle, an advantage of producing somewhat less in the way of metabolic adverse effects. All the antipsychotics will need ECG assessment to detect any abnormalities such as lengthening of the QTc interval; in the case of pemoline, it will need to be repeated. Antipsychotics should be discontinued through a gradual tapering of dosage.

Central adrenergic inhibitors, such as clonidine and guanfacine, act through stimulation of alpha-2 adrenergic receptors in the brain. This results in a reduction of noradrenergic (and therefore sympathetic nervous system) actions. They are not as effective against tics as the dopamine-blocking agents, but they are less prone to dopaminergic adverse effects. Many practitioners therefore use them in milder cases as a first line of medication. They may also hope that such drugs will help to control other behavioural problems such as ADHD, other impulse control problems, and rage attacks.

It may well take weeks before improvement appears with alpha-2 adrenergic inhibitors. Possible adverse effects include sleepiness, depression, headache, and dizziness. They are also used (typically in much higher dosage) for the treatment of high blood pressure. They should not be discontinued suddenly for fear of creating a rebound rise in blood pressure. Monitoring should include an initial ECG to measure QTc interval, and, if abnormal, this should be repeated (especially if the drug chosen is extended-release guanfacine). Tablets come in a wide range of strengths: prescribing errors need to be guarded against.

Monoamine depletors: tetrabenazine acts as an inhibitor of vesicular monoamine transporter 2 (VMAT2). Its use is mostly for severe and refractory neurological problems (including hemiballismus, Huntington's chorea, and tardive dyskinesia). However, it could be considered for very severe tics, especially those leading to self-injury. There are many adverse effects to consider; it can cause severe depression. Specialist consultation would be needed.

Topiramate is an antiepileptic; it enhances GABA-A receptor activity and reduces glutamate activity at some receptor sites. It also blocks the voltage-dependent sodium channels, which may suppress the spread of seizures and tic activity. It is used in the prophylaxis of migraines. Its use in young people with Tourette disorder has some low-quality trial evidence, but no regulatory approval. Additionally, it can cause loss of appetite and cognitive blunting (Yang et al., 2013).

Botulinum toxin injection is used to paralyse or weaken muscles, and therefore is an effective way of reducing tics (or dystonias) affecting single movements. Injection into the vocal cords can reduce vocalizations. Repetitive blinking, grimacing, and head jerking have often been the targets. Systemic adverse effects are not to be expected. A Cochrane review has emphasized the lack of support from good-quality randomized trials (Pandey et al., 2018). The effect typically lasts only 6 to 12 weeks, so repeated injections will be needed.

Deep brain stimulation should also be considered for severe tics involving self-injury.

9.7.2 Complex motor stereotypies

The stereotyped activities accompanying ASD and ID can be reduced by the antipsychotic drugs that are used to control agitation and aggression. There is, however, very little evidence to guide pharmacotherapy in individuals without ASD. Animal models suggest that the movements are associated with high dopamine and low acetylcholine in the brain, but clinical experience does not suggest that corresponding treatments have much benefit in the longer term (Harris et al., 2008).

9.7.3 Other motor problems

The abnormal movement patterns that complicate treatment with FGAs can often be reduced with anticholinergic drugs such as orphenadrine and benztropine. They can also bring their own problems, including confusion, dry mouth, and urinary difficulties.

Cerebral palsy very often includes painful and disabling spasticity of muscles. There are several pharmacological approaches, notably centrally acting muscle relaxants such as baclofen or diazepam. Dantrolene sodium reduces the sensitivity of muscles to nerve signals.

9.8 Pharmacology of drugs to reduce sleep problems

Problems falling asleep and staying asleep are very frequent in children and adolescents with ADHD, ASD, or ID. Indeed, 70–80% of young people with these conditions will have troublesome sleep problems. The reasons are complex and include hypersensitivity to environmental stimuli, hyperarousal, difficulties with self-regulation, high anxiety, changes of body rhythms, and adverse effects of psy-chotropic drugs. The results can be sleepiness and poor concentration in the day-time and family disturbance.

Behavioural treatments and sleep hygiene (see Chapter 8, Section 8.11) are effective for many people and should usually be tried before proceeding to hypnotics. Medical causes, such as obstructive sleep apnoea, restless legs syndrome, and irritating skin conditions, should be considered and if necessary treated.

Most hypnotic drugs (e.g. promethazine, chloral, trazodone, benzodiazepines, and 'z-drugs' such as zolpidem) are sedative and indicated in childhood only for a few days' use. All have their advocates, but the most widely used substance is *melatonin*. This nat-urally occurring hormone is produced by the pineal gland. Its blood levels are controlled by retinal perception of light and endogenous cyclic rhythms. Levels rise after the onset of darkness and are at their highest in the middle of the night. They act on cells in the hypothalamus controlling diurnal and nocturnal body changes.

Modified-release melatonin has a European licence for children and adolescents with insomnia in ASD and Smith–Magenis syndrome, when sleep hygiene measures have been insufficient. Trial evidence supports its use, particularly in ASD (Esposito et al., 2019). A randomized trial in 160 children with ASD aged 2 to 10 years gave sound evi-dence of effectiveness when sleep hygiene measures did not work (Cortesi et al., 2012). Dosage starts in childhood with 1 mg given up to 30 minutes before bedtime. The max-imum recommended is 5 mg for adolescents. Adverse effects are not very common but can include daytime sleepiness, tiredness, and irritability. Treatment can be continued in the long term but needs six-monthly reviews.

The natural levels of melatonin vary from person to person, and have been described as altered in Down and Prader–Willi syndromes. Several mutations of melatonin receptors are known. There is, however, no evidence that either the blood levels or the receptor status condition the response to melatonin supplementation.

Drugs promoting wakefulness (e.g. modafinil, methylphenidate, and amphetamines) are used in conditions of excessive sleepiness. Narcolepsy and sedation from antiepileptics are the commonest indications. Kleine–Levin syndrome may also re-spond. (For episodic somnolence and overeating, see 'Recurrent episodes of sudden transient behaviour change', Chapter 6, Section 6.2.)

9.9 Conclusion

Drug treatments are valuable for overcoming several of the problems affecting young people and adults with neurodevelopmental disorders. With the exception of ADHD, there is too little trial data for recommendations to be based on satisfactory evidence. The way forward should, therefore, be the establishment of better evidence and joint decision making by professionals, families and other caregivers, and young people themselves.

References

Aman, M. G., Smith, T., Arnold, L. E., Corbett–Dick, P., Tumuluru, R., Hollway, J. A., Hyman, S. L., Mendoza–Burcham, M., Pan, X., Mruzek, D. W., Lecavalier, L., Levato, L., Silverman, L. B., & Handen, B. (2014). A review of atomoxetine effects in young people with developmental disabilities. *Research in Developmental Disabilities*, *35*(6), 1412–1424.Angold, A., Erkanli, A., Egger, H. L., & Costello, E. J. (2000). Stimulant treatment for children: a community perspective. *Journal of the American Academy of Child & Adolescent Psychiatry*, *39*(8), 975–984.

Arnold, L. E., Roy, A., Taylor, E., Hechtman, L., Sibley, M., Swanson, J. M., Mitchell, J. T., Molina, B. S. G., & Rohde, L. A. (2019). Predictive utility of childhood diagnosis of ICD-10 hyperkinetic disorder: adult outcomes in the MTA and effect of comorbidity. *European Child & Adolescent Psychiatry*, *28*(4), 557–570.

Benson, K., Flory, K., Humphreys, K. L., & Lee, S. S. (2015). Misuse of stimulant medication among college students: a comprehensive review and meta-analysis. *Clinical Child and Family Psychology Review*, *18*(1), 50–76.

Blader, J. C., Schooler, N. R., Jensen, P. S., Pliszka, S. R., & Kafantaris, V. (2009). Adjunctive divalproex versus placebo for children with ADHD and aggression refractory to stimulant monotherapy. *American Journal of Psychiatry*, *166*(12), 1392–1401.

Bolea–Alamañac, B., Nutt, D. J., Adamou, M., Asherson, P., Bazire, S., Coghill, D., Heal, D., Müller, U., Nash, J., Santosh, P., Sayal, K., Sonuga–Barke, E., Young, S. J., & British Association for Psychopharmacology. (2014). Evidence-based guidelines for the pharmacological management of attention deficit hyperactivity disorder: update on recommendations from the British Association for Psychopharmacology. *Journal of Psychopharmacology*, *28*(3), 179–203.

British National Formulary for Children (BNFC). (2019). https://bnfc.nice.org.uk/

Caraci, F., Enna, S. J., Zohar, J., Racagni, G., Zalsman, G., van den Brink, W., Kasper, S., Koob, G. F., Pariante, C. M., Piazza, P. V., Yamada, K., Spedding, M., & Drago, F. (2017). A new nomenclature for classifying psychotropic drugs. *British Journal of Clinical Pharmacology*, *83*(8), 1614–1616.

Cipriani, A., Zhou, X., Del Giovane, C., Hetrick, S. E., Qin, B., Whittington, C., Coghill, D., Zhang, Y., Hazell, P., Leucht, S., Cuijpers, P., Pu, J., Cohen, D., Ravindran, A. V., Liu, Y., Michael, K. D., Yang, L., Liu, L., & Xie, P. (2016). Comparative efficacy and tolerability of antidepressants for major depressive disorder in children and adolescents: a network meta-analysis. *Lancet*, *388*(10047), 881–890.

Coghill, D., & Seth, S. (2015). Effective management of attention-deficit/hyperactivity disorder (ADHD) through structured re-assessment: the Dundee ADHD Clinical Care Pathway. *Child and Adolescent Psychiatry and Mental Health*, *9*(1), 52.

Coghill, D. R., Seth, S., Pedroso, S., Usala, T., Currie, J., & Gagliano, A. (2014). Effects of methylphenidate on cognitive functions in children and adolescents with attention-deficit/hyperactivity disorder: evidence from a systematic review and a meta-analysis. *Biological Psychiatry*, *76*(8), 603–615.

Correll, C. U., Sikich, L., Reeves, G., Johnson, J., Keeton, C., Spanos, M., Kapoor, S., Bussell, K., Miller, L., Chandrasekhar, T., Sheridan, E. M., Pirmohamed, S., Reinblatt, S. P., Alderman, C., Scheer, A., Borner, I., Bethea, T. C., Edwards, S., Hamer, R. M., & Riddle, M. A. (2020). Metformin add-on vs. antipsychotic switch vs. continued antipsychotic treatment plus healthy lifestyle education in overweight or obese youth with severe mental illness: results from the IMPACT trial. *World Psychiatry*, *19*(1), 69–80.

Cortese, S., Adamo, N., Del Giovane, C., Mohr-Jensen, C., Hayes, A. J., Carucci, S., Atkinson, L. Z., Tessari, L., Banaschewski, T., Coghill, D., Hollis, C., Simonoff, E., Zuddas, A., Barbui, C., Purgato, M., Steinhausen, H. C., Shokraneh, F., Xia, J., & Cipriani, A. (2018). Comparative efficacy and tolerability of medications for attention-deficit hyperactivity disorder in children, adolescents, and adults: a systematic review and network meta-analysis. *Lancet Psychiatry*, 5(9), 727–738.

Cortese, S., Holtmann, M., Banaschewski, T., Buitelaar, J., Coghill, D., Danckaerts, M., … & European ADHD Guidelines Group. (2013). Practitioner review: current best practice in the management of adverse events during treatment with ADHD medications in children and adolescents. *Journal of Child Psychology and Psychiatry*, 54(3), 227–246.

Cortesi, F., Giannotti, F., Sebastiani, T., Panunzi, S., & Valente, D. (2012). Controlled-release melatonin, singly and combined with cognitive behavioural therapy, for persistent insomnia in children with autism spectrum disorders: a randomized placebo-controlled trial. *Journal of Sleep Research*, 21(6), 700–709.

Daviss, W. B. (2008). A review of co-morbid depression in pediatric ADHD: etiologies, phenomenology, and treatment. *Journal of Child and Adolescent Psychopharmacology*, 18(6), 565–571.

De Hert, M., Dobbelaere, M., Sheridan, E. M., Cohen, D., & Correll, C. U. (2011). Metabolic and endocrine adverse effects of second-generation antipsychotics in children and adolescents: a systematic review of randomized, placebo controlled trials and guidelines for clinical practice. *European Psychiatry*, 26(3), 144–158.

De Vries, T. P. G., Henning, R. H., Hogerzeil, H. V., Fresle, D. A., Policy, M., & World Health Organization. (1994). *Guide to good prescribing: a practical manual* (No. WHO/DAP/94.11). World Health Organization.

Esposito, S., Laino, D., D'Alonzo, R., Mencarelli, A., Di Genova, L., Fattorusso, A., Argentiero, A., & Mencaroni, E. (2019). Pediatric sleep disturbances and treatment with melatonin. *Journal of Translational Medicine*, 17(1), 77.

Faraone, S. V., & Buitelaar, J. (2010). Comparing the efficacy of stimulants for ADHD in children and adolescents using meta-analysis. *European Child & Adolescent Psychiatry*, 19(4), 353–364.

Ferrin, M., & Taylor, E. (2011). Child and caregiver issues in the treatment of attention deficit–hyperactivity disorder: education, adherence and treatment choice. *Future Neurology*, 6(3), 399–413.

Fusar-Poli, P., Rubia, K., Rossi, G., Sartori, G., & Balottin, U. (2012). Striatal dopamine transporter alterations in ADHD: pathophysiology or adaptation to psychostimulants? A meta-analysis. *American Journal of Psychiatry*, 169(3), 264–272.

Gordon, C. T., Nelson, J. E., Hamburger, S. D., & Rapoport, J. L. (1993). A double-blind comparison of clomipramine, desipramine, and placebo in the treatment of autistic disorder. *Archives of General Psychiatry*, 50(6), 441–447.

Gormez, A., Rana, F., & Varghese, S. (2014). Pharmacological interventions for self-injurious behaviour in adults with intellectual disabilities: abridged republication of a Cochrane systematic review. *Journal of Psychopharmacology*, 28(7), 624–632.

Graham, J., & Coghill, D. (2008). Adverse effects of pharmacotherapies for attention-deficit hyperactivity disorder. *CNS Drugs*, 22(3), 213–237.

Guaiana, G., Barbui, C., & Cipriani, A. (2010). Hydroxyzine for generalised anxiety disorder. *Cochrane Database of Systematic Reviews*, (12) CD006815. https://doi.org/10.1002/14651858.CD006815.pub2

Hardan, A. Y., Fung, L. K., Libove, R. A., Obukhanych, T. V., Nair, S., Herzenberg, L. A., & Tirouvanziam, R. (2012). A randomized controlled pilot trial of oral N-acetylcysteine in children with autism. *Biological Psychiatry, 71*(11), 956–961.

Harris, K. M., Mahone, E. M., & Singer, H. S. (2008). Nonautistic motor stereotypies: clinical features and longitudinal follow-up. *Pediatric Neurology, 38*(4), 267–272.

Hennissen, L., Bakker, M. J., Banaschewski, T., Carucci, S., Coghill, D., Danckaerts, M., Dittmann, R. W., Hollis, C., Kovshoff, H., McCarthy, S., Nagy, P., Sonuga–Barke, E., Wong, I. C., Zuddas, A., Rosenthal, E., Buitelaar, J. K., & ADDUCE Consortium. (2017). Cardiovascular effects of stimulant and non-stimulant medication for children and adolescents with ADHD: a systematic review and meta-analysis of trials of methylphenidate, amphetamines and atomoxetine. *CNS Drugs, 31*(3), 199–215.

Hirota, T., Veenstra–VanderWeele, J., Hollander, E., & Kishi, T. (2014). Antiepileptic medications in autism spectrum disorder: a systematic review and meta-analysis. *Journal of Autism and Developmental Disorders, 44*(4), 948–957.

Hollander, E., Chaplin, W., Soorya, L., Wasserman, S., Novotny, S., Rusoff, J., Feirsen, N., Pepa, L., & Anagnostou, E. (2010). Divalproex sodium vs placebo for the treatment of irritability in children and adolescents with autism spectrum disorders. *Neuropsychopharmacology, 35*(4), 990.

Hollander, E., Soorya, L., Chaplin, W., Anagnostou, E., Taylor, B. P., Ferretti, C. J., Wasserman, S., Swanson, E., & Settipani, C. (2012). A double-blind placebo-controlled trial of fluoxetine for repetitive behaviors and global severity in adult autism spectrum disorders. *American Journal of Psychiatry, 169*(3), 292–299.

Kennedy, E., Kumar, A., & Datta, S. S. (2007). Antipsychotic medication for childhood-onset schizophrenia. *Cochrane Database of Systematic Reviews*, (3) CD004027. https://doi.org/10.1002/14651858.CD004027.pub2

Kent, J. M., Kushner, S., Ning, X., Karcher, K., Ness, S., Aman, M., Singh, J., & Hough, D. (2013). Risperidone dosing in children and adolescents with autistic disorder: a double-blind, placebo-controlled study. *Journal of Autism and Developmental Disorders, 43*(8), 1773–1783.

King, B. H., Hollander, E., Sikich, L., McCracken, J. T., Scahill, L., Bregman, J. D., Donnelly, C. L., Anagnostou, E., Dukes, K., Sullivan, L., Hirtz, D., Wagner, A., Ritz, L., & STAART Psychopharmacology Network. (2009). Lack of efficacy of citalopram in children with autism spectrum disorders and high levels of repetitive behavior: citalopram ineffective in children with autism. *Archives of General Psychiatry, 66*(6), 583–590.

March, J. S. (2004). Cognitive-behavior therapy, sertraline, and their combination for children and adolescents with obsessive-compulsive disorder: the Pediatric OCD Treatment Study (POTS) randomized controlled trial. *Journal of the American Medical Association, 292*(16), 1969.

March, J., Silva, S., Petrycki, S., Curry, J., Wells, K., Fairbank, J., Burns, B., Domino, M., McNulty, S., Vitiello, B., & Severe, J., & Treatment for Adolescents with Depression Study (TADS) Team. (2004). Fluoxetine, cognitive-behavioral therapy, and their combination for adolescents with depression: Treatment for Adolescents with Depression Study (TADS) randomized controlled trial. *Journal of the American Medical Association, 292*(7), 807–820.

McCarthy, S., Wilton, L., Murray, M. L., Hodgkins, P., Asherson, P., & Wong, I. C. (2012). Persistence of pharmacological treatment into adulthood, in UK primary care, for ADHD patients who started treatment in childhood or adolescence. *BMC Psychiatry, 12*(1), 1–9.

Molina, B. S., Hinshaw, S. P., Swanson, J. M., Arnold, L. E., Vitiello, B., Jensen, P. S., Epstein, J. N., Hoza, B., Hechtman, L., Abikoff, H. B., Elliott, G. R., Greenhill, L. L., Newcorn, J. H., Wells,

K. C., Wigal, T., Gibbons, R. D., Hur, K., Houck, P. R., & MTA Cooperative Group. (2009). The MTA at 8 years: prospective follow-up of children treated for combined-type ADHD in a multisite study. *Journal of the American Academy of Child & Adolescent Psychiatry*, 48(5), 484–500.

MTA Cooperative Group. (2004). National Institute of Mental Health Multimodal Treatment Study of ADHD follow-up: 24-month outcomes of treatment strategies for attention-deficit/hyperactivity disorder. *Pediatrics*, 113(4), 754–761.

National Collaborating Centre for Mental Health. (2005). Section 1.6.6: Depression in children and young people: identification and management in primary, community and secondary care. *Database of Abstracts of Reviews of Effects (DARE): Quality-assessed Reviews [Internet]*, p. 19.

National Collaborating Centre for Mental Health (UK). (2015). Challenging behaviour and learning disabilities: prevention and interventions for people with learning disabilities whose behaviour challenges. National Collaborating Centre for Mental Health, UK—2015.

National Collaborating Centre for Mental Health (UK). (2018). *Attention deficit hyperactivity disorder: diagnosis and management of ADHD in children, young people and adults* (NICE Guideline No. 87). British Psychological Society https://www.ncbi.nlm.nih.gov/books/NBK493361/

National Institute for Care and Health Excellence (NICE). (2013). *Psychosis and schizophrenia in children and young people: recognition and management* (Clinical guideline 155). https://www.nice.org.uk/guidance/cg155

National Institute for Care and Health Excellence (NICE). (2014). *Antisocial behaviour and conduct disorders in children and young people: recognition and management* (Clinical guideline 158). http://www.nice.org.uk/guidance/cg158

Pandey, S., Srivanitchapoom, P., Kirubakaran, R., & Berman, B. D. (2018). Botulinum toxin for motor and phonic tics in Tourette's syndrome. *Cochrane Database of Systematic Reviews*, (1) CD012285. https://doi.org/10.1002/14651858.CD012285.pub

Patsalos, P. N., & Perucca, E. (2003). Clinically important drug interactions in epilepsy: general features and interactions between antiepileptic drugs. *Lancet Neurology*, 2(6), 347–356.

Pearson, D. A., Santos, C. W., Roache, J. D., Casat, C. D., Loveland, K. A., Lachar, D., Lane, D. M., Faria, L. P., & Cleveland, L. A. (2003). Treatment effects of methylphenidate on behavioral adjustment in children with mental retardation and ADHD. *Journal of the American Academy of Child & Adolescent Psychiatry*, 42(2), 209–216.

Penttilä, M., Jääskeläinen, E., Hirvonen, N., Isohanni, M., & Miettunen, J. (2014). Duration of untreated psychosis as predictor of long-term outcome in schizophrenia: systematic review and meta-analysis. *British Journal of Psychiatry*, 205(2), 88–94.

Pliszka, S., & AACAP Work Group on Quality Issues. (2007). Practice parameter for the assessment and treatment of children and adolescents with attention-deficit/hyperactivity disorder. *Journal of the American Academy of Child & Adolescent Psychiatry*, 46(7), 894–921.

Pringsheim, T., Panagiotopoulos, C., Davidson, J., Ho, J., & Canadian Alliance for Monitoring Effectiveness and Safety of Antipsychotics in Children (CAMESA) Guideline Group. (2011). Evidence-based recommendations for monitoring safety of second-generation antipsychotics in children and youth. *Paediatrics & Child Health*, 16(9), 581–589.

Raman, S. R., Man, K. K., Bahmanyar, S., Berard, A., Bilder, S., Boukhris, T., Bushnell, G., Crystal, S., Furu, K., KaoYang, Y.–H., Karlstad, Ø., Kieler, H., Kubota, K., Chia–Cheng Lai, E., Martikainen, J. E., Maura, G., Moore, N., Montero, D., Nakamura, H., . . . & Wong, I. C. K. (2018). Trends in attention-deficit hyperactivity disorder medication use: a retrospective observational study using population-based databases. *Lancet Psychiatry*, 5(10), 824–835.

Rani, F., Murray, M. L., Byrne, P. J., & Wong, I. C. (2008). Epidemiologic features of anti-psychotic prescribing to children and adolescents in primary care in the United Kingdom. *Pediatrics*, *121*(5), 1002–1009.

Reddihough, D. S., Marraffa, C., Mouti, A., O'Sullivan, M., Lee, K. J., Orsini, F., Hazell, P., Granich, J., Whitehouse, A. J. O., Wray, J., Dossetor, D., Santosh, P., Silove, N., & Kohn, M. (2019). Effect of fluoxetine on obsessive-compulsive behaviors in children and adolescents with autism spectrum disorders: a randomized clinical trial. *Journal of the American Medical Association*, *322*(16), 1561–1569. https://doi.org/10.1001/jama.2019.14685

Sagar–Ouriaghli, I., Lievesley, K., & Santosh, P. J. (2018). Propranolol for treating emotional, behavioural, autonomic dysregulation in children and adolescents with autism spectrum disorders. *Journal of Psychopharmacology*, *32*(6), 641–653.

Shaw, M., Hodgkins, P., Caci, H., Young, S., Kahle, J., Woods, A. G., & Arnold, L. E. (2012). A systematic review and analysis of long-term outcomes in attention deficit hyperactivity disorder: effects of treatment and non-treatment. *BMC Medicine*, *10*(1), 99.

Shaw, P., Stringaris, A., Nigg, J., & Leibenluft, E. (2014). Emotion dysregulation in attention deficit hyperactivity disorder. *American Journal of Psychiatry*, *171*(3), 276–293.

Shea, S., Turgay, A., Carroll, A., Schulz, M., Orlik, H., Smith, I., & Dunbar, F. (2004). Risperidone in the treatment of disruptive behavioral symptoms in children with autistic and other pervasive developmental disorders. *Pediatrics*, *114*(5), e634–e641.

Simonoff, E., Taylor, E., Baird, G., Bernard, S., Chadwick, O., Liang, H., Whitewell, S., Riemer, K., Sharma, K., Pandey Sharma, S., Wood, N., Kelly, J., Golaszewski, A., Kennedy, J., Rodney, L., West, N., Walwyn, R., & Jichi, F. (2013). Randomized controlled double-blind trial of optimal dose methylphenidate in children and adolescents with severe attention deficit hyperactivity disorder and intellectual disability. *Journal of Child Psychology and Psychiatry*, *54*(5), 527–535.

Sonuga–Barke E. & Taylor E. (2015). ADHD and hyperkinetic disorder. In A. Thapar, D. S. Pine, J. F. Leckman, S. Scott, M. J. Snowling, & E. A. Taylor (Eds.), *Rutter's child and adolescent psychiatry* (6th ed.) (pp. 738–756). Blackwell–Wiley.

Walkup, J. T., Albano, A. M., Piacentini, J., Birmaher, B., Compton, S. N., Sherrill, J. T., Ginsburg, G. S., Rynn, M. A., McCracken, J., Waslick, B., Iyengar, S., March, J. S., & Kendall, P. C. (2008). Cognitive behavioral therapy, sertraline, or a combination in childhood anxiety. *New England Journal of Medicine*, *359*(26), 2753–2766.

Yang, C. S., Zhang, L. L., Zeng, L. N., Huang, L., & Liu, Y. T. (2013). Topiramate for Tourette's syndrome in children: a meta-analysis. *Pediatric Neurology*, *49*(5), 344–350.

CHAPTER 10

FROM ALTERED FUNCTION TO RESTRICTION OF LIFE

10.1 ADVERSE OUTCOMES

KEY lines of development, and the influences on their pathology, have in previous chapters been based on descriptions of behaviour and cognition. Many of the changes in them could be considered simply as differences between people rather than necessarily as disorders. For them to be considered as disorders, there should also be an impact: that daily life should be affected for the worse. Chapter 1, Section 1.2.8 has drawn out the difference between an inability to carry out desired activities and the extent to which that leads to restrictions on daily life. Life for individuals with altered mental function does not have to be restricted. Unfortunately, it often is. Their families do not have to suffer, but they often do. This chapter describes the pathways that often lead to adverse outcomes and how they might be bettered. They will be conceptualized as a series of encounters between people with neurodevelopmental problems and potentially harmful environmental influences on them.

Adverse outcomes include academic and occupational achievement below what should be expected, unhappy relationships with other people, limitations in self-care and travel, shortened life span, problems in physical health and medical care, emotional distress, institutionalization, drug misuse, and oppressive care.

This chapter has no intention of assuming that the limitations accompanying neurodevelopmental disorders are necessary or constant features of the brain and mental changes. Rather, the massive influences of context will be acknowledged by organizing the routes from symptoms to disability in terms of the situations people will encounter in the course of their development. Reactions to these situations account for much of the fluctuation seen in the courses of the psychiatric syndromes. Many of these contextual influences apply for all neurodevelopmental alterations, so ways of alleviating their impacts can often be considered transdiagnostically.

There are also some kinds of adverse outcome that can be considered as unfolding of the specific impairments of specific conditions, and these aspects have been considered in the sections on 'Course over time' in Chapters 3, 4, and 5. Genetic influences, for instance, operate on course as well as on the initiation of disorders. They can influence both the extent to which people with disorders are exposed to harmful environments and their reactions to them (see 'Gene–environment interactions and correlations', Chapter 7, Sections 7.5.3 and 7.5.4).

10.2 CULTURAL ENCOUNTERS: STIGMA

People with neuropsychiatric conditions encounter a variety of stereotyped, negative perceptions about people like themselves. The details vary from place to place, condition to condition, and time to time.

Sociological formulations generally follow Goffman (2009) in describing *stigma* as a belief, behaviour, or reputation about groups of people which is socially discrediting and devalues people's social identity. Those affected by stigma have a quality that their society sees as undesirable—a discrepancy between the person they might ideally be and the person they are. The discrepancy, in Goffman's words, is between their virtual and actual social identity. Social process disempowers those regarded as *other* than the true members of society. There is an extensive literature on the stigma of mental illness in adults, but rather little on psychiatric disorders in children (Mukolo et al., 2010). It is true that children are already attributed with much less power and status than adults, but the societies which they inhabit (e.g. peer culture, school systems, families) can still exclude or disqualify minorities among them. Children and their parents can still be held to be more or less responsible for their problems and more or less worthy of being helped. The impact of stigma on young people and their families depends on the culture in which they live, the extent to which their problems are visible, and the extent to which they are perceived as uncontrollable.

10.2.1 Stigma in different conditions

Some individuals' problems are visible and cannot readily be hidden except by reclusiveness. Others can be hidden from view, but at a price. Young people with Tourette disorder, for instance, often try to camouflage their involuntary movements by turning them into something apparently purposive. A stabbing gesture may be modified, after it has started, into the appearance of pointing. This may still get a negative reception, but that can be preferred to being seen as out of control. Grand mal seizures, by contrast, evoke strong reactions in people watching them. Parents often think that a child, in a first witnessed attack, is dying. The seizures seem inexplicable and terrifying. They represent human vulnerability and the inability of bystanders to help.

In virtually all cultures, there is strong stigma towards, and felt stigma by, people with epilepsy. The details vary. In traditional Chinese cultures, like many others, seizures can be seen as moral failings, with shame and guilt felt by families as well as by the individuals concerned (Kleinman et al.,1995). Attitudes are changing, but children with epilepsy can still be kept secret and they may not be able to marry. In Africa, supernatural explanations and secrecy about affected family members are still common in rural areas (Jilek–Aall et al. 1997). In many parts of the world, people with epilepsy are legally barred from some kinds of employment such as the police, armed forces, or teaching. In Europe and North America, beliefs that epilepsy is contagious have largely disappeared, but seizures are still regarded by many people as mental rather than neurological disorders (Jacoby et al., 2005).The perceived implications are then of being potentially violent, retarded, weak, and sluggish (Scambler, 1989).

Motor disorders such as cerebral palsy and developmental coordination disorder (DCD) are often readily apparent, even if the full extent of problems is not. Behavioural syndromes such as attention deficit hyperactivity disorder (ADHD) and autism spectrum disorder (ASD) often make it clear, even on first acquaintance, that there is something different about the person. The extent to which stigma is involved is largely a matter of the knowledge and attitudes of the people involved, as indicated in the following sections on parents, siblings, educators, and peers.

Other neurodevelopmental conditions cannot be readily seen. Well-controlled epilepsy will be invisible. Aspects of ADHD and ASD, such as a tantrum in the supermarket or a refusal to greet a family friend may well be conspicuous, but they are likely to be perceived by outsiders as problems relating to mental health or parenting. Different kinds of stigma then apply. The label attached to the condition is an important determinant of reactions to the person. One way of coping is by concealing the label.

10.2.2 Concealment

Families vary in the extent to which they want the information about children's conditions to be shared. For some, the benefits of explicit recognition include clarity, accommodations in education, and provision of health resources. For others, the benefits are outweighed by the likelihood of stigma—for instance, what family, friends, and school personnel will think. Guilt and shame can appear in the family, sometimes even more than in their child. 'Courtesy stigma' involves the extension of stigma from the individual to those associated.

Young people themselves not only find that they are often discriminated against in fact; they also assume, from their general knowledge of other people's attitudes, that they will be devalued and discriminated against. They can sometimes become expert in information control (e.g. about the reasons for clinic appointments). If they cope by using strategies such as secrecy and social withdrawal, they risk distancing themselves from others and reinforcing their own feeling of stigma. Loneliness and distress are frequent results. If young people internalize society's stereotyped and negative beliefs, their self-esteem tends to fall, and they consider themselves unworthy of friendship or love. This form of self-stigmatization is not universal. Many will have the same pride in achievement and satisfaction in relationships as anybody else. The section on cerebral palsy (6.3.3.13) has illustrated how children can be much more positive than their parents about their lives.

Occasionally, society's views are reflected by children acting into them and adopting exaggerated forms of the socially proscribed roles. Children with ADHD, for instance, may take on deliberately clownish styles of boisterousness or intrusive rudeness. Children with a specific learning disorder (LD) may refuse to contribute to classroom discussions. These evasions can preserve their sense of being in control and provide a role in the society of children. Adolescents and adults can adopt a similar front as an excuse for their other failings, or as a disguise for them. The risks are exclusion and the avoidance of challenge. Stigma can then be exacerbated.

10.2.3 Myths

Stereotypical views about disability are complex, variable, and widespread, with both positive and negative attributions. Autism, for instance, is still seen by many as a form of intellectual disability, but by many others as a marker to high but unusually specialist intelligence. Media presentations have helped to form a stereotype of an unworldly person with savant abilities. Parents can be led to unrealistic assumptions about brilliant cognitive achievement or, alternatively, to unrealistically despairing predictions about capacity to learn, or to frustration that their expectations are not being met. All can be harmful, in different ways.

The extent to which myths should be considered as aspects of stigma is complicated by the diversity of prejudice, and the influences on them that come from society at large. Some authorities implicate mass and social media, some the transmission of family and professional views, some the importance of religious beliefs, and some the assumptions of educational policy. Useful theory might guide professionals to understand and interrupt stigma in these conditions.

A transcultural approach to global mental health has identified young people's conditions as suffering crucially from stigma and discrimination (Patel et al., 2007). There is a pressing need for mental health services to be given as much priority as those for physical health and for integration with other youth programmes, including education and social care. In many countries, political action will be needed. This does not have to involve the undue medicalization that could detract from local cultural acceptance of unusual adolescent behaviour. The involvement of young people should be a key part of the process.

10.2.4 Counteracting stigma and discrimination

Common sense has produced many ways of counteracting the toxic effects of stereotypes that regard people with brain-based conditions as being less than fully human or not entitled to help. Consumer advocacy and the voluntary sector have been very important in preventing children from being hidden from public view and excluded from treatment, care, and support.

Health professionals are in a good position to challenge entrenched myths. Childhood disability is sometimes thought to be linked to divine punishment, possession, witchcraft, or more modern types of supernatural influence. Simple contradiction then risks losing all credibility. Professionals may find it helpful to make links with the local leaders who carry power in the community. These leaders may be traditional healers, priests, shamans, broadcasters, media stars, and/or social media influencers. Refusal to recognize their influence and good intentions risks forfeiting opportunities to debate. They may be persuaded that children with disorders are no risk to others or that treatment is possible, even within a framework of prevailing beliefs that will take a long time to change.

Psychoeducation to children of different ages, to their families, and to non-specialist teachers has been helpful in changing attitudes. Bipolar disorder, ADHD, ASD, and Tourette syndrome (TS) are all probable examples of impact reducing when knowledge increases. It is not so clear whether, as hoped, there has been an improvement in emotional acceptance of, and by, disabled people. Yamaguchi et al. (2013) describe studies of conveying non-stigmatizing pictures of mental illness to young people at college through media of puppetry, drama, stories, and the like. The hope is that when they are fully adults, they will make a less discriminatory world.

The effects of remedial efforts can sometimes be paradoxical. Read et al. (2006) reviewed attempts to reduce discrimination against people with schizophrenia through explanation and information. When members of the public were given genetic explanations of the illness, their subsequent attitudes toward people with the illness were actually more negative than when given accounts that focused on family and environmental causes. They were more inclined to regard those affected as dangerous and unpredictable, and therefore to show more fear of them and wishes to keep away from them. Such findings call into question the frequent belief of researchers that biogenetic findings will dispel prejudice and stigma. Physical explanations of cause can have the disadvantages of implying untreatability and fixed outcomes. Perhaps these disadvantages can sometimes outweigh any benefits of diminishing the self-blame that is potentially fuelled by advice that stresses social causes.

Names of disorders can be changed away from those carrying heavily prejudicial connotations. It typically takes a long time, but eventually helps. 'Spastic' came to imply stupidity and to be a playground term of abuse. It has not yet been eliminated as such in England. 'Mongolism', however, is seldom heard any more in that context, perhaps because racism itself is withering. An apparently successful change in Japan has been for the word that translates as 'schizophrenia', 'Seishin-Bunretsu-Byo' (mind-split disease), to be replaced by the new name of 'Togo-Shitcho-Sho' (integration disorder) (Sartorius et al., 2014). An immediate result was an increase in communicating the diagnosis to patients and, in the view of psychiatrists, it has accompanied a widespread shift from fatalistic pessimism to realistic optimism. South Korea, Hong Kong, and Singapore (but not China) have taken similar decisions. It remains to be seen whether the change is permanent, or whether stigma will outrun the exact words used.

Publicity, through journalism and advocacy campaigns, can counteract the images of untreatability and portray mental disorders as events that can happen to anybody. This should indeed reduce some harmful ideas of otherness. On the other hand, stories emphasizing that 'he can't help it' and 'it's not her fault' can inadvertently strengthen the notions that the conditions are uncontrollable and the individuals incompetent— which are themselves key aspects of stigma. Positive role models can have high impact. Sportsmen and performers with ADHD, and artists and IT workers with ASD, have all 'outed' themselves. They have conveyed a powerful message of the possibility of good lives and personal control.

First-hand contact between typically and atypically developing children, and the same for their respective parents, is emphasized by many models of countering stigma. Intuitively, it seems clear that people who interact more with young people labelled as deviant will share more with them, find more in common, and develop more empathy.

A legal framework asserting the rights of all people to attend school or work, to have housing, to family life, and to access healthcare, is enshrined in international conventions of human rights. It can be used to persuade public opinion away from crude forms of stigma and discrimination (Eaton, 2019). In many countries, including England, abuse of disabled people is punishable under the same laws that apply to hate crime, racism, and religious intolerance. By the same token, an empowerment of people who are themselves affected by disability is coming to contribute to policy development about definitions and legal protection. Research could and should address all these approaches. Its lack might indeed be itself a manifestation of stigma.

10.3 Encounters with illness and danger

10.3.1 Mortality

Premature death is more common in people with ASD, learning disabilities, and ADHD than in those developing typically—but for different reasons.

10.3.1.1 *Mortality in ASD*

A large epidemiological study based on a Swedish population register was able to identify 27,122 people who had received a spectrum diagnosis (Hirvikoski et al., 2016). In ICD-9 this meant autism, Asperger syndrome, atypical autism, pervasive developmental disorder not otherwise specified, and childhood disintegrative disorder. They were compared with a matched control group of some 2.7 million. Death rates were higher in ASD, especially in females with low IQ. The commonest association in those with low IQ was epilepsy; in those with ordinary or superior intelligence, suicide.

In both the high- and low-functioning groups there was also greater mortality across a wide range of causes of death. Causes on death certificates included mental and behavioural disorders, and diseases of nervous, circulatory, respiratory, and digestive systems (Bilder et al., 2013). Some in the more disabled group would have had illnesses caused by the conditions causing the ASD (e.g. chromosomal and genetic anomalies); some might well have received a lower standard of medical care than was available to the high-functioning group.

Some more detailed information about risks for suicide in the high-functioning group comes from a survey of 256 men and 118 women recently diagnosed with Asperger's syndrome for the first time, in adult life (Cassidy et al., 2014). Thoughts of, or attempts at, suicide were very frequent—reported at 35%, and depression was rated at 31%. These rates seem very high. They are even higher than those reported in studies of people with multiple physical illnesses or people with psychotic illness. Adults with ASD do have high rates of many adversities that would predict suicide in the general population—including unemployment, few close relationships, and emotional problems.

10.3.1.2 *Mortality in epilepsy*

Epilepsy poses substantial challenges to life. Death rates are increased: in the UK, there are about 1,200 premature deaths a year in people with epilepsy. Some of these deaths are caused by complications during or after a seizure, and accidental falls and drowning play a part. Safety helmets can be used to reduce traumatic injury from falls but are stigmatizing and correspondingly unwelcome to many. There are contributions from underlying neurological problems that have caused the epilepsy, and from coexistent cardiac or respiratory problems.

Sudden, unexpected death (SUD) in epilepsy is a rare event and people will make different decisions about how far to go to reduce the risk. It is possible that it can result, not from the obvious risks of asphyxiation or vomiting, but from autonomic discharges stopping the heart or breathing. The most effective prevention is simply to enhance control of seizures—it is more common in those with very poor control. It can happen in sleep, so people with nocturnal seizures sometimes use a seizure alarm to alert someone who can help. 'Antisuffocation' pillows, which have holes in them for ventilation, probably make no difference. The fear of SUD can motivate high levels of restriction of activity (e.g. by never sleeping away from home).

Undue safety concerns are sometimes imposed on young people with epilepsy for fear of accidental death or failure at tasks. In some places, they may not be allowed to take part in school sports or even some lessons. They may be discriminated against by employers for fear of expensive mistakes, drowsiness, and inattention due to antiepileptic drugs, costs incurred for paid sick leave, or periods of a few hours after a seizure in which they are unproductive. Those fears are not always rational.

10.3.1.3 *Mortality in ADHD*

Mortality in ADHD is also higher than in people developing typically. The reasons for it, however, are different from those in ASD and intellectual disability (ID). Accidents are the leading cause in Europe. A survey from a Danish population register was reported by Dalsgaard et al. (2015a). Out of 1.9 million people of all ages, they identified 32,061 with a diagnosis of ADHD. The mortality rate per 10,000 person years was 5.85 in ADHD, compared with 2.21 in those without. The increase in risk was greater in females than males. The complicating presence of conduct problems and/or substance misuse accounted for some of the high rates in ADHD. However, ADHD by itself was indeed a risk (McCarthy et al., 2009). Unnatural causes of death predominated—especially accidents. The probable reasons are that children and adults with ADHD are more likely to be living in risky areas, and more likely to take hazardous risks, to underestimate danger, and to lack the skills for prevention of injuries, than do peers without ADHD. A study from the UK based on the General Practice Research Database (GPRD) found that the risk of death from accidents was reduced by about half for children and adolescents with ADHD who had been prescribed drug treatments to reduce ADHD problems (Dalsgaard et al., 2015b).

Suicide is also increased by comparison with people without ADHD. In several studies, reviewed by Balazs and Kereszteny (2017), ADHD is a risk for suicidal ideation and action in young people and adults. Scandinavian registers yield enough data—51,707 patients with ADHD in a study by Ljung et al. (2014)—to allow rates of completed suicide to be compared with those in matched controls. Like non-lethal suicidal ideation, self-inflicted death is more frequent in ADHD, with an odds ratio of 5.9 even after adjusting for coexistent psychiatric diagnoses. Much of the risk appears to be mediated either by impulsiveness and emotional dysregulation (rather than the other components of ADHD) or by coexistent disorders (depression in females, conduct disorder and substance misuse in males).

In other parts of the world, including the USA and Taiwan, homicide figures strongly as a cause of increased mortality in ADHD (Chen et al., 2019). Conduct problems, with or without ADHD, also make violent death much more probable. Involvement with antisocial companions could well be a key influence.

Sudden death has been proposed as an adverse effect on the heart of the drugs commonly prescribed for ADHD. However, this plays no substantial part. An examination of the UK's GPRD focused on patients aged 2–21 years with a prescription for methylphenidate, dexamphetamine, or atomoxetine (Dalsgaard et al., 2015b). Out of 18,637 patient years, seven patients died—but none from sudden death with evidence for a drug-related cardiac problem.

10.3.2 Chronic physical health problems

Apart from violent and sudden death, it is likely that the outlook for chronic health conditions will be worsened by neurodevelopmental disorders. In ADHD, risky behaviour exposes young people and adults to conditions (e.g. obesity, smoking, unprotected sex) that are themselves hazards for physical health (Nigg, 2013). The risk is increased by the coexistent presence of conduct problems and substance misuse. It is not always certain how much of the risk is due specifically to ADHD features rather than the conduct problems that frequently coexist.

ASD and ID both come with high rates of known medical problems. A mean of 24% of people in seven population studies had significant disorders of several kinds (Gillberg & Coleman, 1996). Some of them are the effects of the probably causative conditions described in Chapter 7. Many genetic and chromosomal disorders (e.g. Down and 22q11 deletion syndromes) are risks for many physical problems, as well as being associated with autistic features and low IQ. Detailed investigation yields evidence of many serious physical conditions in samples of people with ASD and ID—for instance, respiratory, gastrointestinal, and epileptic events—which lead the causes of fatal illness in these groups (Bilder et al., 2013). A medical workup is therefore indicated as part of routine assessment.

Other medical conditions (see Chapter 6) may be exacerbated by the effects of ASD and ID. Extreme diets in these conditions can lead to constipation, which is often a serious and even a fatal medical problem. Lymphoid hyperplasia in the ileum, which can result from constipation, was responsible for a false but widespread scare that both it and ASD were results of the mumps, measles, rubella (MMR) vaccination (discredited *Lancet* paper by Wakefield et al.; withdrawn, so not cited here). Eating disorders and body dysmorphic disorders are often present in populations screened positive for ASD by questionnaires. Drugs prescribed for people with ASD and/or ID often carry adverse effects for physical health (see Chapter 9, passim). These add to the burden of illness.

Some common physical disorders that are more prevalent in those with ASD than other people (e.g. hypertension, hyperlipidaemia, allergies) are controllable with good medical care. Unfortunately, people with ID or ASD often lack access to such care. They and their caregivers encounter difficulties in travelling to clinics or hospitals, and even when they reach them, there are problems to overcome. Communication problems often leave the explanation of problems and solutions to be a duty for caregivers. Results are frequently that young people with impairments feel excluded from the process and do not participate. The relationship between health professionals and carers can be problematic, especially when constraints of funding and time prohibit time-consuming explanations and adequate support for the carers. Healthcare systems are forbiddingly complicated for many, and often the explanations are in written form, meaning that they demand levels of literacy that exclude those with learning difficulties. Even high-functioning young adults with ASD express dissatisfaction with their access to good service, even when the service specializes in mental health (Lake et al., 2014).

The value of physical medicine for mentally disabled people is increased if general medical services keep a register. They can then be alerted to needs, to make their services more accessible and easier to understand.

Some other common physical disorders may be less common in ASD. Autistic people tend to have lower rates of migraine headaches, sexually transmitted infections, tobacco use, and alcohol misuse than the general population.

10.4 A TURNING POINT IN PHYSICAL DEVELOPMENT: PUBERTY AND THE BRAIN

Puberty consists of three components: adrenarche, growth axis activation, and gonadarche (Dorn & Biro, 2011). They are driven by changes in hormone levels. Staging of puberty is based on Tanner stages of breast and pubic hair development in girls and testicular and pubic hair development in boys (Tanner, 1962). Adrenarche is activation of the hypothalamic–pituitary–adrenal (HPA) axis. It occurs generally around 6–9 years of age for girls and a year later for boys. Axillary hair, breast buds, and body odour are typical early signs. Growth spurt, driven by pituitary growth and hormones, typically starts at about 11 years for females, 12 years for boys. Gonadarche—activation of the hypothalamic–pituitary–gonad axis—starts at around 8–14 years of age for girls and 9–15 for boys.

There is a very wide range of normal variation in the timing of all the bodily changes and the speed at which they take place. In young people with neurodevelopmental disorders, as in everybody else, profound changes take place in brain and endocrine organization. Some of these may be responsible for altered presentations of disorders. Later development of frontal than limbic structures is typical of adolescence, and this could be responsible for enhancing the adolescent tendency to emotional storms. Such changes are sometimes misattributed to a change in the disorder itself or to a change in the quality of care.

In general, earlier timing of puberty is understood to be associated with negative outcomes for emotional life (e.g. depression) and behaviour (e.g. risky behaviours, acting out). The full picture is more complicated. Laitinen–Krispijn et al. (1999) found, in a large epidemiological study in the Netherlands, that depression in boys was less frequent (at least, according to parents' reports) in those who were making more rapid progress in puberty.

Expectations based on gender are in the process of change in several cultures. Young people with difficulties in social understanding can be even more confused than typically developing adolescents about their sexual identity and personal expectations, and about how they should behave. Lesbian, gay, bisexual, and transsexual (LGBT) people who have a neurodevelopmental disorder have an extra set of experiences of discrimination. The hormonal and physical changes of puberty are very similar to those of other young people, but the psychological meaning can differ (Grossman et al., 2014). Feelings of sexual desire can be hard to integrate with self-esteem for LGBT people. Change of body shape and personal expectations can be hard to tolerate for people who resist any kind of change. (See 'Eating disorders in ASD', Chapter 4, Section 4.1.5.5).

10.5 ENCOUNTERS WITH ECONOMIC DISADVANTAGE AND STRESS

Financial costs of disorders are substantial. They are usually estimated separately for each diagnosis. The basis for costing varies, but is usually either the whole cost to society or the burden falling on families specifically. The effect of low incomes as early environmental influences on developing disorders such as ADHD and ASD has been considered previously (see Chapter 7, Section 7.10). Cash poverty can also be an important result of disorders, and consequently an influence on the pathway from impairment to restriction of opportunity.

Buescher et al. (2014) have estimated financial outcomes for autism in the UK. Aggregated national costs of supporting children with ASD are £3.1 billion GBP (US $4.5 billion). These average annual costs of services (especially special education) and support, together with the opportunity costs of lost productivity (mostly by caregivers), make it an exceptionally expensive medical condition. Costs are even higher for those with ASD and ID than for those with ASD alone. The figures given here are for those with ASD assuming a 40% rate of ID. Figures are similar in the UK and USA, in spite of differences in which agencies bear the costs. Costs specifically for families—private ASD services, lost income, and informal care—were estimated in Ireland by Roddy and O'Neill (2019). They amounted to approximately €28,464.89 (£24,630 GBP) a year.

ADHD is also expensive (Russell et al., 2016). Deloitte Access Economics (2019) estimated the total costs for ADHD in Australia, in 2019, as $20.57 billion AUD (£11.3 billion GBP), which translates to $836 AUD (£459 GBP) per capita. Of this total, 63% was attributable to financial costs and 37% to wellbeing costs (including loss of life and loss of life quality). Zhao et al. (2019) costed the economic burden falling on families in Pennsylvania, USA until the children reached the age of 17 years. They included direct costs related to the child's behaviours (excluding treatment expenses) and indirect costs related to caregiver strain. The total was $15,036 per child (c. £11,725 GBP)—more than five times greater than that incurred for young people without ADHD ($2,848 per child). This difference remained significant after controlling for intellectual functioning, oppositional defiant symptoms, or conduct problems.

The impact of low family income on young people will vary from place to place and time to time. It can be gauged from a quasi-experimental study in North Carolina, USA (Akee et al., 2010). There, the Eastern Cherokee community profited from the opening of a casino. Their incomes were increased by about $4,000 a year through a governmental transfer programme that did not take into account parental disadvantage or other needs of the children. Children in those households showed a reduction in behaviour problems, including ADHD, and an increase in school achievement (about 15% more likely to graduate). The study did not focus specifically on the neurodevelopmentally impaired but found that ADHD, although not anxiety, was affected for the better. The ability of parents to better supervise their children probably accounted for much of the change. The study is therefore relevant to the difficulties of poor children with ADHD and poor achievement at school. It supports welfare measures to give parents and others the time and resources to care for and educate children with a disability.

Impoverishment may, therefore, be one strand in the vulnerability of young people with neurodevelopmental disorders such as ADHD to developing coexistent problems of antisocial behaviour or delinquency (Reiss, 2013). It can be hard to understand why there is evidence for a substantial secular increase of adolescent emotional problems and antisocial behaviour in the population of high-income countries (Collishaw, 2015). Despite the absolute increase in income, the gap between low- and high-income groups has widened over time. This disparity might be responsible for the transitions from neurodevelopmental to mental health problems. Both absolute deprivation and relative inequality are probably involved in the transition. There is, however, little reliable knowledge about the balance of the two. Nearly all the research has been carried out in affluent countries. This is a serious limitation on general conclusions about how social influences operate on child development. Any interaction between inequality and neurocognitive impairment is similarly obscure.

10.5.1 'Stress' effects in children's neurodevelopmental disorders

Maltreatment of young children has been described in Chapter 7, Section 7.10 as a potential cause of brain abnormality. Furthermore, suspicion of it contributes to stigma. Fear of being accused of it deters some families from contact with helping agencies. Some professionals' reluctance to admit their suspicions openly deters them from raising the possibility in a clear and matter-of-fact manner.

Several overlapping concepts describe the impact of early and repeated stressors on the development of children with neurodevelopmental disorders.

> *Adverse childhood experiences* describes the events themselves, whether or not they have had a harmful effect.
>
> *Complex post-traumatic stress disorder* is the diagnostic term in the *International Classification of Disease* (draft 11th edition) that defines the impact on the person. Emotional dysregulation, a negative sense of self, physiological reactions, and disturbances of relationships are all included. The application of the concept to children is not fully worked out.
>
> *Developmental trauma* refers to a variable and wide range of negative reactions considered to result from harmful events. The term has the advantage for clinicians of extending more widely than any one conventional diagnosis, and the disadvantage of conflating many processes that may not necessarily represent direct effects

of psychosocial stressors. It has been proposed, but not accepted, as a diagnosis in its own right for DSM-5. Dysregulation of mood, physiological arousal, attention, and behaviour are key aspects, so it will overlap with many other diagnoses, and the grounds for making it (rather than another diagnosis) may be obscure.

10.6 ENCOUNTERS WITH FAMILY: DISTRESS, HOSTILITY, OVERPROTECTION, OVERINVOLVEMENT

Families change when a child develops neurodevelopmental problems. Many parents apply their personal resources, cope well, and find the experience of raising such a child to be rewarding. Many others are challenged to the point of crisis. Children, in turn, are distressed by the problems of their parents. Young people's reactions may include either lessening or worsening of behaviour problems. Siblings share in the emotional and practical challenges.

Parenting distress is the subjective, negative experience of parents and is usually assessed by self-report. It is affected for the worse by many aspects of living with children and young people whose development is non-typical. Burden of care is high for families coping with low-functioning children who need help with daily activities or with severe problems in mobility or continence. The burden falls selectively on the primary caregiver—in most societies, the mother. Time resources are restricted by the needs to interact with schools, attend clinics and benefit agencies, and travel for services. Financial difficulties arise especially when parents must cut down on paid work, provide special diets or mobility aids, and employ care assistants. Worry about the future is exacerbated by chronically poor school performance and children's refractoriness to teaching. Frustration comes from slow rates of progress, and from the unresponsiveness of some children to attempts at relating to or soothing them. Social isolation results from lack of time for activities, and from shame and guilt related to stigma (see Section 10.2).

10.6.1 Dysfunctional parent–child interactions

Nurturing, responsive, and consistent positive interactions between parents and children are vulnerable both to risks arising from the children's difficulties and to associated risks. The latter include poor mental health of a parent, poverty, overcrowding, lack of neighbourhood social capital, and poor parental coping.

Dysfunctional interactions are associated with the presence of emotional and behaviour problems in the children. Child behaviour problems from all causes predict parental distress. ASD and ADHD are particularly potent, especially when there are problems of conduct complicating ADHD (meta-analysis by Theule et al., 2013). This would be true both in studies of the general population and clinical samples. When neurodevelopmental disorders are studied separately, ASD and ADHD seem to have the harshest impact on parental distress (Craig et al., 2016).

The outcomes for parenting distress operate in two directions. Some children's problems can come from qualities in parents that are not caused by their offspring. The influence of the early maternal environment on children's neurodevelopment has been considered in Chapter 7, Section 7.10. Evidence of bidirectional impact comes from studies of the emotional atmosphere in homes. One series of laboratory experiments used volunteer parents and confederate children who were trained either to misbehave in ADHD fashion or to behave compliantly (Pelham & Lang, 1993). The children behaving in a difficult way reliably elicited distress and alcohol consumption by the parents—even those parents who did not have problems of their own. In turn, alcohol use made the parents more ineffective (e.g. more indulgent) in their handling of children's difficult behaviour. There were both child-to-adult and adult-to-child effects. ADHD (impulsive) behaviours were very potent in altering parents' reactions. Conduct disorder (aggressive) behaviours added only a little more.

A proxy measure for the emotional quality of parent–child interaction can be applied in research and clinical practice: expressed emotion. Parents talking about their children's problems will have their speech content and manner influenced by emotional attitudes. From recordings of what parents have said, observers can code the way their comments are influenced. *Hostility* will be reflected in remarks that are unnecessarily critical of the child's personality (rather than just descriptive of misbehaviour) and carry intense criticism in the tone of voice. Lack of spontaneous praise, and spontaneous criticism after mentioning a good quality, can also be detected reliably for research purposes by a trained rater. Clinicians will make similar judgements about the child in the course of an interview, but need to avoid a judgement about hostility based only on descriptions of difficult behaviour. Questions such as 'How have you felt about this problem?' can be very useful.

Emotional overinvolvement can also be rated reliably from the way that caregivers describe their child's difficulties. It is based on evidence of overprotectiveness, marked overconcern, excessively self-sacrificing behaviours, or exaggerated emotional responses when talking about the child. These aspects, however, do not seem to be influential for the development of psychopathology in children. In adults with schizophrenia, by contrast, they do seem to be associated with relapse. Perhaps emotional overinvolvement is not a good way of describing the relationship between parents and dependent children.

High levels of hostility and criticism from the caregivers (high EE) are quite strongly associated with irritability and antisocial behaviour in the child, and with punishment-based or frightening discipline. These associations hold even after controlling for genetic confounding, by studying them in identical twins (Caspi et al., 2004). They probably contribute to the development of oppositional problems in children with ADHD who do not have other neurodevelopmental problems or evidence of brain damage or disease. High levels of critical expressed emotion are also associated with adverse outcomes in young people with schizophrenic, depressive, obsessive-compulsive, eating, and bipolar disorders (Peris & Miklowitz, 2015). Indeed, the measure was originally introduced to monitor the reasons for relapse in adults with schizophrenia after their discharge home from hospital.

High EE levels are associated with adverse outcomes for the children They may reflect direct stresses at home, and such remarks in themselves may heighten emotional arousal in the children. They may also be markers to the absence of protective factors in the parent–child relationship, such as harmony and support, which ordinarily buffer the effects of parental stress on the children. They can also influence young people's reactions to stress. Physiological studies on university students who had previously been depressed found altered brain responses when listening to tapes of their mothers making critical remarks about them. There was, by comparison with never-depressed students, less activation in the dorsolateral frontal cortex and more activation in the amygdala (Hooley et al., 2009). High EE can also represent the effects of child behaviour on adults. Schachar et al. (1987) found that high levels of critical expressed emotion by adults were lowered after medication of the children reduced their difficult behaviour.

Parenting distress and dysfunctional parenting can correspondingly be modified both by interventions directed at children and by help for parents to understand, stay calm, and learn skills of interaction (see Chapter 8). Many programmes of 'parent training' are available (see Chapter 8, Section 8.5) and effect sizes are moderate to large (meta-analysis by Vidal & Connell, 2019).

10.6.2 Parenting in chronic tic disorders

Children with TS are also more likely than those in the general population to have distressed parents. The stresses on parents include those associated with other chronic medical conditions: guilt, shame, and difficulty in coping. Specific problems, however, arise in relation to discipline because of the unpredictability of the condition, and the difficulty in distinguishing deliberate from involuntary misbehaviour.

Perceptions of the controllability of tics can drive unhelpful reactions. Sometimes tics are misunderstood as voluntary naughtiness, and sometimes managed by punishment or humiliation. Such reactions tend to make the tics worse and the child more demoralized. Sometimes, by contrast, they are considered as a disease entity that is responsible for all the other difficulties that may be present. Medical management can then be seen as essential. If so, there is a danger that medication may be started prematurely and continued at excessive doses.

The strongest risk for distress in the parents of those with chronic tic disorders comes if there are other mental disorders as well. Epidemiological studies have confirmed both the frequency and impact of complicating disorders. As an example, 91,642 parents or guardians of children from birth to the age of 17 years were randomly selected, from the entire population of families with a landline telephone number, in the USA National Survey of Children's Health 2007 (Robinson et al., 2013). Parents who said that they had at any time received a diagnosis of TS for their child were more likely than others to report high levels of aggravation. This kind of distress was nearly always related, not to the tics themselves, but to the associated problems—especially (and in order of frequency) ADHD, other behaviour problems, anxiety, depression, and ASD (obsessive-compulsive disorder was not included in this survey).

10.6.3 Protection and overprotection

The risk that hyperactive and impulsive behaviours pose for accidental injuries (see Section 10.3) can be attenuated by alert supervision from parents who have the time to provide it. For instance, Schwebel et al. (2004) reanalysed data from a previously studied group of some 10,000 American 5-year-olds. The temporal resources of the families interacted with the hyperactivity-impulsivity of the children to reduce the association between hyperactivity and accidents requiring medical attention.

The risks to life and physical health from epilepsy can be attenuated—for young children, by wise control of activities; and for teenagers, by engaged discussion about avoidable risks. One parental reaction is to restrict their child's activities in the interests of safety. The balance between undue restrictiveness and dangerous exposure is not easy to achieve, but most families will reach it with good explanation. In epilepsy, for example, some unsupervised activities with risks of injury, danger, or damage to health may need to be avoided. Swimming, cycling, climbing, and driving all carry hazards if the person loses awareness or control in a seizure. If seizures are well controlled with medication, then there is little risk. Most people with controlled epilepsy will reckon to take part in a full range of activities—if necessary, with a responsible person to help in an emergency. Driving and operating heavy machinery, however, are usually under legal restrictions that vary from country to country. In some places, patients are required by law to report themselves and, sometimes, there is a legal duty on parents to ensure that they do.

10.7 SUBSTITUTE CARE AND ACCOMMODATION

If children's needs overwhelm the resources of their families, the local authority has a duty to provide any services necessary to meet the needs of disabled children. In theory, this could mean anything. In practice, it usually means a residential school, a residential or short-term care home, centre-based respite care, a link with another family for regular but short-term respite stays, or a range of play schemes, youth clubs, and other activities outside the home.

Sometimes, special needs such as challenging behaviours are met by long-term health-based accommodation. It may be provided in NHS or private-sector hospitals, or in nursing homes. Hospital care, however, is not usually well organized for promoting long-term development. There have been scandals of neglect and cruelty, often related to inadequately trained staff or an orientation to cure rather than care. The caring professions have a different skill set and organizational culture from therapists. Treatment and care should not be confused.

Short of abusive neglect or cruelty, care can still be oppressive. It can fail to address the recipients of care as individuals. It can deny them the opportunity to make decisions for themselves. It can make excessive use of calming medication—sometimes to make life easier for the carers. It can present an attitude of regarding its recipients as threats or nuisances, and making them feel like that. Assertion of legal rights can help. Advocacy for those who cannot assert for themselves can be provided. The traps of allowing single-issue campaigners to become advocates can be avoided. Oppression can be countered by enough valuing of carers to enable them to value recipients.

10.8 ENCOUNTERS WITH MISUSED SUBSTANCES

For young people in most countries, the relationships they make with alcohol and drugs of misuse are significant determinants of their path to independence. It has been thought, and is still usually said, that ASD acts as protection against both early and late stages of misuse. It may not be entirely true. The belief comes from a time when autism was rare and most autistic people were intellectually disabled and living away from the temptations of ready access and peer pressure. Nowadays, most people diagnosed with ASD are in the normal range of IQ and attending mainstream education. As a result of normalization, several potential risks come into play. High levels of anxiety seem to be putting autistic people at risk for self-medication patterns of substance use.

Social difficulties do not only lead to isolation: they sometimes bring people with ASD into contact with youth cultures that accept eccentricity and may adopt use of substances such as cannabis as part of that culture. ASD very often exists in combination with ADHD, which does have an association with some forms of substance misuse. Compulsive and repetitive behaviour patterns characterize ASD and are also quite frequent in addiction.

Many adults have come through childhood and adolescence with difficulties but without diagnosis. One population study using case registers indicated that people with diagnosed ASD (and an IQ above 100) had higher rates of diagnosed substance misuse (about 4%) than matched controls (1.3%) (Butwicka et al., 2017). Much of the increased risk was attributable to coexistent ADHD, but people diagnosed only with ASD still had a doubled risk.

ADHD has a well-recognized association with substance misuse. Lee et al. (2011) conducted a meta-analysis of 27 studies that had the important qualities of prospective longitudinal designs. In these follows-up, ADHD predicted later substance misuse. Children with ADHD were twice as likely as unaffected children to have a later history of 'ever used' nicotine and were more likely to continue. They were not more likely to have 'ever used' alcohol, but they did have a somewhat increased risk for alcohol use disorder (OR = 1.7). They were nearly three times more likely to have reported 'ever used' marijuana' and approximately one and a half times more likely to develop marijuana abuse or dependence, and they were twice as likely to be using cocaine. Longitudinal data on the use of opiates is lacking.

The prescribed use of stimulants does not seem either to increase or reduce these risks (see 'Adverse effects of stimulants', Chapter 9, Section 9.4.4).

A great part of these worrying associations is attributable to the coexistent presence of oppositional-defiant disorder or conduct disorder. These disruptive problems of conduct raise the risk of substance use disorders even without ADHD, and limited evidence suggests that young people with ADHD only (and no oppositionality) are no more at risk than any other teenager. The exception may be for the risk of tobacco smoking, where observational studies suggest that ADHD, even without comorbid problems, is still a substantial risk. Perhaps the pharmacological anti-ADHD effects of nicotine promote greater use than would otherwise be the case.

Common influences across ADHD, ID, and ASD (e.g. disrupted parenting practices, deviant peer affiliation) may work synergistically with neurodevelopmental changes that are particularly salient in adolescence, including levels of striatal dopamine and its influence on reward sensitivity and risk taking (Galvan, 2013). Finally, some dimensions of anxiety may actually protect individuals with ADHD from risk taking, externalizing behavior, or substance misuse (Levy, 2004).

10.9 ENCOUNTERS WITH SCHOOL AND PEERS

School systems vary in their willingness and ability to accommodate children's impairments. Special needs can arise from children's tolerance of school environments, struggles in learning, communication and attention problems, impulsive and antisocial conduct, movement and sensory difficulties.

10.9.1 Tolerance of school

Starting in school is an unfamiliar experience, and children with special needs may need to adjust more gradually than others. ASD and related features in other disorders often include components that make school environments very unpleasant for them. Specialist schools have evolved ways of making classrooms more bearable for children and young people with ASD. They are often available for consultation for those working in regular classrooms. These days, most autistic children are in mainstream schools and often unrecognized as such. Teachers can, however, use some common-sense approaches that stem from understanding the barriers imposed by ASD and similar conditions. Above all, advice should be to take individualized approaches in line with the pupil's needs.

- Mainstream classrooms are often noisy, and their sound levels can be aversive to children with auditory hypersensitivity.
- Consider a quiet place (not the ones used for time out) to which children can retreat, or try ear plugs.
- There is often a good deal of change in a good classroom. Most children will enjoy plenty of changes of activity, from quiet study to group work to games. Not so those with strong preferences for the predictable. Routine helps to make them feel secure. For them, any change may need to be explained in detail beforehand.
- Simplify communication and allow time for children to process information. Use visual aids like day planners.
- Some autistic children get fixated on one subject—maybe trains or maps or timetables. Teachers can use this to motivate learning—in reading about maps, or calculations about trains, or in learning how to explain their special interest to other people.
- Keep a behaviour diary, or an antecedent–behaviour–consequence (ABC) chart.
- Keep anxiety down: deal with any bullying promptly; maintain safe spaces; and encourage pupils to use an 'escape card' to indicate that their stress levels are rising and they need to leave the classroom.
- Negotiate their curriculum with them: what to learn and when. This is especially applicable to children with high levels of demand avoidance. They need to feel that they are in control.
- Parents can be very helpful—in reassuring their children about their safety, and in explaining their unique profile of strengths and weaknesses to the teachers and assistants.

Besides features associated with ASD, other neurodevelopmental problems may make it desirable to consider modifying the classroom environment. For children with ADHD, remaining still or quiet can be very unpleasant. Days absent from school are more frequent in young people with ADHD. Teenagers with ADHD are much more likely to drop out from school and end their education prematurely. They may need more opportunities than other students for muscular activity. This can sometimes be channelled—for instance, by making them the messengers to take information around the school. It may mean missing some teaching time, but that is usually worth it.

For children with learning difficulties, the fear and experience of failure may make classrooms become settings of conditioned anxiety. Truancy and school refusal result.

10.9.2 Communication problems

Children with ASD, language delays, or ID may struggle to explain the difficulties they are having. Parents and other caregivers can be very helpful interpreters, and wise schools will recognize their value and encourage contact. Misunderstandings between children and teachers add to the time and effort required from teachers. Children's reluctance to speak out—at the extreme, selective mutism—increases the distance between them and their teachers.

10.9.3 Anxiety

High anxiety characterizes many children with ASD, ADHD, and learning disabilities. It is not always immediately apparent what the triggers are. Sensitive enquiry and observation may make it clear—for instance, that there is an unfamiliar scent or a break in routine. Children with impairments are by no means immune to worries about their future, or the reactions of their parents to bad reports from school, or test/exam results, or friendships going wrong, or problems at home, or violence outside the school, or indeed any of the troubles that beset young people. To the contrary, they are more likely to encounter these sources of distress and be less equipped to deal with them. Communication problems may mean that they struggle to express their worries, and therefore be less likely to get relief from counselling or cognitive therapies. Indeed, they may not get access to cognitive behavioural therapy (CBT) because of a mistaken belief that they cannot profit from it. Clinical professionals may need to develop their patience and the simplicity of what they say.

10.9.4 Attention problems

Difficulties in concentrating are a key part of ADHD. As with all children, they can be signs of boredom, or a mismatch between the child's ability and the level of difficulty of the tasks assigned to them. In ADHD, however, the problems take a distinctive form. Teachers will usually be alert to this, but may not always recognize the disorganized attention of ADHD. Increasing the structure in presenting material to be learned usually helps. Experienced teachers also know the value of orientating the child—'now listen and learn how to do this'—before embarking on explanations. In these respects, those with ADHD need to be taught like people younger than themselves. The individual attention that is needed can complicate and slow down dealing with the rest of the class. Teaching assistants can take on much of this individual work. If they are not available, then volunteer parents can help, but may need the support of training in how to break down tasks into smaller parts and reward successful attempts at them.

It can be hard to tell whether failures to learn are the result of poor memory or whether the material to be learned has not been fully registered in the first place. The latter is typical of the attention problems of ADHD. Poor attention can be a powerful cause of failing to learn. In a longitudinally followed cohort, rated inattentive behaviour at the age of 7 years was a good predictor of poor academic achievement at age 16 years (Sayal et al., 2015b). Indeed, there was a linear association between each one-point increase in inattention symptoms and worse outcomes in terms of grades at the English national certificate examination (a two- to three-point reduction) and the probability of attaining the national standard of three good GCSEs (a 10% reduction). These figures applied across the whole range of variation in the population and not only to the extremes associated with an ADHD diagnosis. This important impact of inattention does not only affect children after they have started at school, and is not only because of impulsive conduct. Another cohort study followed English children from the age of 3 years until 10–11 years, the age at which secondary education will begin (Washbrook et al., 2013). It found a similar association between inattentiveness at the outset and learning problems at outcome.

Unfortunately, however, the clear epidemiological evidence for the educational impact of inattentiveness has not so far been matched by evidence of effective interruption of the pathway. Several approaches have been tried (see Chapter 8, Section 8.6). A randomized cluster-controlled trial in schools involving more than 50,000 children found no useful effect on academic outcomes of giving evidence-based advice to the schools on how to intervene for ADHD (Sayal et al., 2015a). Another intervention in the same study involved identifying, to the schools, the children who screened positive for ADHD. This naming, however, was actually followed by worsening in comparison with children who were not identified in this way. Perhaps there were negative effects of labelling and teacher expectations were lowered for the identified cases. This should be a caution against routine screening for ADHD in schools unless and until there is sound evidence for effective interventions.

Programmes of intervention in schools to enhance attention and academic learning have received plenty of research, a thorough systematic review, and meta-analysis (Richardson et al., 2015). It turned out that there were great differences between the outcomes reported from the various randomized controlled trials. Effects of school attempts to improve scholastic achievement in ADHD were small or very small. On other kinds of ADHD outcomes, effect sizes varied greatly, from very small to large. The most promising results came when the outcomes were neuropsychological test scores rather than observable behaviour. The researchers, however, could not find evidence that any particular intervention was better than any other. They included several trials of different ways that schools might help: contingency management; daily report card; cognitive-behavioural self-regulation; cognitive skills retraining; academic study skills; and emotional skills training. None outperformed the others, and there was little evidence that aspects of intervention delivery (context, provider, time, setting, duration, and intensity) made any difference. On balance, the review and, therefore, the current state of the art give some, admittedly doubtful, support for attempts in schools to help children's attention to flourish—but not for any one method over and above any other.

One must add that the extent to which the current trials should guide practice is greatly limited by weaknesses in their methods. None included both random allocation and blind assessment to the level required for clinical confidence. Most of the trials were conducted in schools in North America, which are not representative of international education. It should, therefore, be incumbent on school systems adopting a package for attention improvement in their pupils to include an assessment of whether it is working.

There have been attempts to reduce distractions in the classroom environment or to provide background music. They do not seem to be successful in improving levels of attention in most children, and indeed there is no good reason why they should. Inattentive children do have lapses of attention, but they stem from within, not primarily from being captured by attractive external stimuli.

Experimental attempts to improve cognitive aspects of attention and executive function can also be delivered in school (see Chapter 8, Section 8.6). Systematic review suggests that they have not yet been shown to be effective when their outcomes are rated by blinded assessors (Sonuga–Barke et al., 2013). The possible exception is in working memory, which probably can be improved by systematic training. It has not been proven to improve ADHD outcomes—but this might be because most children with ADHD do not, in fact, have a working-memory problem (see Chapter 3, Section 3.8).

10.9.5 Impulsive behaviour

Impulsiveness, in the longitudinal studies of child populations cited previously, did not have the same effect as inattention in predicting poor academic achievement. Indeed, there is some evidence that higher levels of impulsiveness in the general population of children is associated with higher levels of attainment (Tymms & Merrell, 2011). It may well be that impulsiveness in the classroom, such as calling out answers and questions without being asked to, leads to a richer educational experience. Very impulsive children are at risk for other kinds of classroom problems, in different ways to those whose difficulties are only in attending effectively. They tend to irritate teachers and pupils, and to receive disciplinary action. Oppositional and other problems of behaviour are likely to follow and may amount to the serious problem of conduct disorder.

Behaviour problems such as these are not, of course, confined to those with ADHD or impairments of learning. Whether or not ADHD is present, the management in schools is usually based on similar lines (Pilling et al., 2013). Contingency management and cognitive-behavioural approaches both have some evidence for benefit when delivered in schools (see Chapter 8, Section 8.5). The rewards in a contingency management approach may need to be delivered in an extra rapid and consistent way. The reward systems in ADHD brains are vulnerable to delay between earning the reward and receiving it. ADHD brains may also lose their responsiveness to reward if the effect becomes dulled by repetition. Novelty therefore becomes helpful to reward-based learning: 'Today we are working for points that will make the break start early; to-morrow, for access to art materials.'

A meta-analysis by DuPaul et al. (2012) analysed trial evidence for the efficacy of interventions carried out in schools. It found many North American trials, but few carried out elsewhere. The conclusion was that school-based interventions for students with ADHD yield significant effects for both behavioural and academic outcomes. The evidence was largely based on single-case and within-case designs. Between-case designs, by contrast, did not show useful effect sizes in improving behaviour. The difference is that between-case designs are based on a comparison between a group receiving one intervention and another not receiving it—a strong design, and the one usually used for clinical evaluations, but not always feasible in community work.

10.9.6 Independence

Social and emotional learning (SEL) programmes help children and young people to recognize and manage emotions, set and achieve positive goals, appreciate the perspectives of others, establish and maintain positive relationships, make responsible decisions, and handle interpersonal situations constructively (see Chapter 8, Section 8.7). Schools cannot do it all! However, they can play a part. Like health promotion in other contexts, promoting young people's independence operates by engaging their community and cooperating with it to set goals, plan priorities, and implement them together.

10.9.7 Modifying teaching methods and curricula.

There have been attempts to base teaching methods differentially on the cognitive strengths and weaknesses of individual children as revealed by psychological testing. The usual methods of teaching reading skills, in most European schools, are based on phonics. Some formulations of 'dyslexia' suggest that their core problems are in analysing word sounds, and that, if so, visual methods might work better. There is not much evidence that this kind of 'prescriptive teaching' is better than the usual kind. The debate has often revolved around the teaching of reading to those with specific learning difficulties. The nature of specific reading difficulties is discussed in Chapter 5, Section 5.2.3. Poor readers learn to read in very similar ways to anyone else. In general, their need is for more, and more careful teaching, and enhanced monitoring of their progress; rather than a different approach based on neuropsychological testing and prescription. Enhanced teaching should not be withheld from those with lower non-verbal IQs. Educational need rather than neuropsychiatric diagnosis should be the key consideration.

Children with special needs and disabilities are entitled, in many countries, to special educational help. This may mean a separate class for autism, or a small sanctuary class for pupils with very high levels of anxiety (see Section 10.9.1). It may mean a curriculum to fit in with the highly specialist interests of some autistic pupils. It may mean physical re-structuring of classrooms to allow access to wheelchairs or other mobility aids. Sensory impairments may call for teachers with special skills (e.g. in a sign language). It may mean a structured classroom run on token economy lines for some very impulsive children. It may mean dropping some subjects to allow for more time on individual needs.

In all these specialist accommodations, there are complex issues to consider in individual cases. Clinicians are well placed to act as advocates for the children. They should, however, do so with respect for the competing needs of the schools and other children in them. Specialist placements have disadvantages too. The 'best' school may be so far away that family life is damaged. The most modified curriculum may reduce chances of success in the world after school. A special class may reduce the opportunities for interacting with typically developing students and thereby fuel stigma. The most expensive interventions, such as individual tuition, may have to be subject to political decisions about the impact on school budgets. The balance can be difficult to define; individual judgement is essential.

In some places, such as some states of the USA, a clinical diagnosis of disorder (including ADHD) is enough to mandate special assistance. This can lead to families making strong representations to clinicians of the need for a diagnosis. In other parts of the world, including the UK, provision is not made by clinical diagnosis but by assessment of educational need.

10.9.8   Accommodation in examinations

In places with competitive examinations on which students' later prosperity depends, examination boards are usually keen to ensure flexibility in the interests of equal opportunity. They may well allow 'dyslexia' or motor problems to be a reason for extra time for the examination, or for using an amanuensis. Motor problems will often be met by permission to use a keyboard. If a clinician is making a case to assist a patient in the spectra of ADHD or ASD, it will be advantageous to obtain standardized test scores (e.g. from an educational psychologist or educational consultant). Generalized impairment is often not seen in the same way, so it may be helpful to emphasize the problems imposed by coexistent disorders.

Where school funding is based on the examination results of students, some head teachers will resort to 'gaming' the system. Pupils in the USA may be referred for medication in the hope (probably unfounded) that it will improve their marks. Where this practice holds, medication use may be high. Hinshaw and Scheffler (2014) have used epidemiological figures to hold it to be, in part, responsible for a massive increase in ADHD diagnoses and treatment, which they have termed the 'ADHD explosion'. Similar concerns in the UK may lead some heads to 'offload' children from their school roll. Advocacy from clinicians may be needed to ensure that all children get, as is their right, an appropriate education.

10.9.9 Pastoral care for young people with neurodevelopmental impairments

Children's needs to talk about their predicaments do not disappear just because their difficulties are based primarily on brain dysfunction. On the contrary, they may very well need to discuss those difficulties and any diagnoses they have been given in relation to their school performance. Teachers themselves are often the most trusted as well as the first resource. Impaired children may well not have realized that their teachers have already appreciated that their poor performance is nothing to do with laziness or unco-operativeness. Making this recognition overt is a way to counteract some of the frustration and poor self-image that afflicts children who are trying hard but failing to get good results.

Young people often want support in problems about friendships. Some difficulties in peer relationships can derive from the students' conditions. Social impairment may be making them appear weird or uninterested to other students. Impulsive behaviour can be very annoying to other students, even at the minor levels of noisiness and intrusive fidgeting. Tourette-type involuntary actions (poking other children, kicking chairs, crumpling paper) can be wrongly perceived as aggressive and invite retaliation. A teaching assistant in the classroom can make quick comments when these are happening, encourage a word of apology and correction if necessary, and give positive feedback for prosocial acts. These consequences should come as quickly as possible, to counteract the typical tendency of impulsive children to need very rapid consequences if they are to learn from them.

Social skills groups can be delivered in schools. Children can be helped by them to read facial expressions, body language, and tone of voice. Angry and impulsive children can learn to recognize the first signs of a tantrum developing, and either rechannel it or leave the situation for a short period. Role playing of social interactions is widely used and popular. It can instil alternative patterns of responding and so help pupils to make better relationships with their peers. Creative arts sessions will uncover some pupils' special strengths and provide alternative routes to achievement and social standing. Play therapy should foster senses of capability and being appreciated, and can be useful in directly encouraging abilities such as joint attention, imitation, visual attention, and solving problems (Pittala et al., 2018).

Education about mental health issues can also be undertaken in schools. A programme directed to all students can be a benefit to impaired children as well. The HeadStrong approach was evaluated positively in a cluster-randomized trial (Perry et al., 2014). HeadStrong comprises a booklet for teachers and a slideshow, providing teacher-delivered information on mood disorders and classroom activities over approximately 10 hours of class time. The effects on personal distress among students were not very promising, but the key outcome was mental health literacy, and this improved substantially by comparison with routine personal and social education. The likely relevance for neurodevelopmentally impaired children is to reduce the stigma felt towards them by other children. One can also hope that it will encourage their own knowledge about mental health problems and, therefore, their ability to cope with their vulnerability to anxiety and depression.

10.9.10 Antibullying

Bullying can be any of several repeated, hurtful behaviours. These behaviours can be verbal (e.g. threatening, taunting, spreading rumours) as well as physical (e.g. pushing and kicking), and involve exclusion from social activities. They are part of power relationships, with the stronger, older, and more able young people being the perpetrators over the weaker. Schools are by no means the only places where bullying happens, but their pastoral care is a key way of responding.

The experience of individuals and their families emphasizes that young people with neurodevelopmental disorders are at high risk for being bullied. Epidemiological studies have produced such different figures for the size of the association that it is hard to give an estimate of prevalence that will be generally applicable. A Scandinavian population study was able to consider characteristics of children that placed them at particular risk (Nordhagen et al., 2005). Odds ratios (OR) for being a victim of bullying (by comparison with others of the same age) indicated large increases in those with chronic disorders—the most relevant being hyperactivity (OR = 9.6), psychiatric disorders (OR = 9.1), epilepsy (OR = 4.8), and speech difficulties (OR = 3.2). (Hyperactivity was also a risk for becoming a perpetrator of bullying.)

The specific risk that people with ASD, ADHD, and/or ID carry of being bullied has also been followed in a large, prospective, population study of twins in Scandinavia (Törn et al., 2015). The risk was not confined to those with ASD. Rather, the total load of all the neurodevelopmental problems at the age of 9–12 years predicted whether the same young people at the age of 15 years would report having been bullied. Social interaction and motor problems were notably strongly associated, but not after allowing for the total load of problems. The longitudinal analyses indicated that qualities of the children evoked bullying, rather than the other way around. Perhaps the perpetrators perceived the young people as exploitable with impunity.

The signs of bullying extend beyond disclosure from victims. They can include bruises, broken or missing possessions, becoming solitary and withdrawn, aggression at home, insomnia, bedwetting, somatic symptoms, and worrying or refusing about going to school. Distress and social impairment occur even in children who were previously developing typically. Arseneault et al. (2010) reported the later consequences from a population-based cohort followed over time. In later childhood and adolescence, the victims have higher rates of anxiety and depression, suicidal thinking, and self-harm. The risk even extends to psychotic symptoms (Schreier et al., 2009).

Children with chronic problems of mental health find that the experience of being bullied exacerbates their marginalization, diminishes self-esteem, and hinders their development of friendships. Takizawa et al. (2014) extended the knowledge about risk to later decades of life. At ages 23 and 30, people who as children had been victims of frequent bullying showed higher rates of depression (OR = 1.95), anxiety disorders (O+R = 1.65), and suicidality (OR = 2.21) than their non-victimized peers. Because it was a large study of twins in the general population, it was possible to be clear that the effects are over and above any previous symptoms and any genetic or family influences shared by members of a family.

The impact of bullying by peers on victimized schoolchildren with ADHD or ASD is probably like that on those with other disorders of mental health (Holmberg & Hjern, 2008). Those with ADHD may be even more likely than those with other problems to become victimizers themselves.

Schools are by no means the only sites of peer bullying, but they are a good place to put in countermeasures. School professionals should be alert for the signs (remembering communication problems may make it hard for affected children to speak out) and be ready to invoke protection measures and possibly refer for specialist help (e.g. post-traumatic CBT). Olweus (1993) influenced many educators to recognize the signs of a child being bullied and to bring in sanctions for perpetrators. The specific suggestions in the Olweus programme are intuitively attractive. Recommendations include: a Bullying Prevention Coordinating Committee; setting up an anonymous survey; having a school conference day; explicit classroom rules against bullying, with sanctions; supervision of the indoor and outdoor environments; and regular meetings between teachers and parents (Olweus et al., 1999). Evidence from trials is conflicting about whether such recommendations are effective (Evers et al., 2007). Meta-analysis by Ttofi and Farrington (2011) suggests that the overall effect sizes of controlled trials are small to moderate. Whole-school and multifaceted programmes seem to be the most helpful. They are quite demanding in terms of the amount of school time, especially at secondary level, and perhaps they are not always thoroughly applied.

Nowadays, nearly all schools will have explicit antibullying policies as part of safeguarding. They are not usually tailored specifically to preventing harm for children with disabilities. For them, there might be a need for more specific whole-school goals for increasing empathy and promoting inclusion. Teacher training could include spotting signs in children whose communication problems prevent them from complaining, and listening respectfully to parents who have done so. Activities can be encouraged in which disabled and typically developing children spend time together. Other children can become mentors and be supervised in the role—they are likely to spread the word among other children that bullying those with a disorder is cowardly and unacceptable. If a school has 'drop-in' groups where children can talk with each other about their feelings in the presence of a person with authority, this can encourage awareness about recognizing emotional problems in bullied children (and others) and telling them where help is available.

Much can be done in partnership between school and home. Parents may need to moderate their natural suggestions to hit back—on the often false belief that 'all bullies are cowards'. Victims who do fight back may well find that it makes matters worse or gets them into trouble with authority. Parents should ask their children what they would like to have done about it and encourage telling a teacher or school counsellor or nurse.

10.9.11 Physical activities

Physical exercise that raises the heart rate is good, as for most children. Very competitive sports such as football may be unrewarding for children who struggle to remember multiple directions, dislike physical contact, or are less well coordinated than other children. They might be better suited to a less competitive atmosphere such as (some kinds of) swimming or cycling. Martial arts are sometimes recommended to 'channel their aggression', but it depends very much on the tutor whether it does that or in fact glorifies aggression. Time taken to find what suits the individual child is well spent.

Low levels of physical activity contribute to the medical problem of obesity. In the USA, and to a lesser extent in many other Western countries, obesity is a crisis of public health. Neurodevelopmental disorders play a part.

- A nationally representative study from the USA reported on obesity in adolescents with ASD (Phillips et al., 2014). A rate of 32% in ASD contrasted with 13% in those without developmental disabilities. Adolescents with ADHD and learning disabilities were also at risk.
- An over-representation of high body mass in ADHD by comparison with typically developing young people was found in a systematic review of studies, mostly of clinic attenders (Cortese et al., 2016). There are several plausible mechanisms. Dietary indiscretions such as snacking, binge eating, and junk food could represent impulsive patterns of eating. Delay aversion could lead to rapid intake overcoming satiety mechanisms. 'Reward deficiency' might encourage compensatory overeating for emotional gratification. There could be a biological association between ADHD and large body size if measured before stimulant medication. However, medication can then cause growth decrement (Swanson et al., 2007).
- A nationally representative study of 45,897 young people aged from 10 to 17, in the USA, reported that those with a combination of learning disabilities and ADHD were more likely to be obese than those without the combination (Cook et al., 2015). Children with ID are less physically active than their contemporaries when movement is measured with accelerometers (Einarsson et al., 2015). Ng et al. (2017) provided a systematic review of physical exercise programmes applied to ADHD. Moderately positive effects on health could be seen for those with ADHD and ID. This may reduce the risk for obesity.

10.10 ENCOUNTERS WITH THE INTERNET AND VIDEO SCREENS

The internet is changing society fundamentally. New cognitive and social challenges are appearing for young people. We know little about whether the challenges are appearing in a different form for those with differently developing brains. Firth et al. (2019) have reviewed the challenges from a perspective of typically developing people. There are several possibilities of how the exposure might produce brain changes that could, in principle, worsen the features of ADHD, ASD, and learning disabilities.

- The rapid flow of information requiring attention to be divided across multiple sources could be reducing the capacity for sustained attention. Teachers often refer to their impression that young people do not sustain interest as once they did. This impression, however, has often featured in the past, at times of historical change such as the advent of television use and that of mass reading of popular literature. More empirically, individuals who make heavy use of multitasking, by comparison with more sparing users, do tend to be more susceptible to distraction (Ophir et al., 2009). The causal association is not clear, but there is a little longitudinal evidence that adolescents who multitask extensively have poor attention in other settings (Baumgartner et al., 2018).
- The accessibility of large amounts of information could be discouraging the use of personal stores of information or helping those with low stores (Sparrow et al., 2011).
- The increased cognitive demands of social interaction—such as keeping abreast of a very large number of contacts—might be making it harder for those with cognitive impairments to have a full role in modern friendships.
- The very explicit feedback from current social media on one's social standing (e.g. through 'likes') could be having a negative effect on self-esteem in young people who are not socially successful. On the one hand, social media may make social contacts easier for those who are isolated. On the other hand, cyberbullying is hard to avoid.
- Screen time, of all types, is widely perceived as an enemy of attention and learning, and several researchers have studied the issue in school and preschool children. The case for a direct effect is not yet made. Emotional and behaviour problems may be somewhat more noticeable in children who use screens heavily from an early age and have them in their bedroom, but even if that is the case (studies differ), it may be due chiefly to a reduction in hours of sleep (Lin et al., 2019).
- On the other hand, there may be benefits for impaired young people of the increased use of social media. They may be a route to friendships for those who are constrained from physical meetings by immobility or overprotection or phobic avoidance. Those who are exceptionally skilled in the electronic world may have a pathway to high es-teem and occupation.

10.11 ENCOUNTERS WITH EMPLOYMENT

Many developmentally impaired people have skills that should enable them to thrive in jobs, yet cannot find them. In ASD, paid employment of any type is found by less than one-third of those who seek it. They are often disadvantaged at job interviews because of difficulties with social communication and interaction, other people's lack of understanding, and sensory issues. In ADHD, the difficulty is more often with keeping a job than with getting one. Problems arise when executive function is needed. Inconsistency, distractibility, and an appearance of chaotic disorganization create problems with other employees. They may well make rapid changes of employment, affecting their reputation in the workplace. Their salaries are lower than those of their contemporaries and they are less likely to be promoted (Klein et al., 2012).

Nevertheless, those with neurocognitive alterations can have much to offer. Entrepreneurs, artists, entertainers, IT specialists, and executives (with people to whom they can delegate routine administration) have all reached the heights of their professions. Managers can help those starting in employment in several ways:

- Clarifying the expectations of their role and providing detailed training in it— including the etiquette and the unwritten rules.
- Making the work environment better suited to them, for instance by removing excessive interruptions or sensory distraction.
- Reviewing performance regularly with brief, frequent assessments; instructions that are concise, focused, and specific.
- Letting other employees (with consent) know about their disability and how it may affect them.
- Being prepared to give advice and reassurance in crises, with emphasis on honesty, directness, and support.

10.12 LEGAL ISSUES

People with impairments come into contact with the law as defendants, witnesses, litigants, and as people in need of protection.

The legal court system does not map neatly on to medical considerations. Criminal responsibility starts at 10 years of age in England. Until the age of 10, children cannot be arrested or tried in court, but they can be given a Child Safety Order or taken into the care of the local authority. This is very much younger than in most European countries, where it ranges widely: from 12 years (Scotland), 14 years (Germany, Italy, Spain), 15 years (Denmark, Sweden, Norway, and Finland), to 18 years (Belgium and Luxembourg). Children who are too young for criminal responsibility may be valuable to organized criminals who believe that they will be immune to prosecution.

Children in England between 10 and 17 years can be arrested and taken to court if they commit a crime, but they are treated differently from adults. They will be dealt with by a youth court, given different sentences, and will not go to an adult prison (there are special secure centres for young people). Youth offending teams are part of the local authority, not the police or the courts, and offer interdisciplinary advice.

The forensic rules are based on chronological, not developmental, age. Jurisdictions vary in how they cope with individuals who lack the cognitive abilities to understand the laws or the volitional abilities required to follow them. The presence of mental disorder or impairment is unlikely to be a consideration in whether a person is guilty of a bad act or culpable intent. It is therefore unlikely to be a part of evidence in a trial. Nevertheless, the presence of disorder can be very influential on considerations of sentencing and fitness to plead. Fitness to plead will explicitly involve understanding the nature and object of the proceedings, the possible consequences of the proceedings, and the ability to communicate with legal representatives.

Courts may well accept that the moral responsibility for outrageous actions can be altered by several types of neurocognitive change as well as ID. Sexual assault can occur in the context of the inability of a person with limited social understanding to interpret that the victim is not consenting to sexual overtures. Arson can follow from an obsessive preoccupation with flames and fire, rather than a deliberate wish to damage life or property. Violence to other people can come from intolerance of closeness and lack of appreciation of the motives of the victim who may be oblivious to the perpetrator's intense need for distance from others. The court is, however, likely to require more evidence that the abnormality is present consistently than the mere fact of a diagnosis. A mental health condition is considered a disability under the Equality Act 2010 only if it has a long-term effect on normal day-to-day activity.

'Diminished responsibility' is a feature of English law, but only as a partial defence against a charge of murder that allows reduction of the charge to manslaughter.

Young people with mental impairments may also be involved with the courts as witnesses. False confessions by people with ADHD can result from an extreme of delay aversion and a need to escape the prolonged questioning of a police interview. They may not be able to handle multiple questions. People with ASD may misinterpret the import of questions. Witness support may be needed at police interviews. Judges may need to instruct counsel on what is an acceptable style of questioning.

The law also governs consent to treatment. As with criminal responsibility, adult status comes at the age of 16 years. From that point, a young person is presumed to have the capacity to make their own decision on whether or not to accept offered treatment. Before that age, they can still be considered 'Gillick competent', following a case centring on a decision about birth control in which the young person was considered able to agree in spite of parental opposition. In practice, and in case of dispute, the courts will expect attempts to have been made, in good faith, to resolve disagreements. If unsuccessful, they will make their own decisions. In practice, UK courts have been broadly sympathetic to teenagers wishing to consent unilaterally, but more cautious in cases of their wishing to refuse when parents and medical opinion are in favour.

When a person's condition impairs their ability to consent, yet involves risk of harm to others or oneself, the law sets out ways by which assessment or treatment can be made compulsory. In England, the Mental Health Act includes several 'Sections' that can be implemented by mental health professionals and overseen by the law courts to preserve individuals' rights. It has applied both to people with mental illnesses and those with disabilities. It has recently been reviewed, especially about whether people with ASD or ID should be excluded from its scope. The result of applying it to those neurodevelopmental conditions can be long periods of forced residence in hospitals and inappropriate medical treatment or oppressive care.

10.13 ENCOUNTERS WITH DIAGNOSIS

10.13.1 Diagnosis of ASD

For adults with ASD, and for parents, the experience of diagnosis is very variable (Powell & Acker, 2016). It can be a positive experience. People often describe a sense of relief. Not only does it clarify the uncertainties they have previously felt about themselves, it dispels notions that their problems are their own fault, or that they represent a personality failing. The diagnostic term provides an external attribution for their problems.

The experience can also be unsatisfactory (Crane et al., 2016). Long delays from requesting advice to the confirmation of an ASD diagnosis (typically 3.5 years in the UK) and limited post-diagnostic support are the rule. There are also problems for those who are told that they have some features of autism, but not the full set necessary for a diagnosis. To them, it can come over as an arbitrary matter (and, indeed, there are arbitrary features about the cut-off chosen). Their reaction emphasizes the value that is attached to a label with the connotation of a medical condition. It is in some contrast to the more negative experiences of those given a diagnosis of ADHD.

There are other negative features, too. Adults with a new diagnosis can feel angry with professionals who have missed it in the past, or with those who have not given the support and sympathy appropriate to an illness. The connotation of lifelong impairment is a deeply unwelcome aspect for some.

Many people with the clinical features of the autism spectrum will nowadays want to reject vigorously any suggestion that they have a disorder rather than a difference. Instead, they see themselves as being in a minority that is discriminated against. Indeed, many feel dismay at the involvement of clinical scientists whom they perceive as trying to find the causes, in order to cure, rather than the means of removing the obstacles that society has put in their way (Pellicano & Stears, 2011). For others with similar views, the label can be perceived as a help to understanding the nature of their difference. The positive aspects of external attribution and relief of guilt remain.

There are illogical aspects in current diagnostic practice. I have encountered highly intelligent people who have been flummoxed by the implication that, if they overcome disability but retain some of the characteristic symptoms and signs, they lose the right to the label. They would say, by analogy, that a person does not cease to be 'hearing impaired' because they have overcome all the disability imposed by deafness. Others would say that the only disability is the uncomprehending attitudes of other people that confuse diversity with disorder. Overcoming stigma and self-stigmatization is one of the tasks for personal development.

Physicians may find themselves in some internal conflict if they regard the dimension of autism as a continuum of human diversity; yet acknowledge both the positive effects on some of their clients of regarding high levels as a discrete diagnosis and the negative effects on others in enhancing discriminatory attitudes. It is often helpful, though time-consuming, to enter a discussion about diversity, impairment, and disability. The tendency of autistic people to prefer precise black-and-white concepts can indeed be an obstacle to constructive understanding, and may itself need to be recognized and explained.

It should be possible, eventually, to develop consensus even among groups within the autistic community who are on opposite sides of the argument. There is no prospect, for the moment, of a ready or universally accepted formulation of how to reconcile the views of autism activists (that society must change) with those of others (especially those who show, or look after those who show major disability) that society has a duty to pursue for cures of the condition. The approach of some agencies, such as Autistica, to develop such a consensus within the community deserves the involvement of scientists and clinicians.

10.13.2 Other disorders

In the case of ADHD, ID, LD, and chronic motor disorders, the controversies over a diversity approach are not yet as intense as in ASD. They are perhaps increasing as the voices of capable adults become more widely attended.

Already, the system of developing guidelines for practice usually involves members of the communities as well as authoritative experts. The whole idea of 'authority' is problematic in a culture that gives high value to self-determination. The standards of good practice are not to be set only by medical or psychological pronouncement but also by consensus from those who are living with it, informed by public scientific knowledge. There is a tension if guidelines are developed with the participation of individuals from the community who have very different approaches to diagnosis from each other. Respectful debate will be needed before a community can offer an undivided voice. This is not unique to neurodevelopment, but a usual part of the relationship between medicine and society.

References

Akee, R. K., Copeland, W. E., Keeler, G., Angold, A., & Costello, E. J. (2010). Parents' incomes and children's outcomes: a quasi-experiment using transfer payments from casino profits. *American Economic Journal: Applied Economics, 2*(1), 86–115.

Arseneault, L., Bowes, L., & Shakoor, S. (2010). Bullying victimization in youths and mental health problems: 'much ado about nothing'? *Psychological Medicine, 40*(5), 717–729.

Balazs, J., & Kereszteny, A. (2017). Attention-deficit/hyperactivity disorder and suicide: a systematic review. *World Journal of Psychiatry, 7*(1), 44.

Baumgartner, S. E., van der Schuur, W. A., Lemmens, J. S., & te Poel, F. (2018). The relationship between media multitasking and attention problems in adolescents: Results of two longitudinal studies. *Human Communication Research, 44*(1), 3–30.

Bilder, D., Botts, E. L., Smith, K. R., Pimentel, R., Farley, M., Viskochil, J., McMahon, W. M., Block, H., Ritvo, E., Ritvo, R–A., & Coon, H. (2013). Excess mortality and causes of death in autism spectrum disorders: a follow up of the 1980s Utah/UCLA autism epidemiologic study. *Journal of Autism and Developmental Disorders, 43*(5), 1196–1204.

Buescher, A. V., Cidav, Z., Knapp, M., & Mandell, D. S. (2014). Costs of autism spectrum disorders in the United Kingdom and the United States. *Journal of the American Medical Association: Pediatrics, 168*(8), 721–728.

Butwicka, A., Långström, N., Larsson, H., Lundström, S., Serlachius, E., Almqvist, C., Frisén, L., & Lichtenstein, P. (2017). Increased risk for substance use-related problems in autism spectrum disorders: a population-based cohort study. *Journal of Autism and Developmental Disorders, 47*(1), 80–89.

Caspi, A., Moffitt, T. E., Morgan, J., Rutter, M., Taylor, A., Arseneault, L., Tully, L., Jacobs, C., Kim–Cohen, J., & Polo-Tomas, M. (2004). Maternal expressed emotion predicts children's antisocial behavior problems: using monozygotic-twin differences to identify environmental effects on behavioral development. *Developmental Psychology, 40*(2), 149.

Cassidy, S., Bradley, P., Robinson, J., Allison, C., McHugh, M., & Baron–Cohen, S. (2014). Suicidal ideation and suicide plans or attempts in adults with Asperger's syndrome attending a specialist diagnostic clinic: a clinical cohort study. *Lancet Psychiatry, 1*(2), 142–147.

Chen, V. C. H., Chan, H. L., Wu, S. I., Lee, M., Lu, M. L., Liang, H. Y., Dewey, M. E., Stewart, R., & Lee, C. T. C. (2019). Attention-deficit/hyperactivity disorder and mortality risk in Taiwan. *Journal of the American Medical Association: Network Open, 2*(8), e198714–e198714.

Collishaw, S. (2015). Annual research review: secular trends in child and adolescent mental health. *Journal of Child Psychology and Psychiatry, 56*, 370–393.

Cook, B. G., Li, D., & Heinrich, K. M. (2015). Obesity, physical activity, and sedentary behavior of youth with learning disabilities and ADHD. *Journal of Learning Disabilities, 48*(6), 563–576.

Cortese, S., Moreira–Maia, C. R., St. Fleur, D., Morcillo–Peñalver, C., Rohde, L. A., & Faraone, S. V. (2016). Association between ADHD and obesity: a systematic review and meta-analysis. *American Journal of Psychiatry, 173*(1), 34–43.

Craig, F., Operto, F. F., De Giacomo, A., Margari, L., Frolli, A., Conson, M., Ivagnes, S., Monaco, M., & Margari, F. (2016). Parenting stress among parents of children with neurodevelopmental disorders. *Psychiatry Research, 242*, 121–129.

Crane, L., Chester, J., Goddard, L., Henry, L., & Hill, E. (2016). Experiences of autism diagnosis: a survey of over 1000 parents in the United Kingdom. *Autism, 20* (2), 153–162. https://doi.org/10.1177/1362361315573636

Dalsgaard, S., Østergaard, S. D., Leckman, J. F., Mortensen, P. B., & Pedersen, M. G. (2015a). Mortality in children, adolescents, and adults with attention deficit hyperactivity disorder: a nationwide cohort study. *Lancet, 385*(9983), 2190–2196.

Dalsgaard, S., Leckman, J. F., Mortensen, P. B., Nielsen, H. S., & Simonsen, M. (2015b). Effect of drugs on the risk of injuries in children with attention deficit hyperactivity disorder: a prospective cohort study. *Lancet Psychiatry, 2*(8), 702–709.

Deloitte Access Economics. (2019). *The social and economic costs of ADHD in Australia.* www.deloitte-au-economics-social-costs-adhd-australia-270819.pdf

Dorn, L. D., & Biro, F. M. (2011). Puberty and its measurement: a decade in review. *Journal of Research on Adolescence, 21*(1), 180–195.

DuPaul, G. J., Eckert, T. L., & Vilardo, B. (2012). The effects of school-based interventions for attention deficit hyperactivity disorder: a meta-analysis 1996–2010. *School Psychology Review, 41*(4), 387.

Eaton, J. (2019). Human rights-based approaches to mental health legislation and global mental health. *British Journal of Psychiatry International, 16*(2), 37–40.

Einarsson, I. O., Olafsson, A., Hinriksdóttir, G., Jóhannsson, E., Daly, D., & Arngrímsson, S. A. (2015). Differences in physical activity among youth with and without intellectual disability. *Medicine & Science in Sports & Exercise, 47*(2), 411–418.

Evers, K. E., Prochaska, J. O., Van Marter, D. F., Johnson, J. L., & Prochaska, J. M. (2007). Transtheoretical-based bullying prevention effectiveness trials in middle schools and high schools. *Educational Research, 49*(4), 397–414.

Firth, J., Torous, J., Stubbs, B., Firth, J. A., Steiner, G. Z., Smith, L., Alvarez–Jimenez, M., Gleeson, J., Vancampfort, D., Armitage, C. J., & Sarris, J. (2019). The 'online brain': how the Internet may be changing our cognition. *World Psychiatry, 18*(2), 119–129.

Galván, A. (2013). The teenage brain: Sensitivity to rewards. *Current Directions in Psychological Science, 22*(2), 88–93.

Gillberg, C., & Coleman, M. (1996). Autism and medical disorders: a review of the literature. *Developmental Medicine & Child Neurology, 38*(3), 191–202.

Goffman, E. (2009). *Stigma: notes on the management of spoiled identity.* Simon and Schuster.

Grossman, A. H., Foss, A. H., & D'Augelli, A. R. (2014). Puberty: maturation, timing and adjustment, and sexual identity developmental milestones among lesbian, gay, and bisexual youth. *Journal of LGBT Youth, 11*(2), 107–124.

Hinshaw, S. P., & Scheffler, R. M. (2014). *The ADHD explosion: myths, medication, money, and today's push for performance.* Oxford University Press.

Holmberg, K., & Hjern, A. (2008). Bullying and attention-deficit–hyperactivity disorder in 10-year-olds in a Swedish community. *Developmental Medicine & Child Neurology, 50*(2), 134–138.

Hooley, J. M., Gruber, S. A., Parker, H. A., Guillaumot, J., Rogowska, J., & Yurgelun–Todd, D. A. (2009). Cortico-limbic response to personally challenging emotional stimuli after complete recovery from depression. *Psychiatry Research: Neuroimaging, 171*(2), 106–119.

Hirvikoski, T., Mittendorfer–Rutz, E., Boman, M., Larsson, H., Lichtenstein, P., & Bölte, S. (2016). Premature mortality in autism spectrum disorder. *British Journal of Psychiatry, 208*(3), 232–238.

Jacoby, A., Snape, D., & Baker, G. A. (2005). Epilepsy and social identity: the stigma of a chronic neurological disorder. *Lancet Neurology, 4*(3), 171–178.

Jilek–Aall, L., Jilek, M., Kaaya, J., Mkombachepa, L., & Hillary, K. (1997). Psychosocial study of epilepsy in Africa. *Social Science & Medicine, 45*(5), 783–795.

Klein, R. G., Mannuzza, S., Olazagasti, M. A. R., Roizen, E., Hutchison, J. A., Lashua, E. C., & Castellanos, F. X. (2012). Clinical and functional outcome of childhood attention-deficit/hyperactivity disorder 33 years later. *Archives of General Psychiatry, 69*(12), 1295–1303.

Kleinman, A., Wang, W. Z., Li, S. C., Cheng, X. M., Dai, X. Y., Li, K. T., & Kleinman, J. (1995). The social course of epilepsy: chronic illness as social experience in interior China. *Social Science & Medicine, 40*(10), 1319–1330.

Lake, J. K., Perry, A., & Lunsky, Y. (2014). Mental health services for individuals with high functioning autism spectrum disorder. *Autism Research and Treatment*, 2014(502420). https://doi.org/10.1155/2014/502420

Laitinen–Krispijn, S., van der Ende, J., & Verhulst, F. C. (1999). The role of pubertal progress in the development of depression in early adolescence. *Journal of Affective Disorders, 54*, 211–215.

Lee, S. S., Humphreys, K. L., Flory, K., Liu, R., & Glass, K. (2011). Prospective association of childhood attention-deficit/hyperactivity disorder (ADHD) and substance use and abuse/dependence: a meta-analytic review. *Clinical Psychology review, 31*(3), 328–341.

Levy, F. (2004). Synaptic gating and ADHD: a biological theory of comorbidity of ADHD and anxiety. *Neuropsychopharmacology, 29*(9), 1589–1596.

Lin, J., Magiati, I., Chiong, S. H. R., Singhal, S., Riard, N., Ng, I. H. X., Muller–Riemenschneider, F., & Wong, C. M. (2019). The relationship among screen use, sleep, and emotional/behavioral difficulties in preschool children with neurodevelopmental disorders. *Journal of Developmental & Behavioral Pediatrics, 40*(7), 519–529.

Ljung, T., Chen, Q., Lichtenstein, P., & Larsson, H. (2014). Common etiological factors of attention-deficit/hyperactivity disorder and suicidal behavior: a population-based study in Sweden. *Journal of the American Medical Association Psychiatry, 71*(8), 958–964.

McCarthy, S., Cranswick, N., Potts, L., Taylor, E., & Wong, I. C. (2009). Mortality associated with attention-deficit hyperactivity disorder (ADHD) drug treatment. *Drug Safety, 32*(11), 1089–1096.

Mukolo, A., Heflinger, C. A., & Wallston, K. A. (2010). The stigma of childhood mental disorders: a conceptual framework. *Journal of the American Academy of Child & Adolescent Psychiatry, 49*(2), 92–103.

Ng, Q. X., Ho, C. Y. X., Chan, H. W., Yong, B. Z. J., & Yeo, W. S. (2017). Managing childhood and adolescent attention-deficit/hyperactivity disorder (ADHD) with exercise: a systematic review. *Complementary Therapies in Medicine, 34*, 123–128.

Nigg, J. T. (2013). Attention-deficit/hyperactivity disorder and adverse health outcomes. *Clinical Psychology Review, 33*(2), 215–228.

Nordhagen, R., Nielsen, A., Stigum, H., & Köhler, L. (2005). Parental reported bullying among Nordic children: a population-based study. *Child: Care, Health and Development, 31*(6), 693–701.

Olweus, D. (1993). *Bullying at school: what we know and what we can do*. Blackwell.

Olweus, D., Limber, S., & Mihalic, S. F. (1999). *Blueprints for violence prevention, book nine: bullying prevention program*. Center for the Study and Prevention of Violence.

Ophir, E., Nass, C., & Wagner, A. D. (2009). Cognitive control in media multitaskers. *Proceedings of the National Academy of Sciences, 106*(37), 15583–15587.

Patel, V., Flisher, A. J., Hetrick, S., & McGorry, P. (2007). Mental health of young people: a global public-health challenge. *Lancet, 369*(9569), 1302–1313.

Pelham, W. E., & Lang, A. R. (1993). Parental alcohol consumption and deviant child behavior: laboratory studies of reciprocal effects. *Clinical Psychology Review, 13*(8), 763–784.

Pellicano, E., & Stears, M. (2011). Bridging autism, science and society: moving toward an ethically informed approach to autism research. *Autism Research*, 4(4), 271–282.

Peris, T. S., & Miklowitz, D. J. (2015). Parental expressed emotion and youth psychopathology: new directions for an old construct. *Child Psychiatry & Human Development*, 46(6), 863–873.

Perry, Y., Petrie, K., Buckley, H., Cavanagh, L., Clarke, D., Winslade, M., Hadzi–Pavlovic, D., Manicavasagar, V., & Christensen, H. (2014). Effects of a classroom-based educational resource on adolescent mental health literacy: a cluster randomised controlled trial. *Journal of Adolescence*, 37(7), 1143–1151.

Phillips, K. L., Schieve, L. A., Visser, S., Boulet, S., Sharma, A. J., Kogan, M. D., Boyle, C. A., & Yeargin-Allsopp, M. (2014). Prevalence and impact of unhealthy weight in a national sample of US adolescents with autism and other learning and behavioral disabilities. *Maternal and Child Health Journal*, 18(8), 1964–1975.

Pilling, S., Gould, N., Whittington, C., Taylor, C., & Scott, S. (2013). Recognition, intervention, and management of antisocial behaviour and conduct disorders in children and young people: summary of NICE–SCIE guidance. *British Medical Journal*, 346, f1298.

Pittala, E. T., Saint–Georges–Chaumet, Y., Favrot, C., Tanet, A., Cohen, D., & Saint–Georges, C. (2018). Clinical outcomes of interactive, intensive and individual (3i) play therapy for children with ASD: a two-year follow-up study. *BMC Pediatrics*, 18(1), 165.

Powell, T., & Acker, L. (2016). Adults' experience of an Asperger syndrome diagnosis: analysis of its emotional meaning and effect on participants' lives. *Focus on Autism and Other Developmental Disabilities*, 31(1), 72–80.

Read, J., Haslam, N., Sayce, L., & Davies, E. (2006). Prejudice and schizophrenia: a review of the 'mental illness is an illness like any other' approach. *Acta Psychiatrica Scandinavica*, 114(5), 303–318.

Reiss, F. (2013). Socioeconomic inequalities and mental health problems in children and adolescents: a systematic review. *Social Science and Medicine*, 90, 24–31.

Richardson, M., Moore, D. A., Gwernan–Jones, R., Thompson–Coon, J., Ukoumunne, O., Rogers, M., Whear, R., Newlove–Delgado, T. V., Logan, S., Morris, C., Taylor, E., Cooper, P., Stein, K., Garside, R., Ford, T. J. (2015). Non-pharmacological interventions for attention-deficit/hyperactivity disorder (ADHD) delivered in school settings: systematic reviews of quantitative and qualitative research. *Health Technology Assessment*, 19(45), 1.

Robinson, L. R., Bitsko, R. H., Schieve, L. A., & Visser, S. N. (2013). Tourette syndrome, parenting aggravation, and the contribution of co-occurring conditions among a nationally representative sample. *Disability and Health Journal*, 6(1), 26–35.

Roddy, A., & O'Neill, C. (2019). The economic costs and its predictors for childhood autism spectrum disorders in Ireland: how is the burden distributed? *Autism*, 23(5), 1106–1118.

Russell, A. E., Ford, T., Williams, R., & Russell, G. (2016). The association between socioeconomic disadvantage and attention deficit/hyperactivity disorder (ADHD): a systematic review. *Child Psychiatry & Human Development*, 47(3), 440–458.

Sartorius, N., Chiu, H., Heok, K. E., Lee, M. S., Ouyang, W. C., Sato, M., Yang, Y. K., & Yu, X. (2014). Name change for schizophrenia. *Schizophrenia Bulletin*, 40(2), 255.

Sayal, K., Merrell, C., Tymms, P., & Kasim, A. (2015a). Academic outcomes following a school-based RCT for ADHD: 6-year follow-up. *Journal of Attention Disorders*, 1087054714562588.

Sayal, K., Washbrook, E., & Propper, C. (2015b). Childhood behavior problems and academic outcomes in adolescence: longitudinal population-based study. *Journal of the American Academy of Child & Adolescent Psychiatry*, 54(5), 360–368.

Scambler, G. (1989). *Epilepsy*. Tavistock.

Schachar, R., Taylor, E., Wieselberg, M., Thorley, G., & Rutter, M. (1987). Changes in family function and relationships in children who respond to methylphenidate. *Journal of the American Academy of Child & Adolescent Psychiatry*, 26(5), 728–732.

Schreier, A., Wolke, D., Thomas, K., Horwood, J., Hollis, C., Gunnell, D., Lewis, G., Thompson, A., Zammitt, S., Duffy, L., Salvi, G., & Harrison, G. (2009). Prospective study of peer victimization in childhood and psychotic symptoms in a nonclinical population at age 12 years. *Archives of General Psychiatry*, 66(5), 527–536.

Schwebel, D. C., Brezausek, C. M., Ramey, S. L., & Ramey, C. T. (2004). Interactions between child behavior patterns and parenting: implications for children's unintentional injury risk. *Journal of Pediatric Psychology*, 29(2), 93–104.

Sonuga–Barke, E. J., Brandeis, D., Cortese, S., Daley, D., Ferrin, M., Holtmann, M., Stevenson, J., Danckaerts, M., van der Oord, S., Döpfner, M., Dittmann, R. W., Simonoff, E., Zuddas, A., Banaschewski, T., Buitelaar, J., Coghill, D., Hollis, C., Konofal, E., Lecendreux, M., … & European ADHD Guidelines Group. (2013). Nonpharmacological interventions for ADHD: systematic review and meta-analyses of randomized controlled trials of dietary and psychological treatments. *American Journal of Psychiatry*, 170(3), 275–289.

Sparrow, B., Liu, J., & Wegner, D. M. (2011). Google effects on memory: cognitive consequences of having information at our fingertips. *Science*, 333(6043), 776–778.

Swanson, J. M., Elliott, G. R., Greenhill, L. L., Wigal, T., Arnold, L. E., Vitiello, B., Hechtman, L., Epstein, J. N., Pelham, W. E., Abikoff, H. B., Newcorn, J. H., Molina, B. S. G., Hinshaw, S. P., Wells, K. C., Hoza, B., Jensen, P. S., Gibbons, R. D., Hur, K., Stehli, A., … & Volkow, N. D. (2007). Effects of stimulant medication on growth rates across 3 years in the MTA follow-up. *Journal of the American Academy of Child & Adolescent Psychiatry*, 46(8), 1015–1027.

Takizawa, R., Maughan, B., & Arseneault, L. (2014). Adult health outcomes of childhood bullying victimization: evidence from a five-decade longitudinal British birth cohort. *American Journal of Psychiatry*, 171, 777–784.

Tanner, J. M. (1962). *Growth at adolescence* (2nd ed.). Blackwell.

Theule, J., Wiener, J., Tannock, R., & Jenkins, J. M. (2013). Parenting stress in families of children with ADHD: a meta-analysis. *Journal of Emotional and Behavioral Disorders*, 21(1), 3–17.

Törn, P., Pettersson, E., Lichtenstein, P., Anckarsäter, H., Lundström, S., Gumpert, C. H., Larsson, H., Kollberg, L., Långström, N., & Halldner, L. (2015). Childhood neurodevelopmental problems and adolescent bully victimization: population-based, prospective twin study in Sweden. *European Child & Adolescent Psychiatry*, 24(9), 1049–1059.

Ttofi, M. M., & Farrington, D. P. (2011). Effectiveness of school-based programs to reduce bullying: a systematic meta-analytic review. *Journal of Experimental Criminology*, 7, 27–56. https://doi.org/10.1007/ s11292-010-9109-1

Tymms, P., & Merrell, C. (2011). ADHD and academic attainment: is there an advantage in impulsivity? *Learning and Individual Differences*, 21(6), 753–758.

Vidal, S., & Connell, C. M. (2019). Treatment effects of parent–child focused evidence-based programs on problem severity and functioning among children and adolescents with disruptive behavior. *Journal of Clinical Child & Adolescent Psychology*, 48(Supp1), S326–S336.

Washbrook, E., Propper, C., & Sayal, K. (2013). Pre-school hyperactivity/attention problems and educational outcomes in adolescence: prospective longitudinal study. *British Journal of Psychiatry*, 203(4), 265–271.

Yamaguchi, S., Wu, S. I., Biswas, M., Yate, M., Aoki, Y., Barley, E. A., & Thornicroft, G. (2013). Effects of short-term interventions to reduce mental health–related stigma in university or college students: a systematic review. *Journal of Nervous and Mental Disease, 201*(6), 490–503.

Zhao, X., Page, T. F., Altszuler, A. R., Pelham, W. E., Kipp, H., Gnagy, E. M., Coxe, S., Schatz, N. K., Merrill, B. M., Macphee, F. L., & Pelham, W. E. (2019). Family burden of raising a child with ADHD. *Journal of Abnormal Child Psychology, 47*(8), 1327–1338.

Epilogue

....

THIS epilogue is being written during the Covid-19 pandemic and the consequent lockdown. At this point, it seems probable that education, mental health and research methods will be markedly influenced in the longer term. It is too soon to estimate the full impact, but one expects both desirable and unwelcome changes:

Late neurological complications can be expected to emerge, as after other waves of infections causing neuroinflammation in young people.

Closer family ties might result from closure of schools and centres. On the other hand, domestic disharmony has increased for some families, from being cooped up together, and will have consequences for the mental health of those who have lived through it. Reduced access for young people to school life and peer society is unlikely to benefit their mental development.

Increased remote teaching could penalize pupils lacking internet access because of poverty or inability to use it.

The temporary shift to non-residential services that has been forced by pandemic conditions could become permanent. This could well be beneficial. It is, however, also possible that health and care services will become even more stretched than they used to be, particularly in crisis care.

An increased emphasis on remote professional input has altered patterns of service. This seems likely to become permanent. On the positive side, the travel burden for families with multiple needs should reduce. It seems likely that reliance on caregivers to alert clinicians to needs will increase, and this could entail greater empowerment of families in discussions about assessment and treatment plans. On the other hand, increased reliance on reports of informants (for instance, in assessing results of medication) might be at the cost of emphasizing changes that benefit carers rather than the experience of young people.

Remote home observations to guide monitoring of medication has become necessary. The ability for professionals directly to observe psychosocial interactions at home could lead to important influences on behaviour (such as timing, quality, and consistency of reinforcement) becoming accessible to understanding.

Global recession and increasing unemployment will probably reduce the opportunities for people with a disability in adult life, at least unless government subsidy changes the incentives for employers. If economic privation increases, mental health problems are likely to increase, too.

New methods of digital communication could accelerate conversation between different professionals dealing with the same case. The frustration of 'team meetings' being unable to reach a consensus decision because of the absence of a key member could be ended.

Use of social media has increased and could come to make interactive professional advice more accessible for young people and caregivers.

Whether or not the immediate effects of the pandemic subside, we can hope for scientific developments to advance some long-hoped-for practical changes.

Schools should be an excellent place for meeting the special needs of mental health. There are many fine individual examples. There is still much to do, however, in achieving integration of health and education services, at a scale that can contribute effectively.

There is also much to do in reducing the cost of specialist services and, therefore, access to them. Assessment can often be shortened, for instance by integrating specialist approaches that are now disparate. A more focused approach for matching the individual to the intervention could replace the rather cumbersome current systems of using clinical diagnosis for this purpose. Modern methods of direct assessment of impaired functions could complement or, if successful, replace current reliance on caregivers' impressions. The statistical methodology of computerized adaptive diagnosis and testing, based on multidimensional item response theory, already offers hope of efficient approaches to characterizing individuals. As the field moves to 'personalized' interventions that are driven by better application of knowledge about groups to individuals, mathematical approaches to prediction could well advance and make more use of artificial intelligence (AI) methods. At present, the value and uptake of AI is limited by the opacity of the results—a great amount of information can be incorporated by the machine after it has learned what predicts, but it is not in a form intelligible to human clinicians. Even if this situation continues, increasing use of computing devices in clinical settings could give accurately quantified estimates of probable outcomes.

Reduction of cost will also be crucial for the development of services in low- and middle-income countries (LAMIC). Interventions that work in trials in affluent parts of the world will need to be complemented by increasingly rigorous cost-effectiveness assessments in poorer areas. Development of applications in order to be relevant to LAMIC will probably need recognition of strengths, as well as weaknesses, in those societies. The strengthening of research and development in such regions will best be served by training innovators there, rather than only exporting interventions from the developed world.

In the longer term still, fundamental research seems likely, if allowed to proceed, to extend public understanding and reduce stigma.

Rapid advances in genetics are likely to enhance our ability to make predictions about course, response to interventions, and outcomes for individual people. Polygenic profiles are already increasing the scope—for example, in predicting the risk of autistic people to develop anxiety and, thereby, to allow early intervention. There could well be spectacular advances in the ability to modify individual genes (mostly rare) that have a large effect on cognition and behaviour. Gene-editing methods (e.g. via clustered regularly interspaced short palindromic repeats, CRISPR) could become useful and acceptable.

Neuroscience will continue to clarify the translation from biochemical processes to altered brain function. Clarification of neural circuits ought to lead to practical applications such as new targets for drug actions and neurofeedback, and for more logical classification. For instance, it seems likely that we shall see more effective methods for enhancing cognition. When that comes, a new kind of service will need to emerge. Ethical difficulties will then include fairness of access, and how much responsibility should be given to individuals and families to decide what is best for them. Left to themselves, carers' decisions could, for instance, accelerate rates of psychotropic medication in order to service perceived needs for competitive academic excellence at the expense of broader personal development. As ever, clinicians will need to know a great deal about the range and effects of different interventions, and have the wisdom not always to use them.

Index

For the benefit of digital users, indexed terms that span two pages (e.g., 52–53) may, on occasion, appear on only one of those pages.

Abbreviations used in the index can be found on pages xiii–xviii

Tables, figures and boxes are indicated by *t*, *f* and *b* following the page number